# BEYOND COMMON SENSE

This innovative volume approaches Japanese culture and society from a new angle. An ethnographic study, it is concerned with lifestyles in Japan that have hitherto remained largely unreported. The main research categories are gay men, lesbian women, single men and women and feminist men and women Transvestites, transsexuals and hermaphrodites also receive attention. Using participant observation, in-depth unstructured interviews and experiential research, Lunsing connects with all aspects of his informants lives and relationships to explore this underlying question - *how do people whose feelings, ideas or lifestyles do not agree with heterosexual marriage cope with life in a society in which everyone is expected to marry?* Four main themes emerge in the course of the work: 1) space, gender and sexuality, 2) constructions of homosexuality, 3) selves and self-constructionand 4) the isolation of elements that contribute towards a wider international comparative study.

After discussing the position of marriage in Japanese society, including political and legal aspects, Lunsing discusses how people in the various research categories attempt to fit in with the idea that one should marry by entering into marriage, and the problems that arise. Different forms of alternative lifestyles are examined, in the context of dealing with an outside world that has little understanding of people with alternative lifestyles, feelings or ideas. Lunsing then looks at the ways in which the various categories are regarded and relate to each other, especially the relations between gender and sexuality and the discourses of sex and sexual activities, as well as debates within and between individuals and circles consisting of people from the various categories.

In pursuing this investigation, Lunsing goes beyond what anthropologists usually do; instead of merely establishing standard lifestyles in a particular culture, he examines lifestyles that are at variance with prevailing norms.

**The Author** Wim Marinus Lunsing received his PhD in Social Anthropology from Oxford Brookes University and has been Research Fellow at Tokyo University.

**Japanese Studies**
**General Editor: Yoshio Sugimoto**

The titles in this series are listed at the back of this volume.

# BEYOND COMMON SENSE

## SEXUALITY AND GENDER IN CONTEMPORARY JAPAN

*Wim Lunsing*



KEGAN PAUL

London • New York • Bahrain

To Furuhashi Teiji,

who suddenly passed away at the age of 35 in the week I received my doctorate

First published in 2001 by
Kegan Paul Limited
UK: P.O. Box 256, London WC1B 3SW, England
Tel: 020 7580 5511 Fax: 020 7436 0899
E-mail: books@keganpaul.com
Internet: http://www.keganpaul.com
USA: 61 West 62nd Street, New York, NY 10023
Tel: (212) 459 0600 Fax: (212) 459 3678
Internet: http://www.columbia.edu/cu/cup
BAHRAIN: bahrain@keganpaul.com

Distributed by
John Wiley & Sons
Southern Cross Trading Estate
1 Oldlands Way, Bognor Regis
West Sussex, PO22 9SA, England
Tel: (01243) 779 777 Fax: (01243) 820 250
E-mail: cs-books@wiley.co.uk

Columbia University Press
61 West 62nd Street, New York, NY 10023
Tel: (212) 459 0600 Fax: (212) 459 3678
Internet: http://www.columbia.edu/cu/cup



ISBN: 0-7103-0593-1

**British Library Cataloguing in Publication Data**
Lunsing, Wim.
Beyond common sense: sexuality and gender in contemporary Japan
1. Sex –Social aspects – Japan 2. Gender identity – Japan
I. Title
306.7'0952
ISBN 0710305931

**Library of Congress Cataloging-in-Publication Data**
Applied for.

# Contents



In the text, Japanese names are given in the Japanese order, i.e. first the family name and then the given name.

# Acknowledgements

This project has been supported by the Austrian Ministry for Research and Science, the Japanese Ministry for Education, the Japan Foundation Endowment Committee, Erasmus and the Japan Society for the Promotion of Science. Further I am indebted to my dear friend Tik Ho Ong, my parents Ria and Henk Lunsing and my brother Jan Lunsing.

In a project like this, one becomes indebted to many people whose cooperation and support is of vital importance. Most of all I wish to thank the many people who participated in the fieldwork, by letting me share their lives, ideas and feelings. Since many of them must remain anonymous I will not mention any of them here but let it be known that I am very grateful to all the people who find something of themselves in this book.

For professional support I wish to thank Dr Jan van Bremen, Professor Wim Boot, Dr David Groth and Professor Sepp Linhart who helped getting this project off the ground. Important roles during the fieldwork were played by Professor Fujieda Mioko and Professor Ueno Chizuko, both of whom agreed to be my supervisors in Japan. In the writing up stage I was greatly helped by the advice and support of my supervisors in Oxford, Professor Joy Hendry and Professor Michael Argyle. My examiners, Dr Lola Martinez, Dr Roger Goodman and Dr Jeremy McClancy, offered valuable advice as to what improvements could be made when the thesis was to become a book. Professor Ueno Chizuko offered me the valuable opportunity to return to Japan in 1996 so that I could discuss my thesis with her students, people working in my area and people who participated in the research project. I also wish to thank Sam Dear and Sylvia Erikkson for their valuable assistance in improving my English.

So many are the people who offered advice and help that I cannot begin to mention them all. I wish, nevertheless, to express my gratitude to all who showed interest and supported me in any way.

# 1 Introduction

My first visit to Japan took place in 1986. I was 25 years old and stayed in Japan for one long hot summer. Contrary to my expectations, from the moment I descended from the plane I felt familiar with the people and the environment, almost as if I had come home. It was the clearest example of *déjà vu* I ever experienced. This did not mean that everything about Japan was unproblematic. One of the things I found disagreeable was that people frequently asked whether I was married and when I said I was not, whether I had a girlfriend. Since I was openly gay in the Netherlands, such questions were as good as new to me and I had difficulty dealing with them without upsetting those who asked them. This made me wonder how Japanese people in comparable situations deal with such questions and, indeed, how they cope with an environment in which everyone is expected to marry. Since there was an almost complete lack of material on homosexuality in contemporary Japan, I limited my MA thesis to discrimination against women based on a readers' column in a Japanese women's magazine, *Fujin Kōron,* called 'Watashi no Kokuhatsu' (My complaint), which refers to the magazine's request that readers write about sex discrimination. Marriage was the major focus of the complaints (Lunsing 1989).

After my graduation I visited Japan again in 1988. I contacted gay groups and spoke with lesbian and feminist women. In gay circles it was thought that most gay men in Japan marry, which was seen as detrimental to the formation of a gay movement. Among feminist women I found that marriage was a much-discussed theme, regardless of whether they were married themselves or not. My research theme was determined by such meetings: I would investigate how gay and lesbian people, women's and men's liberationists, singles and other people, such as transsexuals, transvestites and hermaphrodites, whose ideas, feelings or lifestyles are at variance with Japanese constructions of marriage and inherently the construction of life, live in Japan.

## Common Senses

Common sense is a cultural construction which differs from one culture to another (Geertz 1983). Many people think that common sense is a matter of using one's brain and that as a result thereof sensible people will come to the same conclusion. If one questions this viewpoint, one may encounter reactions varying from ridicule to aggression, something I experienced often in England where common sense is held in high esteem. An example of common sense is the idea that milk bottles are ecologically more friendly than milk cartons, as the *Guardian* wrote not long ago (May 1995). Dutch research, however, proved that the amount of energy and chemicals used to transport and clean the bottles for re-use is more polluting than the total pollution caused by the manufacture, transport and discarding of cartons, as a Dutch newspaper, *NRC Handelsblad*, reported about a month earlier. Since many people perceive common sense as a manifestation of intelligence, it is little questioned. Common sense is a cultural phenomenon, liable to change.[1] Geertz wrote that:

> perhaps it is an inherent characteristic of common-sense thought precisely to deny that [it is a cultural phenomenon] and to affirm its tenets are immediate deliverances of experience, not

> deliberated reflections upon it. (Geertz 1983: 75)

The Dutch equivalent of common sense is *gezond verstand,* which literally means healthy sense. This made me aware at an early age of common sense's potential lack of sensibleness. My mother said: 'Why don't you go and play outside like a healthy Dutch boy?' Upon this I thought: 'I don't want to be a healthy Dutch boy.' As Geertz writes, the idea of naturalness is one of the features characterizing common-sense thought (ibid.: 85). Instead of common sense, Ohnuki-Tierney uses the term

> naturalization to refer to a historical process whereby culturally determined values and norms acquire a state that makes them seem 'natural', not arbitrary, to people. (Ohnuki-Tierney 1993: 6, borrowing from Bourdieu)

Naturalized ideas are part of common sense. Durkheim's 'normal' sociological phenomena, phenomena that can be found in all or at least a majority of individuals in a society (Durkheim 1964: 55), are, when it concerns collective thought, common-sense ideas. He calls variations present in minorities 'morbid' or 'pathological' (ibid.) and writes that the healthy is by definition normal (ibid.: 58). This view denies the possibility of alternative ideas with a positive value.

In England the concept of nature appears to play a prominent role in deciding what is 'normal' and what is not. Marilyn Strathern wrote a book that discusses the way that the naturalized view of life, which stems from the Victorian age, exerts influence on the way people relate to each other (Strathern 1992b). Seeing discussions on British television, I noticed many times that in

England common sense is closely related to ideas of what is normal or natural. To give an example, I watched a television programme in which the audience participated in a discussion about the question of whether lesbian women should be allowed to have children by artificial insemination. Some people remarked that it was 'not natural' and 'not normal' for lesbian women to have children in this manner, to which lesbian women replied that they were 'natural' and 'normal', which was repeated a number of times until the programme came to an end. Such discussions are about common sense. The lesbian women adapted their argument to the idea that it is important to be natural and normal and failed to question what these terms mean. By stressing that they are natural and normal, they adhered to the common-sense idea that such a thing exists and thereby failed to achieve something that might have become a discussion instead of a fight in which one party says 'yes' and the other 'no'.

Some lesbian and gay scholars are among the foremost questioners of common sense, even if they do not always realize it (Butler 1993, Probyn 1993, Weeks 1991a: 16). There is much more advanced thinking about sexuality and relationships within some lesbian and gay circles than within academia (Butler 1993: 239–40). This thinking is often at variance with common-sense ideas about sexuality and relationships and may lead to constructing alternative visions of what is common sense. As this thinking is not academic in the sense that it does not find its base embedded in existing academic discourse but rather in individual or group thought, it may be difficult to relate to existing academic work, but that does not mean that it is less interesting or valid. An example concerns prejudice against homosexuality in academic circles. Carol Warren, who conducted research on gay men, wrote that in the social sciences people are generally more tolerant of homosexuality than elsewhere (Warren 1988: 63). Is it possible to tolerate something one does not have negative feelings towards in the first place? Tolerance implies prejudice. When I was 19 years old, in my environment in the Netherlands, we established that nobody has the right to tolerate (which implies discriminate against) homosexuality. It seems that common sense within academic circles never arrived at this understanding and that many scholars think that tolerance is acceptable.

Few scholars mention common sense as an important organizing principle in Japan. Although many must be aware of its existence, it is seldom explicated. The Japanese language has a number of terms that might be translated as common sense (Aoyama 1988: 191-2), rhetoric (Lock 1992a, 1993a, b, Martinez 1992), or generally prevalent ideas. The most all-encompassing is *jōshiki*, others include *ippan tsūkan* and *ippan tsūnen*, whereby the first translates as common sense and the last two as general feelings or general concepts. *Jōshiki* is a word many informants used to explain what they had to deal with when relating to people who are not familiar with lifestyles and ideas other than 'normal'. At the same time *jōshiki* is used in the meaning of practical knowledge, which, unlike in England, is frequently questioned. Marriage is a prime example of a concept supported by common-sense ideas. This is illustrated by the fact that marriage is widely believed to be 'natural' (Evans 1993, Strathern 1992b, Weeks 1983 and 1991b) – or in Japanese *shizen* – notwithstanding anthropological evidence that shows that the meaning of the concept of marriage varies from one culture to another to the extent that there are cultures in which there is hardly anything resembling marriage as it is known in Europe, North America or Japan (Riviere 1971, Leach 1991).

Much research on Japan concentrates on the household or family in history (e.g. Kanjō 1992, Neuss-Kaneko 1990, Takamure 1991); changes which occurred recently (e.g. Fuse 1984, Kanei 1988, Mōhwald 1990, Sasabe and Katsura 1990); or on women (e.g. Imamura 1987, Robins-Mowry 1983, Schooler and Smith 1978,

Smith and Wiswell 1982, Vogel 1978) and changes in their position (e.g. Condon 1986, Geddes 1970, Lenz 1990). In this work marriage is considered to be of central importance to people's lives. The fact that for many people it constitutes a problem rather than being a self-evident part of their life course is usually overlooked. Almost all research related to marriage concentrates on those who marry; seldom is attention given to those who do not. If attention is given it is little, as in Lebra (1984), who discusses unmarried women among her sample of 100 women but gives them a coverage that compares in no way to that of married women. This is a bias. There is no reason to assume that those greater in number are necessarily more important for the understanding of societies and cultures than those fewer in number. Like Lebra, most researchers appear not to be aware of this bias or, if they are, to be happy to ignore it.[2]

An obvious cause of this bias in Japan is that the number of those who never marry has been extremely small, especially from the 1950s to the 1980s. Until the late 1970s 98 per cent of Japanese women married at least once in their lifetime (Higuchi 1984: 106, Imamura 1987: 24, Lunsing 1989, Keizai Kikakuchō ed. 1992: 29). This figure suggests that those whose feelings or ideologies do not comply with expectations of marriage are in an awkward position. As Weeks (1991b) indicates, this is not much different from the central position of marriage in Europe and North America until the 1970s: other ways of life were hardly recognized. Considering the fact that most Western scholars grew up before the 1970s, the fact that most tend to overlook other ways of life is not all that surprising. As a result, a picture of Japan has been painted that is largely coloured by 'normality', which makes everything that deviates from an extremely restricted norm implicitly anomalous. As de Lauretis writes, the 'normal' does not exist independently and she claims that Freud was adamant that homosexuality was not necessary pathological (de Lauretis 1994: 17–28). Of course there is a notion of 'normal' in people's minds but this is an impossible construction because who is to decide what is normal?[3]

Recently Japanese books have appeared on alternatives to marriage, including what is called *jijitsukon* (common-law marriage, Ninomiya 1991), being single (Ebisaka 1986, Aoki 1987, Kamisaka 1991, Matsubara 1988, Tanimura 1990, Yoshihiro 1987, 1988) and even same-sex relationships (Fushimi 1991, Itō, S. 1993). A rare article by Ueno (1991b) discusses singles and same-sex relationships in terms of alternative forms of households. In European languages work discussing these topics in Japan is very rare and even in Japan, while there has been a virtual explosion of research in recent years, the main stress of scholarly material related to marriage deals with changes in the more or less standard, or 'normal', marriage and household (Meguro 1987, Kamihara 1992, Itamoto 1992a), rather than with those who do not marry. It seems that common sense discourages scholars from investigating topics that are different from those that are established, simply because not much research has been conducted on them.

Overlooking people whose lifestyles and behaviour are 'not normal' entails the great danger of overlooking people themselves. There are not likely to be many people who actually live in agreement with ideas of what is 'normal'. As Rosaldo wrote in his critique of Evans-Pritchard's work on the Nuer, in which Evans-Pritchard describes what a man is supposed to do in a particular situation:

> only someone pathologically oversocialized could follow such programmed normative commands without exception or contextual gratification. (Rosaldo 1986: 94)

What people actually do is likely to be at variance with rules set by their culture and therefore it makes little sense to describe the rules without looking at the behaviour that is supposed to be governed by them. The investigation of exceptions is crucial when establishing the importance of what people say is 'normal' or common sense.

Anthropology makes progress by refining debates about themes (Geertz 1993) as well as by accumulating knowledge. We all need to be critical and question our own and each other's findings in order to help us avoid developing our own version of unthinking common sense which leads to stagnation. The thesis that 'the description of other cultures is to some extent the projection of the common sense which is part of the researcher's own culture' (Kempny and Burszta 1994: 133) seems to be an understatement. Is it not obvious that common sense concerning the centrality of marriage in society, stemming from scholars' native common sense, has prevented them from looking beyond Japanese 'normality'? This is frustrating for those who do not endeavour to be 'normal' and as students try to relate to a subject in which people like themselves are systematically neglected. Like black people and women who are said to have more than the one worldview which white heterosexual male scholars may have owing to their particular background (Whitehead and Price 1986), I have worldviews, some of which are little reflected in existing academic work.

## Sex, Gender and Sexuality

This brings me to a major theme of this book: categorizations of people. Mary Douglas wrote that 'the primary social distinction' of human beings is that of the two sexes, the female and the male. This she associates with 'primitive cultures' (Douglas 1992: 140), which according to later scholars do not exist and never have existed (Ohnuki-Tierney 1987: 4). I know of no culture in which the first question when someone is born is not: 'Is it a boy or a girl?' People are divided into male and female, which is a division requested on most forms one has to fill out and which is the only feature each person has that is expected to remain unaltered throughout his or her life. Height varies with age, eyes may change colour and hair most likely does, names can change, but one's sex remains until death – so says common sense. As de Lauretis writes, however, ticking the box of female or male on a form is entering a sex-gender system. Rather than marking an existing feature of oneself on the form, this process can be regarded as one in which the chosen category marks itself on the person who fills it out (quoted in Moore 1994a: 85). Filling out forms may socialize people into regarding themselves as belonging to one category or another.

What is sex? Is it not merely having a particular type of genitals, i.e. either a penis or a vagina? Why is such a big point made of some small body parts that are usually kept covered up when in company? Attached to sex as genitals are a large variety of attributes, known as gender attributes, which are constructed to be either feminine or masculine. Being a man or a woman has gained in significance far beyond the mere genitals. From 'men do not cry' to 'real men do not eat quiche' and from 'women are intuitive' to 'women have babies', common-sense notions are heavily loaded with limitations as to how someone born with one set of genitals or the other behaves with regard to dress, food, hobbies, employment and speech.

It has been a long time since Simone de Beauvoir wrote her treatise on the second sex, which states that one is not born a woman but educated to be one (1976a, b). This implies that socialization forces people into 'a mould that does not take their authentic form' (Strathern 1992a: 67). Anthropologists have spent much effort mapping out gender structures in different societies, i.e. ideal types of behaviour of men and women. This brought proof that gender structures are not the same in every society (Ardener 1978, Sanday 1990). Features that are seen as masculine in one culture can be seen as feminine in another. Whereas in Western cultures and in Japan emotionality is seen as feminine, in Iran it is seen as masculine (Gudykunst and Ting-Toomy 1988: 48–9, quoting Hall). This does not necessarily mean that Iranian men are more emotional than, for instance, American men but that their culture constructs them as more prone to emotional outbursts. Discourses vary, even if features of real life may be similar. Cultural variation of what is seen as masculine and feminine abounds (Cornwall and Lindisfarne 1994). Within anthropology work in the area of gender socialization:

> has frequently been very functionalist, especially in the past, in that it tended to imply a situation in which society had need of particular sorts of acculturated persons, who were rather uncomplicatedly female or male. Gender identity was certainly thought to be culturally constructed, but it was conceived of, in the end, as little more than a self-evident outcome of sexual differentiation. (Moore 1994a: 43)

The line of thinking Moore questions can be related to the idea that nature is to culture as woman is to man (Ortner 1974), which, notwithstanding its close resemblance to constructions of the sexes according to Nazi ideology (Badinter 1986: 184), seems to have been quite popular. This idea failed not only to question whether women see themselves as closer to nature (Moore 1994b) but also to foresee the possibility that people might not socialize as is expected in line with their sex, might not become male men or female women. This idea, then, supports sexist ideas concerning the nature of the sexes. If gender is seen as a set of attributes that is not only assigned to a sex but also is one that necessarily accompanies a sex, much of the value of making a distinction between gender and sex is lost. The self-evidency or naturalness of men being men and women being women is reinforced. In the American academic world in particular, the term 'gender' is often used instead of sex. The chapter on homosexuality in *Sex in America* consequently uses gender instead of sex (Michael *et al.* 1995: 169–83), which in this case is particularly awkward. Are we to understand the attraction feminine men may feel towards masculine men as heterosexuality? The authors do not even venture to discuss the problem.[4]

Following de Beauvoir's line of thought, Monique Wittig wrote an essay in which she concludes that lesbian women are not women because they are not socialized as women (Wittig 1992). This alters the meaning of the term 'woman' in the sense that it does not refer to sex, to genitals, but to female gender attributes, which according to Wittig include loving men. Therefore lesbians are not women. Sexuality may, indeed, be regarded as a gender attribute and thus as something that has been socially and culturally constructed, as Margaret Mead concluded many years ago (Mead 1963).

Many people think that an important distinction between men and women is that women can bear children, and they define women in such a way (Callaway 1993). When looked at more closely, this implies that a majority of those with female genitals fall outside the category. The age at which most women can bear children is limited. Furthermore, there are women who are barren throughout their lives and women who do not wish to have children. Are they not women also? In all human societies, women who are sexually accessible are constructed as belonging to a category different from those who are not (Needham 1979: 18). Women who have passed the menopause also may constitute a different category from those who can become pregnant (Lock 1993a, b). Can all these categories of women be assigned to the same gender? If they are, it leads to their construction as abnormal women. If they are not, it implies that there are at least two genders of the female sex which leads to the assumption that there are probably more.

Another common-sense idea concerning the sexes is that physically men are strong and women weak. When measuring averages such a result might be obtained, but what about weak men and strong women? What about women who do body-building[5] and men who hardly move about except when in their car? When constructions of gender are taken strictly, it is most likely that the vast majority of people are anomalous in one way or other. Seeing a society's gender ideology as some monolithic construction and therefore the category of the woman as unitary and opposed to the category of the man is over simplistic. There are hardly any people who totally fit either the female or the male gender. Multiplicity, complexity and the context have to be taken into account (Lepowsky 1990, Meigs 1990), but does that mean that we need more than two genders?

Lately the idea of seeing gender as two sets of attributes linked to sex is questioned by people like Judith Butler (1990, 1993). Her conclusion, that people cannot simply be divided into two genders, was my starting point. Freedom from gender limitations was a theme I discussed with many friends in the early 1980s. We did not endeavour to invent more genders but rather to destabilize the rigidity of gender constructions by combining existing gender attributes in different ways. In that way, attributes that are seen as female can remain female and those that are seen as male can remain male. They are dissociated from people's sex, i.e. genitals. We saw gender not as wholes but as sets from which people can take parts to assemble any possible combination, which agrees with the view of Amadiume (1987), who found in Nigeria that gender attributes do not necessarily coincide with sex.

Pat Caplan suggested that homosexuality might be of particular interest for investigating the relationship between gender and sexuality, which she attributes to 'our' ethnocentrism (Caplan 1987: 22). I do not see why this should be so, unless homophobia is part of that brand of ethnocentrism. Otherwise heterosexuality would surely be of equal interest as homosexuality. She also writes that when discussing homosexuality we are implicitly discussing heterosexuality, 'which is equally socially constructed' (ibid.). While I agree that gender and sexuality are socially constructed, I think we must not forget that individuals deal with existing constructions in their own personal manner and that they may come up with something that did not previously exist as a social construction. There is no one social construction per society but many. Seeing sexuality as a gender attribute comparable to clothing might help to understand the variety that is possible in sets of attributes people may choose. The extraordinary position sexuality is given compared to other attributes could be the result of nothing more than a sensitivity acquired through 'our' particular cultural background.

All my research categories consist of people who fail to fit Japanese common-sense constructions of either female or male gender. Gay men and lesbian women are not primarily sexually attracted to the category they are supposed to be attracted to, single heterosexuals are not married and thereby fail to meet the idea that all people marry, and feminist women do not adhere to their assigned gender expectation which says that they should defer to men. It has been pointed out that structurally the only humans are men and that women are derivative of them (Melhuus 1993, referring to Dumont). In the case of Japan this point was made by Kawashima Takeyoshi, who wrote that women were not seen as humans but as objects (1974: 36). The feminist scholar Ueno Chizuko extends this, using Marxist-feminist theory, to children (1990a: e.g. 65, 103–6) and a further extension is made by gay writer Hashimoto Osamu, who includes unmarried men (1988: 20–8, 62). Women, children and unmarried men are all outside the category of the fully human. Hashimoto's reasoning includes all my main research categories, except for married homosexual men, in the case of whom, however, sexual desire conflicts with assigned gender attributes.

## Finding Selves

How people who perceive their personal attributes as differing from the ones assigned to them live their lives in Japan, how they see and relate to Japanese society and how they construct their selves in relation to society and for themselves, are central questions of this book. They may choose to try to adapt as much as possible to society's demands by suppressing their feelings (passing; Goode 1960); they may choose to divide their lives into a public part in which they conform to assigned gender attributes and a private part in which other characteristics are expressed (compartmentalization, ibid.; or segmentation, Tuan 1982); or they may choose to think that society is wrong and that their problems are nothing but the result of a society that has ordered things 'the wrong way' and try to change that, rather than themselves. They may try to alter common sense.

These methods are known within Western scholarship concerning gender and sexuality. All three methods are seen as conflict-ridden. The first and second produce conflict within the individual concerned, the third with society. The question of which is the more effective and less stressful way to deal with the problem depends on personal qualities as well as one's surroundings and therefore answers to it are likely to show cultural variation. Within lesbian and gay studies in Western countries it is usually implicitly expected that the first two are psychologically harmful and that the third is the only way that can lead to a satisfactory lifestyle. These lifestyles are then dealt with in terms of communities and groups of gays and lesbians with gay and lesbian identities (e.g. Moses 1978, Signorile 1994, Schuyf 1994), but we should not forget that gay and lesbian life also exists outside of such contexts, blending with people other than gays and lesbians. Feminists rarely discuss their special position within society but if they do, their reasoning is similar: feminist women should not be afraid to use the label of feminist and positively assume a feminist identity (Davis 1977, Probyn 1993).

Arguing differently, one can switch identities to suit oneself whenever one feels like it and still be positively gay, lesbian, feminist, single or whatever, because it is after all a personal matter. Similar attitudes have been reinvented lately by American queer theorists like Judith Butler (1990, 1993), who argues that identities are not the same as roles. Butler wrote in an essay that she was 'off to Yale to be a lesbian' (Butler 1991: 18), which means not that she does not see herself as a lesbian otherwise, but that posing as one is something different. Butler and other Americans seem to find this idea disconcerting (Creet 1995), possibly because they are so used to identifying themselves as lesbian or gay that they feel that their identity is at stake when they do not. The strong identification with labels such as gay and lesbian seems to be particular to the American and English cultural contexts. It is, however, an illusion to think that by identifying with a label one can make people see one as one wants to be seen. Whatever label one assumes, how one is perceived depends upon the other.

An angle that is frequently used in discussing lesbians, gays and feminist women is that of counter-culture or counter-values (Davis 1977, Ueno 1988b). An example of counter-culture might be the lesbian and gay communities in major American cities. Their values, however, are often not very different from mainstream culture (Murray 1992a) and people appear to have little difficulty leaving these communities and returning to mainstream lifestyles, suppressing their homosexuality (Lynch 1992). Gay communities are, by and large, not intentionally counter-cultural and often do not have counter-values other than that it is good to be gay, which is often contradictorily combined with the idea that it is better to keep the expression of homosexuality within the boundaries of gay and lesbian communities (Weeks 1983: 224, Signorile 1994). Counter-values may be more prominent in feminist circles but feminists also may decide that it is time to get on with life and adapt to general values and express their counter-values only within feminist circles.

Deviance, a word that is often used in relation to the categories of this book, is itself a term the use of which suggests that scholars are themselves constrained by notions of 'normal'. Only in common sense does normality exist. People may try to appear as normal, which means that they try to make others see them as such, but this does not mean that they really are. People present a part of themselves rather than show what they really are in all its aspects. This theme is discussed by people such as Goffman (1987) in his work on 'the presentation of self', and he and others liken it to playing roles in a drama (Lyman and Scott 1975) and adopt terms like 'mask' (Psathas 1980, Hollis 1985, Goffman 1987) and 'role', which are related to Mauss's concepts of *personne* and *personnage* (Mauss 1985). A common way of presenting oneself is that of what is seen as normal in a given context. This presentation of oneself as 'normal' makes others whose presentation differs come to be seen as deviant and are possibly labelled in a negative sense: they are stigmatized (Goffman 1980).

This interactionist approach has been widely used in explanations of Japanese behaviour, albeit often implicitly. Japanese are said to make a distinction between *tatemae* (face) behaviour and their *honne* (real feelings). There are contexts in which they show their *tatemae* and others in which they show their *honne,* roughly overlapping with what are called *soto* (outside) and *uchi* (inside) contexts (e.g. Bachnik and Quinn eds 1994). Both *honne* and *tatemae* are interactional concepts. Japanese are taught the ability to switch between different forms of behaviour and between different situations from an early age (Hendry 1984, 1986a, Tobin 1992) and learn to be able to distinguish situations in which each type of behaviour is appropriate, an ability, called *kejime,* that is thought to be essential to the maintenance of Japanese social order (Bachnik 1992). If this is so, one might expect that Japanese lesbian, gay and other people with characteristics that disagree with gender ascriptions find it relatively easy to switch between different presentations and to order their feelings in agreement with the demands of a situation. This hypothesis is investigated in this book.

Dorinne Kondo uses the term 'multiple selves' to refer to Japanese selves (Kondo 1992). While, from a particular point of view, the case for Japan may be evident, it makes me wonder whether she thinks that Americans only have one self. Given the notions of gay and lesbian identity, discussed above, it does, indeed, seem that Americans tend to regard their selves as one and whole. Goffman's work, however, suggests that Americans also have a variety of presentations of themselves to employ in various situations. How are Kondo's 'multiple selves' different from Goffman's various presentations of self? Perhaps Americans are not as sophisticated as Japanese in understanding themselves and try to hold on to a notion of individual oneness that is impossible in real life but may be comfortable to hold on to, even if it is an illusion.

The interactionist approach towards the self has a major flaw. It says that people adapt their presentation to social structures (Carrithers 1985, Taylor 1985) which have been made by people. The individual self tends to be neglected. Durkheimian thought holds that the individual self-aware self only exists in modern Western societies (Mauss 1985) and that all other peoples are implicitly less developed. This stance is impossible. All peoples have some form of self-awareness and some form of individuality, which may differ from that in Western societies and therefore be misunderstood by Western scholars but, nevertheless, must not be ignored (Cohen 1994). The Japanese, just as any other people, consist of individuals with their own individual views (Hendry 1992c). Cultural limitations may make it difficult or even impossible to express personal views openly and even when expressed people may not understand them as intended but fit the expressions to their understanding. This does not, however, mean that they are not important for the understanding of people. While it may seem impossible to investigate this inner self, also called self-awareness or self-consciousness, ignoring it does not help to understand people. It must be taken into account (Cohen 1994, Moore 1994a).

In the Japanese case the inner invisible self, that part of the conscious self that people regard as private and do not discuss or show in other ways, is much larger than in America (Barnlund 1975), which might imply that it is also more important to the individual's sense of self. Lebra (1992) postulates an inner self from which everyday behaviour is organized. This inner self is felt to be more important than the interactional self. She also postulates the importance of *muga*, the non-self, raw nature without reflection, which is obviously related to the Buddhist *anatma* or non-soul (Morris 1994: 49–69). She thinks this is the part of the self Japanese value most (Lebra 1992). In this book, the relation between inner self, *muga* and the ways people cope with being 'not normal' is also investigated. After all, it may for instance be possible for gay men to act as if they were heterosexual in most contexts, but where does that leave their inner self? How and why do people combine roles that are at odds with each other and what happens if they do not?

## Historical Developments and Constructions

To provide some background on how the major research categories are discussed in academic circles, the historical material that exists on constructions of them, and a history in the light of which they may be seen, I discuss here feminism, female homosexuality and male homosexuality as constructed from Japanese history. One should keep in mind that these academic and historical constructions may not have much to do with the actual behaviour or constructions of those concerned.

### Feminism

While most Japanese feminists who think about their origins place the beginning of feminism in Japan at the emergence of the Seitōsha (Blue Stockings Society) in 1911 (Sievers 1983: 163) and with people like the poetess Yosano Akiko and the politician Hiratsuka Raichō who became active at the beginning of this century, others place it earlier. Some think that for instance Sei Shōnagon, writer of *Makura no Sōshi* (The pillow book) who lived about 1,000 years ago, could be seen as a feminist *avant la lettre*. She writes, for instance, of irritating habits of lovers who do not get up quietly in the morning but bustle around flapping with their fans for a long time, waking her up before they finally leave (Sei Shōnagon 1962). Since I use the term 'feminist women' to represent women who do not comply with gender assignations, Sei Shōnagon could be regarded as one of them, just like many other historical and mythical figures, such as Hōjō Masako, who appropriated supreme power in Japan in her time (Sansom 1961) and, indeed, Amaterasu Ōmikami, the sun goddess, from whom the imperial family is said to stem in a direct lineage (Sansom 1978, Gōssman 1990). Hiratsuka Raichō referred to Amaterasu in her opening article in the first issue of *Seitō*, which criticizes the dwindling power of women that characterizes much of Japanese history (Hiratsuka 1991).

Sharon Sievers places the beginning of feminism in Japan with Kishida Toshiko, who toured Japan in the 1870s and 1880s to talk to women about their civil rights (Sievers 1983: 33–41). When I proposed Kishida as the starting point to one of the women who started the *ūman ribu* movement in the 1970s, she was amazed. She regarded Kishida as a politician who was not particularly involved in women's issues. As she and most contemporary feminists implicitly see it, feminism in Japan did not exist until Japanese women made contact with feminists in Europe and America. Feminism as presented in Japanese historical treatises parallels developments in Europe and America, including criticizing pre-war movements as bourgeois women's movements which merely tried to obtain the vote for women without promoting the enormous changes that are considered necessary to change societies, to change common-sense concepts of sexuality and gender (Millet 1977: 84–5, Fujieda 1983, 1990, Ueno 1988b, Ehara 1992b). Rhetorics concerning this 'bourgeois feminism (*burujoa feminizumu*)' are that it may have been successful in getting the vote, or even equal opportunities for women on the condition that they meet the same criteria as men, but that it does not question the structure of society as such, which may be the very reason why it has been successful (Ehara 1992b).

The mass media in the beginning of this century treated Seitō women as *nyū ūman* (new women). Seitō members were not always happy with the use of this term. Itō Noe thought that the term should be reserved for women like herself, who were real pioneers by virtue of their experimental lifestyles, and that other women should not appropriate the term because they were mere followers, including some of the women involved in Seitō (Itō 1913). In the mass media the term referred increasingly to young women who dressed differently from how women used to dress, regardless of their ideology or lifestyle. Within Seitōsha, they were criticized for appropriating the term *nyū ūman* (Hasogabe 1913).

The Japanese women's liberation movement that started in the early 1970s was from the beginning strongly influenced by American developments, evidenced by the fact that initially one of their major activities was the translation of American feminists' work. The Urufu no Kai (Wolf's Group), the name of which refers to the wolf that raised Romulus and Remus, the mythical founders of Rome, translated American material into Japanese in order to promote discussion of feminist issues. When the group dispersed in 1974, some members continued activities as journalists, among other things publishing the magazine *Onna Erosu* and preparing for the International Year of the Woman in 1975 (Akiyama 1992). The idea that feminism in Japan is a Western import is criticized by feminists who claim that there are reasons inherent in the Japanese situation leading to the formation of a women's liberation movement there. These reasons are similar to the reasons that led to women's liberation movements in Western countries (Ueno 1988b), which makes it plausible that feminism in Japan is often similar to that in Western countries. Even if feminism is seen as an import, it must be remembered that it was imported by people who found something in it they could relate to. Not everything that exists in Western countries is automatically imported to Japan: a selection is made, as are adaptations, and these reflect existing values and ideas.

In Europe, America and Japan women's liberationists united in the wake of student movements and the characteristics of the movements at that time were similar. The protagonists tended to be highly educated, from middle- or upper middle-class backgrounds and left-wing on the political spectrum. They were strongly anti-authoritarian and concerned with issues like pornography, sexual violence and divisions of tasks based on sex, i.e. gender. The results of the movements varied. While in Western countries the idea that men and women should be treated equally evolved into the idea that they are in fact equal (Komter 1985, 1989), in Japan this did not happen. Most Japanese think that women and men are not treated equally and do not need to be treated equally. In a government survey carried out in 1989 only 5.5 per cent thought that men should take equal shares with women of household tasks, even though about half of them thought that men should do something (Keizai Kikakuchō Kokumin Seikatsukyoku ed. 1992: 103). Unequal treatment is also evidenced by the wage-gap (Saso 1990: 11, 67–71, Naoi 1994), the existence of which is widely recognized and visible in all sectors of employment apart from the service industry, in which wages are relatively low overall and a majority of workers are women (Mori 1992).

It is sometimes suggested that Japanese feminists, unlike their Western counterparts, strive for a feminization of society by adapting labour circumstances to women's, especially mothers', needs, instead of women adapting to the needs of employers (Iwao 1994, Ueno 1988b). While Ueno attacked Illich's ideas concerning vernacular gender (Illich 1982), which were embraced by many feminists in Japan (Katō 1990), she also sees women in the first place in relation to their role as mothers, not because she thinks that women should be mothers but because she sees it as an objective reality that most women become mothers at some stage in their lives (Ueno 1990a, 1991a: 120–7). A tendency to neglect women without children remains. The major change that took place in the 1970s and 1980s is that many women took up part-time work, while mainstream full-time employment remained largely the domain of men (Lam 1993, Naoi 1994, Saso 1990: 53–80). It became more acceptable for women to work outside the house but the choice of work remains limited. An Equal Employment Opportunity Law was adopted in 1986 but it is, amongst other reasons, criticized because it lacks sanctions and offers no protection for those who wish to take legal action (Lam 1993, Mori 1992, Weber 1990). Its major positive result is a small increase in the number of women who are employed in mainstream careers, something that is impossible for most women who wish to marry and have children (Lam 1992, 1993).

## Female Homosexuality

Japanese women had to rediscover lesbian feelings generation after generation. Recently knowledge of lesbian life in foreign countries has played a role in supporting feelings of women for women. Again, translating of foreign writing is a major activity among politically engaged lesbian women in Japan (e.g. Watanabe *et al.*, transl., ed. 1990). While there are reports of lesbian activities in the Edo period (1603–868;[6] Morishita 1991, Bornoff 1992: 639) and before, dating back as far as the Nara period (646–794), very few Japanese are aware of them. The evidence I found is scant. There are *ukiyoe* (pictures of the floating world) depicting women in sexual positions with women from the Edo period (Morishita 1991). Other evidence consists of *harigata* (dildos) from the Nara period onwards. Those found in the Nara period are longer than later ones and it is assumed that this indicates that they were used for masturbating oneself (Kokuhaku Rezu Kurabu 1992b), which makes the link with lesbian feelings tenuous, while those of the Edo period could be strapped around a woman's hips so that she could satisfy another woman (Morishita 1991).

There are also references to lesbian feelings in the feminist magazine *Seitō* in the Taishō period (1912–26), with a description in the form of a letter to an anonymous friend by Kawada (1915), and Hiratsuka (1914) referring to being the object of lesbian admiration in an introduction to the translation of an article by Havelock Ellis on female homosexuality and even writing about her efforts to build a relationship with a woman (Wada 1991). These are wholly neglected in discussions of *Seitō* (Taudin Chabot 1981, Sievers 1983, Hane 1988) and omitted in compilations of discussions in the magazine (e.g. Horiba 1991). At a meeting of Sōtaikai, which is a group that was recently founded to study sex and sexuality in Japan, at Kyoto University in 1996 Furukawa Makoto gave me some insight into the prevalence of young women being quoted in newspapers talking of their admiration, amounting to erotic attraction, for strong women, in particular sportswomen, in the Meiji and Taishō periods. It appears that much research remains to be carried out by historians.

Lately it has been suggested that a number of women in Japanese history loved women, such as Murasaki Shikibu, writer of *Genji Monogatari* (The tale of Genji) around the year 1,000, who, according to Komashaku Kimi, could never have written so sensitively if she had not loved women (Komashaku 1982), the writer Yoshiya Nobuko, who also wrote for *Seitō* (Higuchi 1993b, Wada 1991), and Yuasa Yoshiko and Miyamoto Yuriko (ibid.), whose correspondence has been published (Sawabe 1990). Yoshiya, especially, is associated with the idea of *shisutāfuddo* (sisterhood), or *S* in short, which she described in romantic novels about intimate female relationships. Sex is not explicitly part of this construction (Honda 1991). There are no known examples of sisterhood communities in Japan as there are in China and

Chinese communities abroad (Sankar 1986, Wieringa 1987: 9, 48–68), but that does not necessarily mean that they did not exist.

The 1970s saw the advent of lesbian organizations. The Wakakusa no Kai (Group of Young Girls), founded in 1971, was probably the first lesbian circle in Japan (Hirosawa 1991). It was a nationwide organization of lesbian women who enjoyed hiking and *gasshuku* (overnight group trips)[7] in a lesbian context. They also produced a magazine, *Eve & Eve* (*Ibu & Ibu*), but this was discontinued because of lack of readership (ibid.), which also seems to have happened with other magazines.[8] The radical feminist magazine *Onna Erosu* has some discussions by lesbian women, which are characterized by separatism (Kawara 1981) and by activism against pornography and sexual violence, usually following developments in America (Rezubian Feminisuto Sentā 1981). The mid-1980s saw something called a *rezubian būmu* (lesbian boom) in the media, in which lesbian women were constructed in peculiar ways such as masculine women and women of the all-women musical theatre, based near Osaka, the Takarazuka Revue (Robertson 1992, Shiba 1993a), but it was not until 1987, when a volume in the Bessatsu Takarajima series was devoted to lesbian women, that many lesbian women discovered that they were not alone (Bessatsu Takarajima 1991).

## Male Homosexuality

In contrast, there is abundant material on male homosexuality in Japanese history, knowledge of which was brought to Europe as early as the sixteenth century by the Spanish Jesuit missionary Francis Xavier, who wrote about the prevalence of sodomy (Hirschfeld 1914: 618). It is unlikely that he actually saw men having anal intercourse but it seems that men did little to hide their sexual interest in each other. One of Japan's oldest writings, the *Nihongi*, which is thought to have been completed around AD

720, contains an episode of what has been interpreted to concern the love relationship of two priests (ibid., referring to Karl Florenz's translation), but it could just as well be interpreted differently (Leupp 1995: 22–3).

Three features characterize constructions of male homosexuality in Japanese history. The first is that of homosexuality as practised among Buddhist monks, before they were allowed to marry. The typical construction is that of young novices being used for sexual relief by older monks. A female Buddhist priest said that the marriage ban for Buddhist monks in Japan was first countered by Shinran, founder of the True Pure Land Sect (Jōdō Shinshu) in 1224 (Kitagawa 1990), who was the first Buddhist monk to marry (Wōss 1981), encouraging others of his sect to follow his example (Sansom 1978: 333) in order to bring the clergy closer to the laity (Saunders 1964: 200). According to the female priest, Shinran advocated marriage because the monks of the Tendai sect, the headquarters of which are on Mount Hiei near Kyoto, were continually sneaking out to the pleasure districts of Kyoto to have sex with female prostitutes and often raped women in the woods of Mount Hiei.[9] Even today, there are signs on Mount Hiei warning women not to walk alone (*Hitori aruki o yamemashō*) but this is a common admonition in the Japanese countryside. She was amazed when I told her of literature on homosexuality among monks and said that she had never heard of it. Nevertheless, the stories of *chigo*, the beautiful novices who were the partners of monks, may reflect actual behaviour, albeit probably exaggerated (Childs 1980).

A second frequently mentioned feature is that of love among *samurai* (warriors), which is largely based on Ihara Saikaku's *Danshoku Ōkagami* (The great mirror of male love), written in the seventeenth century (Ihara 1976, 1990). It was a bestseller in its day. The third feature of homosexuality in historical Japan concerns the love for the future *onnagata* (men who play female parts in *kabuki* theatre), for the *wakashu*, or *kagema yarō* (Yamauchi 1991), which is a combination of a cross-generational form and one in which difference in acquired gender plays its part. Thus, Japanese culture knew two major constructions of homosexuality simultaneously, that of cross-gender homosexuality and that of cross-generation homosexuality (Furukawa, M. 1994, 1996).

Homosexual activity used to be called *danshoku* or *nanshoku*, as opposed to *nyoshoku* or *joshoku*, which referred to heterosexual activity, and it is assumed that homosexuality was regarded as accessible to all men who could afford it (Watanabe and Iwata 1987), although prostitution by *wakashu* was ruled illegal at various times, as was prostitution by their female counterparts (Schalow 1989). *Danshoku* is usually translated as pederasty and *nyoshoku* might also be translated by pederasty, for women involved in sex work are also preferably young. In both cases, it concerns adult men being attracted to either young men or young women (Watanabe and Iwata 1987, Furukawa, M. 1992, 1993, 1994, 1996). Female sexuality did not exist in this division, which may partly account for the scarcity of constructions of female homosexuality. Homosexuality was constructed as involving an active masculine man having sex with a passive, younger or feminine man, i.e. the *chigo* or the *wakashu*.

Who made these constructions and what do they have to do with real life? While Saikaku's work includes a love relationship between adult men lasting a lifetime (Ihara 1990: 180–3) as well as stories of men who love men who clearly are not boys, scholars usually regard it as an example of pederasty, or love of adult men for boys, which figures dominantly in it (Watanabe and Iwata 1987, Furukawa, M. 1992, 1993, 1994, 1996). In *The Actor's Analects* plays are discussed in which the major theme is homosexuality between men of about the same age (Dunn and Torigoe transl., eds 1969: 41–4) and as Leupp points out there is, indeed, ample evidence of homosexual activity taking place between adult men

(Leupp 1995: 137–44). The construction of homosexuality in Japanese history as only pederasty is unsustainable.

Nonetheless, love of boys remains a major theme in descriptions of homosexuality today in Japan (Inagaki 1986, Nakajima 1990, Saeki 1992). Benedict wrote that it was the only form Japanese thought to be acceptable (Benedict 1977: 131), similar to constructions in ancient Greece (Foucault 1978, 1988a, Greenberg 1988). The construction of homosexuality as sex between a masculine and a feminine man is also alive today. It appears that there has to be a difference in power relations for people to envisage the idea of people having sex. This, however, does not prove that homosexual activities between two adult men whose age and gender are not much different do not occur. It may just as well indicate that most Japanese have no idea of what goes on.

According to Hirschfeld, homosexuality existed extensively in Japan in the Meiji era and was said to be especially flourishing in the southern province Satsuma, a regional aspect he treated with much circumspection (Hirschfeld 1914: 611). He claims that homosexual activity did not essentially differ from homosexuality as he found it in Egypt, England, France, Germany, the Netherlands, or anywhere else (ibid.: 528). While constructions concerning homosexuality in China similar to those in Japan exist (Furth 1993, Hinsch 1990), they have also been implicitly criticized as not being representative of existing literature and actual behaviour by a Chinese author who found examples of homosexual activity between adult men without a cross-gender component (Xiao 1984). A recent novel describes homosexuality in Taiwan in a manner that should be familiar to gay men in Western countries (Pai 1990).

Mishima's gay novels *Kamen no Kokuhaku* (Confessions of a mask: 1949) and *Kinjiki* (Forbidden colours: 1953) and other gay novels (Senya 1986a, b) give some insight into the period directly after the Second World War, in which homosexuality was much hidden from the everyday life of most people. Watanabe (Watanabe and Iwata 1987: 126–7) writes even of a renaissance of homosexuality in the 1960s, as if it did not exist for a period. Ample material indicates that male homosexual activities continued throughout that time, with reports of widespread homosexual activity among students in the Meiji era (Yamauchi 1991) and of gay groups in the 1950s (Ōta 1987, Karasawa 1992). Homosexuality during the Second World War is a recurrent theme in pornography in especially the gay magazines *Barazoku* and *Sabu* (e.g. Nonomura 1986).

The idea of a renaissance of homosexuality seems to refer to the fact that it became more visible once again, which also may have led to a growth in the number of homosexually active men, simply because they knew where to find others. This development has been furthered by the advent of nation-wide gay magazines since 1971, through which gay men could contact each other and find addresses of gay bars and other gay establishments. A pioneer of gay politics was Tōgō Ken who began running for elections as a gay candidate in the early 1970s. Gay networks existed throughout the 1970s and in the 1980s contact was made with Western groups and more comprehensive political activities started. The questions remain to be answered whether there is anything particular about homosexual practice in Japan compared to elsewhere and to what extent constructions of homosexuality influence actual behaviour.

## Ethnography and Scholarship

This book aims first at filling the gap in ethnographic material about the themes and categories under discussion. Rather than drawing my data into an existing theoretical framework, I try to present my findings in a manner that leaves space for readers to interpret and analyse in their own way. Of course my analysis is present throughout: more or less implicitly in the way themes are ordered and explicitly in conclusions. Culture is not linear but it is unavoidable to write in sentences, thereby transforming reality into a logical form comprehensible to others (Bloch 1991). Bloch thinks that we should not lose ourselves in what he calls 'quasi-theories' of structuralism and transactionalism but be much more descriptive (ibid.). An ethnography is always a choice of what one writes and what one does not (Clifford 1986). I have chosen to let many voices have their say, which Tyler (1986) calls polyphony, and to pay attention to the changes that took place in Japanese society before, during and after the main fieldwork period.

Many of my informants are quite anti-academic. This is not surprising because the few papers, books and remarks scholars have seen fit to write about them have often been extremely biased, not to say homophobic.[10] Since the voice of gay and lesbian people was not heard much, Japanese scholars could write whatever came to mind, a problem that has also been noticeable in Western science, with examples such as Freud and his Oedipus complex, which, according to some Japanese, was something he made up from his own dreams, or possibly nightmares. While Japanese psychologists discuss Freud seriously, gay informants typically had little patience with his theories. Gay writer Hashimoto even argues that Freud was a latent gay man with many psychological problems (Hashimoto 1986: 130–78).

Although I present a hypothesis and some questions above, they were of little importance while I was conducting fieldwork. One traditional anthropological way of looking at people was with me all the time. It is looking at the differences in the ways people say they act, the way they say they should act and the way they actually act. Anthropologists who base their research mostly on participant observation may find themselves confronted with questions like: 'What is your hypothesis?' or: 'What is your research question?' (Agar 1980: 12–13), both of which often are not very important to anthropological work. Robertson (1991: 2) explicitly questions the value of hypothesis-testing for anthropological research and Moeran (1985: 3) even writes that anthropology is not a science but a humanity. Lebra, defending her lack of empiricism, writes:

> what matters is 'experiential' plausibility, not 'empirical' validity, a position that might be justified anthropologically in that stories and narratives provide sources for cultural interpretations. (1993: 22)

To some anthropologists it may seem unnecessary to defend plausibility as a valid goal but many scholars think differently. I would argue that qualitative research is likely to be more reliable than quantitative because quantitative research depends greatly on interpretations by scholars of interpretations by informants, and there is not so much control over what these interpretations are, as there is when doing qualitative fieldwork. That numbers look more academically acceptable is merely a result of the received view of science as impenetrable. Resulting prejudices like: 'If it does not look difficult it cannot be right', are in my eyes a mere mystification of science. I am not much concerned with asking what is most common or how most people act. This book is more concerned with identifying a variety of lifestyles and ways of thinking about them, whereby I maintain that even a lifestyle that is only enjoyed by one person is relevant in that it shows something about the latitude open to Japanese people in carving their own individual ways of life. If one person can maintain a particular lifestyle, it is most likely that more could do so. While results of available surveys are presented, it must be remembered that they are, in most cases, very biased, which makes their significance limited.

The next chapter describes features of the fieldwork and provides some insight into the numbers of interviewees and the spread of informants. Chapter three deals with common-sense ideas concerning marriage and what position marriage has in Japanese culture, both socially and legally. Chapter four investigates how members of my research categories may try to adapt themselves to common sense by marrying and the problems that may entail, after which chapter five investigates alternative lifestyles. Chapter six is concerned with relating to one's surroundings while maintaining an alternative lifestyle or alternative ideas and chapter seven with discourses concerning my research categories as they exist within the circles constituted by them. After this basically ethnographic work, I shall return to the questions brought up here and investigate what they can tell us about Japanese society in relation to human life and its constructions.

## Notes

1 See for example Lock (1993a, b) who describes that among physicians in Japan the notion existed that men had more trouble with menopause than women and, on the other hand, that North American women became very upset when Lock so much as suggested that menopausal problems such as hot flushes might be culturally induced rather than a natural phenomenon. In Japan, in the meantime, the prevalence of menopausal problems among women has gained ground, as has the idea that it is common for women to have them: common sense regarding menopause in Japan has changed.

2 The choice is political in the sense that there is of course just as much to discuss about the lives of single women as there is about married women. This is not related to their numbers. The mere fact that married women are in the majority in a given sample does not, on academic grounds, automatically lead to paying more attention to them. It would make perfect sense to pay as much attention to single women as to married women because variety is likely to be equally wide in both cases.

3 Dorothy Smith expanded on this theme in a discussion of who establishes whether a person called 'K' is mentally ill or not, which leads to the conclusion that this depends wholly on the view of whoever happens to assume the power to decide, in this case flatmates (1990).

4 Ueno Chizuko relates the defeat of the Equal Rights Amendment (ERA) to a strong essentialist tendency among American feminists (Ueno 1995). This essentialist tendency can be related to the idea that woman relates to nature as man to culture and to the blurring of the distinction between sex and gender.

5 Body-building lesbian scholar Marcia Ian describes her body as masculine and compares it to an erect penis (1995).

6 My division into historical periods follows Sansom (1978), with the change of the start of the Edo period from 1615 to 1603. This follows Ohnuki-Tierney (1987), who writes that 1603 is the year most commonly used in Japan, something that is also my experience.

7 Gasshuku is also used for school trips and company trips. Essential is the sleeping together, which is the meaning of the word.

8 Shiba (1993b) mentions Bara no Koheya (Small room of roses) and Watanabe (1990) mentions Subarashii Onnatachi (Splendid women), Za Daiku (The dyke), by a group of lesbian

carpenters, and Hikariguruma (The shining car), all of which appeared in the 1970s but quickly went out of print.

9 As LaFleur (1992) amply clarifies, the fact that Buddhism, apart from the Jōdō Shinshū, persisted in its adherence to celibacy, by no means signified that monks did not engage in sexual activities with women. Furthermore, he writes that there was a gradual increase in monks of all sects marrying and setting up households with sons succeeding them as abbots of their temples during the Edo period.

10 See for instance Ueno (1988a: 13–14), who writes that homosexuality is unnatural and a manifestation of narcissism, or Doi (1975), who deals with homosexuality under the heading of pathology. The manner in which Japanese heterosexual scholars deal with homosexuality is generally marked by gratuitous prejudice. Most do not conduct serious research on the subject and those who do, like Oikawa (1993), tend to investigate extreme samples and then analyse these without much concern about the question of representativeness. Work on transsexuality also tends not to make clear how it should be distinguished from homosexuality (Kuroyanagi 1992).

# 2 Methods and Ethics

This chapter discusses my methods of research and the people and groups I worked with. Further, it discusses sampling techniques and methods of interviewing, as well as the circumstances in which interviews took place. Attention is also given to questions of ethics: of protecting informants and of complying with their wishes. Personal relationships between the fieldworker and informants are discussed, as are the ways informants perceived me, the researcher, and the various personae and roles I came to have. Some sections about myself may seem very private and personal but they are quite public in the research context, for they inform the quality of the data. Since I agree with Rabinow that experiential, reflective and critical activities are 'the very strength of anthropology' (Rabinow 1977: 5), I discuss them in detail in order to provide insight into how the material on which this book is based is composed, including biases, advantages and disadvantages.

## Participant Observation

Participant observation is a method that occupies a central position in the field of social anthropology but otherwise it is not widely understood or recognized. In participant observation a rigidly structured research outline that determines what questions are to be asked and hence what questions are to be overlooked, may be counterproductive. An example of this is the work of Pharr (1981) who investigated political women in Japan and apparently started out from the hypothesis that their being political women was a result of their upbringing. The major finding of her research is that the role of the parents is of little importance. This is of course an important finding but, if she had not been constrained by her hypothesis, her findings could have been more interesting because she could have diverted her focus to what the women she worked with brought forward as important.

Participant observation offers the possibility of finding out what is important to informants, rather than imposing a theoretical structure on how they are seen. It aims more at 'understanding' (Agar 1980: 69–70, Cesara 1982: e.g. 13, 59) informants than at fitting them into existing academic theories. This entails testing findings again and again before anything resembling hypotheses may be drawn up (Agar 1980: 9, 202). In my research this appeared to be the only way to attain valid results because very little research had been conducted on those concerned. This made it imperative to go into the field and discover there what the important questions are.

One research goal was to investigate the variety of life in Japan, rather than what, for instance, most gay men do. For this purpose questionnaires are futile. Uncommon cases are not likely to find the right answer in a multiple choice questionnaire and therefore they are likely not to respond. Questionnaires are extremely problematic in relation to research concerning boundaries like those investigated here. Even the simple categories of 'male' and 'female' are rather offensive for those who have not decided on either, or those who do not want to be categorized in a way they feel does not fit them. The use of 'male' and 'female' in questionnaires does not simply refer to what genitals someone has and, since a definition is never given, it remains vague what is meant. My own experience in the Netherlands and in England has shown me that the answers pre-printed in questionnaires usually do not allow me to give the right answer,[1] simply because it is not there. This is very similar for my Japanese counterparts.

Malinowski's diary is generally believed to have shocked many people because he described his sexual desires (Malinowski 1989). Geertz, however, writes that the underlying cause of the shock was that it showed that doing participant observation is ultimately leading one's life and that, as a consequence, a fieldworker leads 'multiplex lives' (Geertz 1988: 77). Most of the background in research methods I had before going into the field stems from feminist anthropology, which holds that it is important to identify, even side, with those one conducts research with (Mies 1983, Duelli Klein 1983). Empathizing with informants is considered to be necessary on ethical grounds as well as in order to obtain data. Experiencing what informants experience is the best way to further the ability to relate as well as possible to informants (Reinharz 1983). Ultimately this entails living a life similar to the informants' lives. In a highly literate culture like Japan, reading what people read is of great importance. Informants express themselves in writing and are influenced by the writings they read (Clifford 1986). Since reading is part of life it is also part of participant observation. The research included reading written sources such as gay magazines,[2] *minikomi* (small-scale magazines) of the different research groups and novels informants thought to be of interest.

Of course one leads one's life in the field, not necessarily multiply but not the same as that before and after. The idea that leading 'multiple lives' is something unusual strikes me as futile:

most people live their lives in more than one context. Living a life in participant observation is somewhat different from any other life because the fieldworker usually does not want to disturb the usual flow of events. This may seem rather passive but it does not need to be. One can be an active agent as long as one either places oneself outside the group or acts in a way that others in the group may also act. My lives in the field combined to result in living in the fullest sense of the word. They were, however, not 'multiple' but integrated with my lives before and after and they continue today. The only difference between participant observation and other 'living' is that it is professional living, aimed at a goal that directs choices of how one lives.

Feminist anthropologists often have the wish to make a contribution to the improvement of the lives of those they conduct research with and, if they work in Third World countries for which development aid is available, this may be successful (Schrijvers 1985). Even in their own country it is possible to envisage that they might be successful in acquiring funding for projects to improve women's lives. While I would have liked to improve the lives of my informants in Japan, this idea seemed increasingly paternalistic and even ridiculous. They know ways of furthering their interest much better than I and they have greater access to economic means. All I could do was to be present at court cases and discussions with authorities where I, as a foreign researcher, was believed to give extra weight to our argument, and to write and speak my mind. Further, I introduced some informants to others or to networks. This was not different from what any one of them could do. The most useful thing I could do is what I am doing now, i.e. to write about our life in Japan, so that it becomes again a little harder to ignore us. I use 'our' and 'us' because the writings concern my life in Japan as well as that of the informants.

## Groups

Gay groups were located through gay magazines, in which the international gay and lesbian social group Out & About, the gay network of Sōka Gakkai and others advertised. I also contacted directly both Occur[3] and JILGA (International Lesbian and Gay Organization Japan),[4] the major political gay and lesbian organizations in Tokyo of the period. Networking between different groups also widened my scope. Through Out & About I established contact with YLP (Yancha Lesbian Power, now OLP), Kansai's major lesbian group. This contact was consolidated at the Asian Women's Conference in April 1992 in Osaka. They introduced me again to lesbian groups in Tokyo. Women's groups were mostly found through *Onnatachi no Benrichō*, a reference book on women's groups in Japan (Josei no Jōhō o Hirogeru Kai ed. 1991).

The total number of groups with which participant observation was conducted is not easy to establish because in many cases they overlap. This makes it difficult to determine boundaries between groups and whether some groups should be counted as subgroups or not, but the total number amounts to about twenty. Of these, nine consist exclusively of gay men, one is gay and lesbian and one is exclusively lesbian. OGC (Osaka Gay Community) is dominated by gay men but its meetings are open to anyone who wants to discuss personal matters related to sexuality and many non-gay people participate. Menzu Ribu Kenkyūkai (Men's Lib Study Group) excludes women except for infant daughters of participants and also draws people who go to other groups such as the singles' network (Shinguruzu Netto), of which the formal name is Kakushinhan? Shinguru (Crime of Conviction? Single). A group of single women with whom I participated marginally is Dokushin Fujin Renmei (Single Women's League), attended mostly by women aged over 50. A cluster of five related gay groups, whose activities varied from sports events and sightseeing to personal discussions, the manufacture of cassette-tapes and politics were followed throughout my fieldwork period in Japan. These groups are discussed more extensively in following chapters. In the summer of 1992 I took part in a *gasshuku* (an overnight trip) of one of these groups.

Groups that were less directly related to my research were met at a number of research seminars in Kobe, Osaka and Kyoto. I attended meetings of Hitori Aruki no Kai (Group of People who Walk Alone), a group of varied individuals who meet for lectures on subjects related to emancipation and autonomy. They invited me to give a lecture on the reasons for the lack of human rights for women in Japan because they knew I had been working on the topic. I used this opportunity to try and have a discussion about sexuality. Umechika Fōramu (Umechika Forum) is a group that originally was founded to support the case of newspaper salespersons who were forcibly removed from their selling position in Umechika, Umeda's underground pedestrian area (Umechika Fōramu 1990). The group is involved in issues like the environment and architecture and invited me twice to talk about environmental issues because the Netherlands is thought to be an advanced country in this field, which made me a specialist in their view. This offered the opportunity to establish contact with people who did not all belong to my research categories but, being progressive, might have a positive attitude towards the issues.

Occasionally other meetings were attended, especially the series of meetings called Renai no Tatsujin Kōza (Course for becoming Successful in Love) presided over by the feminist scholar Uemura Kuniko. These were interesting because they covered subjects very closely related to my research, such as 'transgender'[5] phenomena, homosexuality, how to deal with being a feminist and loving men and with having more than one lover at the same time. Another meeting I attended was that of the Toshi Minzokugaku Kenkyūkai (Study Group for Urban Ethnology), to which Saeki Junko, author of a book on male homosexual culture, was invited (Saeki 1992). This group includes many participants who are not involved in academic pursuits.

An occasional group was created to protest to the authorities of Osaka city and prefecture about their (lack of) AIDS policies and I was asked to join in order to add weight as a foreigner. I participated in activities on International AIDS Day in Tokyo in December 1992. Invited by Onitsuka Tetsurō, who will be discussed later, I gave information about homosexuality to a network of young volunteers, mostly involved in voluntary work related to the physically disabled. Occur's Gay Rights Rally[6] was attended in the autumn of 1991, as was a session of their court case in Tokyo and the meetings afterwards. I attended JILGA's annual meeting in the summer of 1992 and the event on homosexuality in November 1992 at Osaka University, organized by Puapua, a political gay group based in the Kansai area. Further, I went to the yearly Women's Festival in Kyoto in March 1993 and to a number of other feminist meetings, organizations and spaces managed by feminist organizations.

Participant observation in less formalized contexts, such as at parties and in bars, when riding the underground or train, when having a bath in the local *sentō* (public bath) or washing my clothes in the laundrette, proved to be very relevant to my research aims. My research activities expanded speedily, so that only in the beginning did I spend much time with people who were not directly related to my research categories but who nevertheless provided important information on general attitudes towards marriage and sexuality and the extent of their pervasiveness. With some of them, however, I kept contact throughout my stay in Japan and thereafter.

Many of these informal venues were the parties held by those my research centred on and especially two wider networks of friends proved to be valuable sources of information. One is based in the area where I lived in Osaka. Most people involved share left-wing political beliefs and many Japanese Koreans participate. The other is based in Kyoto. Here political beliefs played a less explicit role, although the atmosphere was extremely progressive, especially towards sexuality and gender. They included the high-tech performance group Dumb Type, in whose *Seminar Show for S/N* on sexuality and AIDS I participated as a gay man, and the drag group Diamond, with whom I visited many clubs. While art was the main connecting factor, issues of gender and sexuality gradually became the major topics. The parties of this network often lasted until dawn. When I related this to my Japanese supervisor, she retorted: 'But that is perverse! (*Sore wa pabāsu!*),' which suggests that such parties are unusual in Japan. Parties were of vital importance as occasions for informal discussions about my research topics.

This description of various examples of participant observation is by no means exhaustive but I hope it gives some insight into the scope of the various sections of the research. Groups are discussed in more detail in following chapters and they are listed in Appendix B.

In most cases at least some of the participants knew that I was doing research and on what, although they may not always have expected me to do participant observation with them. Many (even social science graduates) were not familiar with the idea of participant observation in an urban environment. In this connection an interesting book was written by Satō Ikuya (1992), which is presented as an introduction to fieldwork but reads more like a desperate plea for the recognition of participant observation as an acceptable method for research. Interestingly, Satō calls the book *Fiirudowāku* (Fieldwork) and then sets this method in opposition to quantitative research, including questionnaires. Fieldwork as used by Satō means participant observation.

On hearing that I was doing anthropology (*jinruigaku*) people advised me to go to remote areas like Tōhoku, North Eastern Honshū, which was deemed to be the place to go for anthropologists. In other cases I said I was a sociologist (*shakaigakusha*), which led to people volunteering to assist with the distribution of questionnaires. Participant observation and in-depth interviews seemed not to be acknowledged as methods of research suitable for a sociologist. Satō (1992) writes that he has great difficulty explaining the value of non-quantitative research to his students. According to him, they do not feel secure when they do not produce something quantifiable. They do not perceive work without tables, charts or diagrams as scientific.

In less formal contexts, such as parties, people usually knew about my research and volunteered to give their opinions, often leading to extensive discussions. Notes were taken mostly after the events because it would have been difficult to listen, talk and write at the same time and because it would have been terribly disruptive to take notes at a party or while, for instance, ice-skating. At seminars and such I often took notes because that is normal behaviour. Even though they knew to some extent what my research was about, the other participants were not likely to have appreciated that the contents of my notes, at times, concentrated on the proceedings of the meetings rather than on the contents. This is where I came closest to covert work.

## Finding Informants and Determining Biases

With a research theme dealing with such people as homosexuals, feminists and singles the easiest and most obvious method of finding informants is through groups of gay men, lesbian women and single and feminist women and men. An obvious result of limiting the research to informants from these groups only is that the results are bound to be biased. Many people attending singles' meetings are very different from the majority of unmarried people because they make a positive issue of it and tend to choose to be single, whereas the majority would rather be married or at least say they would. Similarly, women who join feminist or women's liberation groups are more outspoken about feminist ideas than women who act in accordance with feminist ideas but do not consider themselves as feminists or even denounce feminism.

For gay men and lesbian women the picture is somewhat different because there are major differences between various groups, from politically active to purely social. People joining purely social groups are different from the majority of the gay population in the sense that generally they are more assertive about being gay, while those who do not participate in any groups are more negative about being gay themselves as well as about homosexuality in general, although gay men who are negative about homosexuality can also be found in social groups and even in politically oriented ones. Particularly in politically oriented groups there was a relatively large proportion of people with Christian, Marxist or Christian-Marxist backgrounds, something that is visible throughout voluntary organizations in Japan. This is undoubtedly linked to humanism and to the fact that Christians and Marxists are traditionally outside the mainstream of Japanese social organization, which used to revolve around Buddhist temples.

A second method of finding informants was through the gay bar circuit and by contacting people who place advertisements in gay and other magazines,[7] a method I used to a small extent, mainly in the initial stage of my research. This was not very productive but contacts with a woman married to a homosexual man, contacted through the personal advertisement section of a gay magazine, and gay men met in bars and in, at the time, Japan's only gay club in Osaka, proved very informative. The bars and club were good for conducting participant observation and short directive interviews. These are not included in the count of interviewees because it would ultimately include everyone I spoke with. Men frequenting gay bars, again, are a specific section of Japan's gay population and relatively free and financially well-off. Others never or rarely go to them.

To a limited extent the snowball method was used. I asked some people to introduce me to single friends, which in some cases resulted in interviews with totally isolated gay men and lesbian women, who had never before spoken to anyone about their homosexuality. One interviewee at least seems very unlikely to speak of it ever again. In another case I was introduced to someone who according to my introducer had never been married, while it turned out that she had. This method served to show how little Japanese may know those they call friends (*tomodachi*), as regards their private life and sexuality, and the attendant limitations of being able to discuss such matters at both personal and professional levels. I also interviewed heterosexual singles outside networks, which provided insight into differences between networkers and isolated singles.

A problem I expected to arise before starting the research and that eventually materialized, was that the possibility of carrying out interviews was limited by the time available to informants. Particularly those who worked in companies usually could only make time at weekends, when I was busy running from one meeting to another because almost all of the meetings were held on weekend days, which made it very difficult to meet up. This initially seemed to lead to a bias towards those who have more freedom, i.e. those who work at universities, who have freelance or independent occupations or who are unemployed or studying.

This was compensated for by making an extra effort in a later stage of my research to find mainstream company employees. The time at which they might be available for an interview was hard to predict because they usually did not know when they would finish. The circumstances at their company meant that they were unable to predict when they had to work overtime or when they had to go to a bar with colleagues after office hours, while they could not very well excuse themselves because they were going to be interviewed by me. Since this made making an appointment virtually impossible, in the end I interviewed some of them by phone, usually around midnight because that turned out to be the only time they would be certain to be available. Another mainstream company employee was interviewed while working on the newsletter for the singles' network in Osaka. He was quite happy having all the others present listening in and expressing their, often negative, reactions to his tales.

Regionally, informants are concentrated in the Kansai and the Kantō (the areas around Osaka and Tokyo respectively), while about 10 per cent live in small towns or rural areas, thus providing insight into the question of whether circumstances in the *inaka* (countryside) are much different from those in the *daitokai* (metropolis). On a smaller scale it can be said that some categories concentrate in particular parts of cities, although they can be found all over. Well-known and often mentioned examples are Shibuya and Meguro, two wards of Tokyo that are known to have a relatively large proportion of relatively affluent single women (Yoshihiro 1987). In Osaka my interviewees tended to live either in towns to the north of Osaka, or in the north or the south of Osaka city. The towns to the north of Osaka, such as Suita, Minoo and Toyonaka, are relatively progressive and affluent,[8] two factors that combined to offer a greater amount of freedom. The southern part of Osaka city, on the other hand, is cheap to live in, as was the northern part where I lived myself. In both areas I found a relatively high prevalence of single-parent households.

In particular the members or participants[9] in the activities of the cluster of five interrelated gay groups came predominantly from the relatively rich area north of Osaka and west of Kobe, such as Nishinomiya, while others lived in Kobe, Osaka, Kyoto and even as far away as Himeji and Fukui. In Tokyo many informants lived in the western part of the city, including Nagano, Shinjuku, Setagaya and Shibuya wards, as well as the northern part, including Bunkyō, Tōshima and Kita wards, which are cheaper areas to live. In Kyoto the same dichotomy was noticeable, participants living on the one hand in expensive *manshon* (concrete apartments) and, on the other, in cheap wooden rented apartments, often in southern parts of the city.

Informants from Kobe generally lived in *manshon*, while those from the area east of Osaka tended to live in cheap housing.

## Interviewees

The total number of informants who were interviewed in depth, is 109. Of these, 69 interviews were recorded on tape, resulting in approximately 110 hours of cassette-tapes, and 40 were recorded in written notes. Here I make a breakdown in sex and sexual preference to provide some idea of the numbers concerned, notwithstanding my explication in the introduction and above about the problematic nature of these categories. There were 56 female interviewees and 53 male. One was in the process of a sex change and preferred to be identified as a lesbian. Another interviewee was male, as in having male genitals, but identified himself as female. She/he thought of her/his brain and heart as female and had had a career as a transvestite artist. The former was counted as female and the latter as male. Many informants described themselves as masculine while being female or as feminine while being male, which underlines the problematic nature of the seemingly natural division into female and male.

To give a rough idea of the numbers of homosexual interviewees, 38 male interviewees can be categorized as gay and 21 female interviewees as lesbian. While most of them identified themselves as gay or lesbian, a small number are less decided. If someone is bisexual, he or she can still be categorized as homosexual because it can be used not in the meaning that someone is homosexual and nothing else but in the meaning that someone has homosexual desire, which is an attribute that does not preclude another, such as heterosexual, desire. There are of course men whose sexuality is quite ambivalent in that they are not sure whether they are gay or heterosexual, or who engage in homosexual activity while maintaining that they are heterosexual. Homosexuality may be seen more as an activity than as an identity by some people, while at the same time there are those who regard homosexuality as an emotional attraction which does not necessarily need to be consumed sexually.

Some interviewees who said that they were not gay have been counted as gay because they were clearly attracted to men or because, although they identified themselves as heterosexual, in the interview it became apparent that they had no sexual interest in their wives whatsoever. Their sexual attraction was very obviously towards their own sex. In all these cases, other informants also regarded the men in question as gay. In one case an informant, not an interviewee, said that he was not gay but was unclear about what he was and a woman commented that he was 'a mere narcissist'. I regarded him as gay. Two years later, though, he called himself unequivocally gay. What changed was that by then he had a boyfriend. The figures for the number of gay interviewees are very rough but they are only given as an indication and hence of limited importance. Moreover, not only interviewees are discussed throughout this book but also hundreds of informants.

In the case of women it was more difficult to establish whether someone should be considered lesbian or heterosexual because there is even greater ambivalence about what 'lesbian means'. The word *sōsharu rezubian* (social lesbian), mostly used in feminist circles who follow in the steps of Adrienne Rich and her lesbian continuum (Rich 1993), helped to explain part of the problem. The word 'lesbian' may be used to refer to an intimate relation with a female friend. Popular media are somewhat clearer with their *chotto rezu* (a little bit lesbian), which is used to indicate women who are heterosexual but prefer not to become involved with a man because they find them uninteresting and may ultimately become involved in homosexual activities. On reading and hearing about this phenomenon, I found it rather suspect, because it reminded me of the prejudiced view that lesbian women could not find the right man, but women who said that their feelings agreed with this made me conclude that it has more validity than I expected. They are not counted as lesbian.

Lesbian writer Kakefuda Hiroko was astounded to see me write *rezubian* instead of 'lesbian' in an otherwise English text and complimented me on it because she felt that the English word did not fit the Japanese connotations *rezubian* has. Another writer, Matsuo Hisako, said that she disagreed with Jennifer Robertson's (e.g. 1992, 1993) use of the word 'lesbian' in connection with some women of Takarazuka's all-women revue because she felt that it was not appropriate in the case of relationships between women of Takarazuka, which, according to Matsuo, often end when they leave the revue and marry. For the convenience of the reader, I will, nevertheless, use 'lesbian' hereafter. A problem that emerged with English supervisors was that I used 'lesbian' attributively, in phrases like: 'She became lesbian'. I was told that it should be 'a lesbian'. According to my dictionary (Hannay ed. 1993), however, the way I used it is correct also, although it may be less common in England. I have decided to persist in using 'lesbian' as an adjective indicating an attribute similar to the way 'gay' may be used. 'A lesbian' often suggests a connotation of identity and oneness, which may not be appropriate in the contexts I am dealing with. These matters are further discussed in chapters five and seven.

Easier to establish is the marital state of the interviewees. There were 40 men and 35 women who were single in the sense that they had never been married. Among the women, there were 9 divorcees, of whom 6 were lesbian and among the men 5, of whom 4 were gay. There were 6 married men, of whom 3 were gay, and 10 women, including one who became lesbian and eventually divorced after I left Japan and one who said that she would prefer to live with a woman, which she, however, did not equate with having a sexual relationship. The former is counted as lesbian, the latter not. Ideally, a third category would be that of cohabiters, who socially may not be very different from married people, up to the point that their superiors at work may believe that they are married. However, in the classification given here I decided to stick to the legal definition of marriage, as the question of cohabitation is again a different story, which will be discussed in chapter three.

Ages varied between 20 and 67, with the majority aged between 25 and 45, of which those aged 27 to 33 and 39 to 44 again represented a majority. This is due to several factors. Between 27 and 33 years of age lies the period in which marriage becomes a pressing issue and as a result people of that age were more likely to want to be interviewed; they loved the chance to talk about their problems and also wanted the world to know about their existence. They found my research important for themselves and were eager to participate, with some travelling up to three hours to make the interview possible. At the same time it is my own age group. Being 30 years old on arrival and 32 on leaving Japan, I could relate to this group on a very equal basis. The great number of those aged between 39 and 44 must be attributed to the fact that this is the generation of the student revolts of the late 1960s and early 1970s. Although most of those who were active in the student movement eventually adopted mainstream lifestyles, a relatively high number of this generation is politically active in one sense or another or refused to marry because they saw it as a way to oppose the *kanri shakai* – literally the administration society but used by some informants in a way reminiscent of *Nineteen Eighty-Four*'s big brother (Orwell 1949) – in which marriage is seen as occupying a central position.

The selection of interviewees was highly controlled. They were selected from 20 different groups and through several social networks. Attention was given to not interviewing too many people from one group or network but to spreading interviewees as much as possible over the different groups, while taking into account their age, sex, education and occupation. An expected limitation of the interviews was that the interviewee had to be someone who thinks about things and knows how to express him- or herself. This was to some extent a criterion for selection. In order to obtain as wide a range of different attitudes towards life as possible, interviewees were rather chosen for being particular than for being representative. It may seem contradictory but I believe that as a result the outcome is highly representative, not in numbers but in scope.

Speaking of a sample in this context is misleading, as the word 'sample' is taken too often to indicate quantitative representativity. Like Lebra's research on Japanese nobility (1993) the research does not provide for that but for experiential plausibility instead. Unlike Lebra I did not conduct a survey by questionnaire and any quantifications used are based on my informants and what they conveyed to me in participant observation and interviews combined with statistics as they are produced by governmental and other organizations. I do not present numbers of categories of interviewees in tables because when I did this people started to interpret them in an absolute quantitative manner, which is not only ridiculous but also potentially harmful to my research categories.[10] Like Lebra I insist that my informants must all be regarded as key informants, who by their accounts and their activities give insight into not only their own particular lives and ways of thinking but also into those of the rest of those living in Japan.[11] When below I use the plural 'informants', it usually includes interviewees.

## Setting and Content of the Interviews

Interviews were conducted in various locations, varying from coffee shops to restaurants, parks, offices, shops and private living quarters. Usually I let the interviewee decide. Some came to my apartment and others were interviewed in an apartment that was at my convenience to use in Kyoto or in their own apartment. A setback with interviews in public locations was that the music, the waiters and other customers often caused disturbance, which was especially true for some interviews, the recorded tapes of which were difficult to understand due to background noise. Often it was not possible to find a quiet location, and it was anyway preferable not to conduct the interview in a quiet location because others might overhear, which is less likely in noisy circumstances.

One interview was recorded first in a restaurant, then outside a shopping centre and finally in a coffee shop. While we kept looking for a place to talk undisturbed, we were harassed into leaving two locations, first a restaurant, where noise became too loud to talk, then a park bench, where a man started interfering. Another was conducted in the car of my interviewee, since he seemed to be unable to find a suitable coffee shop in Kobe. One interview was recorded by the Asahi Broadcasting Corporation of Osaka, at the request of my interviewee, Hirano Hiroaki, of whose life a documentary was being made in the week I contacted him. In the end the documentary did not include this interview, although I did appear briefly on screen in a take from a meeting of OGC.

The interviews were essentially open-ended but there were a number of subjects I planned to be discussed, such as the interviewee's relation to the family, the work environment, friends and lovers, thinking about the politics of gender and sexuality, feminism and gay movements, attitudes towards marriage and having children, and instances of discrimination. The order of the topics was undetermined and often they came up quite naturally, without me having to steer. Often I began by asking the age of the interviewee, which is a somewhat impolite question and at times worked as an icebreaker. Usually I had no difficulty at all in getting my informants to talk. Within 5 minutes my role became limited to asking a question or proposing a new topic when one was exhausted. Most questions were of the following nature: '*Tomodachi wa dō?* (How about friends?)', '*Kekkon wa dō omou?* (How do you think about marriage?)' or '*Anata ni yoru to feminizumu tte nani?* (What is feminism according to you?)'.

The language I used was as much as possible direct speech – which is considered rude in some circles or circumstances – and to my pleasure interviewees who initially used more distant and polite manners of talking, usually followed me after a while, thus entering the language level I thought to be most appropriate for my purposes: direct speech is used between people who confide in each other. I made major efforts to stop using the politer *masu* endings, let alone polite verbs and other words, which I had been taught to use in Leiden but which maintain or even create distance and therefore are not very useful for relating to people in the way I needed to for my research.

Four interviewees started commenting on my methods during the interview. One thought I was not prepared properly because I had no prepared questions, which I never had for the sake of spontaneity. This was my most difficult interview experience. Both he and I were not feeling very well and the conversation just would not develop. Another wondered why I asked about lesbian bars and such, thinking I knew about them by then. I knew they existed but wanted some more information about them and she was very well informed. The last two thought interviews as a method of research were totally useless because people would give the answers they expected me to appreciate or answers that are generally acceptable.

Indeed, in some cases I could not help wondering whose words the interviewee was recounting but in most cases the accounts were very personal. However, even if they were recounting something they learned at a meeting, from a book or from teachers, friends or parents, that is also relevant to the aims of the research. Accounts of attitudes towards homosexuality by heterosexuals were sometimes suspect. Some were very positive, even if they clearly did not know what they were talking about. In general, though, interviewees frequently disagreed with propositions I put forward. As will be discussed in chapter seven, negative views were also voiced, about homosexuality as well as feminism. Participating in people's daily lives and in the activities of the many groups provided a check and balance with regard to these problems.

I also asked questions that were directed at finding out what interviewees thought to be acceptable behaviour. One of them almost became angry when he could not reply honestly as to why he married. Instead he started telling me that this question was not right and that I could never get the true answer by just asking it because people would just say something they thought appropriate. Of course he was right and I agreed with him but maintained that it still was interesting to know what people answer, which made him feel even more threatened. Instead of answering any more questions, he started to lecture me on research methods. Many other interviewees were very clear about the reasons for their marriage and they were often different from those generally appearing in Japanese government surveys, where answers are pre-printed and the complexity of decision-making cannot be expressed.

## Ethics

Most scholars I discuss my research with believe that it is highly sensitive and that it is important to be very careful in using the data generated. Ethics are thought to be related to morals which prescribe that one should not hurt one's informants (Sieber 1993). As stated, this is a reason to avoid quantifying results. Covert research is thought to be ethically more problem-ridden than overt because informants are not aware of who they are talking with (Burgess 1984: 47–8). Since my research was essentially overt, there is little worry in the area of using information informants might want to remain secret. Even if I write things that groups do not like to see printed about themselves they knew who they were dealing with and in some cases I have asked them to criticize findings that they might see as harmful. A problem that is important, however, is the question of the extent to which the anonymity of informants must be protected.

The word 'morals' in a Western academic context is related to Christian doctrines concerning human relationships, even among people who have long abandoned religion. Therefore the personal relationships a researcher in the field engages in are likely to become a focus of concern. Christian morals in the end proscribe having sex outside marriage and some researchers have tried to avoid having sex with informants, sometimes at great pains (Whitehead 1986). After discussing the protection of anonymity of informants, I discuss my relationships with them and how I dealt with ethical questions in that context.

## Anonymity

In the section on interviewees I have already mentioned some cases of people who will inevitably be recognized in some circles, even if I do not mention names, places, occupations and other information that would facilitate an easy identification. Many people did not really care much whether I mentioned their name or not, especially if I was going to write about them in English. In those cases I pointed out that Japanese increasingly can read English and that I could not promise that there would be no translation into Japanese, which made some change their opinion. Others were more concerned, but keeping their identity from being detected was easier because they did not talk about being interviewed by me to anyone else.

In this sense, much of the power over being recognized or not lies in the hands of the informants themselves for, except where people are publicly known in Japan, I do not use names and when necessary I alter or do not mention details like locations, occupations and such. In other cases I cut the stories of informants up and have them appear under different guises, in order to protect parts of their lives which may be generally known in one circle from becoming known in another, where they might not want them to be known. Since interviews comprised more than one area of people's lives and the ways people combine living in different areas is a focus of interest, my descriptions of this phenomenon are either more general or various details of actual examples are changed, cut up or mixed in order to make them unidentifiable. I believe that this makes it perfectly possible not to distort my findings without endangering the anonymity that may be desired.

Some people seemed to see my research as an opportunity for them to come out. This I felt was inappropriate. I decided to protect them against the uncontrolled exposure that writing their names could bring. Although I do not make much effort to hide their identity, I do not present their full names, even if they said I could, but I may use nicknames under which they are known in particular networks, in which the contents of the interviews are largely known. I believe it to be useful for those who can read English to be able to recognize people who participated in my research. Since this can only happen with people they know well, this does not raise much of an ethical problem. This concerns informants who said that I could use their full name. If they still want to come out, they can do so, as some have in the meantime. This made me increasingly use full names during the process of writing.

Thus, the protection of the anonymity of informants is dealt with on a case-by-case basis. Guiding principles are the importance of mentioning an informant's name for explication and clarity and the indications given by informants on their wish to remain anonymous or not. Informants who have been very open about being interviewed by me will want to see something identifiable as themselves in anything that is published about them to show the friends they told about it. I am certain that I cannot provide for this in all cases, however much I would want to. Here the power is in my hands and I have to make my choices for the sake of the research project. In giving names and protecting anonymity I endeavour to err on the safe side, while being well aware that people may feel disappointed because they are not mentioned.

Never did I tell other people about those I interviewed. In a few cases, though, I confronted interviewees with findings of other interviews, without saying anything about the identity of the former interviewee. Nevertheless, those who were in groups and networks almost invariably talked about the interview to anyone who would listen, something that even led to jealousy among those who were not interviewed. In some groups being interviewed gave status: one had been taken seriously and was thought to be important and interesting enough to be chosen as an interviewee. I would have loved to interview everyone who wanted to be interviewed but that was impossible because there was a time limit on my work. It would also have been superfluous because even now so much material has been gathered that constructing a valid analytical view is extremely difficult.

The same can be said about interviewees who suggested I conduct follow-up interviews because their life and their thinking would be different on another day. The interviews represent only what they were and thought at the time of the interview. This is of course true but, except for a considerable number of interviewees whom I met more often for more in-depth research, it was not feasible to conduct follow-up interviews with everyone, however interesting they would have been. Nevertheless, I gave all interviewees my telephone number and address, so that they could always contact me if they wished to talk more. In the beginning I had two interviewees who had shortly before attempted suicide, which made me apprehensive of that possibility. I felt the least I could do was to try and be available. Although it was difficult to reach me because I was often away from home, many informants phoned, which added valuable data.

## Friends, Love and Sex

Many individuals taking part in the research became good friends; some became lovers. Three visited me in the first six months after I left Japan for Europe, a gay man, a lesbian woman and a feminist woman, and many followed later. These friends all knew what I was doing and supported my research to the extent that they bared their souls for me, something I did in return for them. Mostly they know one or more of my lovers and know roughly how I feel about Japan and the rest of the world. This was beneficial for building the confidential kind of relationships I wanted. As a result the relationships ended up being much more than research relationships.

As I was overt from the beginning about myself and my research with people in connection with my research categories and they usually understood that they were of interest for my research, I did not experience problems met by Joy Hendry, who describes a long-term friendship being disrupted when the friend agreed to be involved in participant observation (Hendry 1992a). The nearest example was when I told a friend that I wrote notes after parties and he was somewhat shocked. He said: '*Kowai*', which literally means frightening but in this context is an expression of shock or surprise.[12] I explained my point of view, which was that having to be *kowai* (shocked) or not depended on the way I would present findings. This he found fully acceptable and his trust in me was apparently sufficient to let this have no influence on our relationship whatsoever. Unlike Hendry, I found no conflict between friendship and research (ibid.). Nor did I find any difficulty with lovers also being informants, as did Ralph Bolton initially, although eventually he also came to see his lovers as informants (Bolton 1995). In my case, it occurred that informants became lovers and lovers informants. Lovers were, like friends, generally eager to participate in my research activities.

An American scholar, whose opinions I value highly, advised me not to fall in love with informants because it might produce a bias towards them. I thought about this and came to the conclusion that it was not a problem. As stated above, I am biased towards all the people I conducted research with and having a love relationship with one or another does not make me less critical of them. On the contrary, having a love relationship inevitably confronts one with less desirable aspects of a partner's character. Nevertheless, I think the advice from my American friend was very interesting because it points at widely held common-sense ideas about love. Love is supposed to make one blind and vulnerable. That did not happen with me and therefore I saw no reason to avoid falling in love with informants.

Indeed, amorous relationships greatly expanded the scope of participant observation. Ideally participant observation should include love and sex, for just like eating, which is a logical part of participant observation, love and sex are important aspects of culture that should not be ignored, especially if the research is on a theme in which love and sex play a major role. The feelings of the researcher may produce problems but this only happened when I had to leave. Of course, separation may bring pain (Dubisch 1995) but it makes little difference whether it concerns a relationship started in fieldwork or any other sphere. The pain of separation was much lessened when I learned that my life in Japan, including love relationships, would continue. When I visited Japan in the winter of 1993–4 and in 1996 it was as if I had not been away and many phone-calls and visits by informants when I am in Europe make me stay in touch with developments. The ethical idea that researchers should not hurt informants cannot be extended to informants with whom the researcher engages in personal relationships. I hurt some by not being the lover they wanted me to be. I also hurt informants by refusing to be their friend and by turning down requests for dating. In personal relationships people do hurt each other.

Initially I tried to prevent people from getting hurt and I used it as an excuse for not getting involved, especially with young men who I thought might be more vulnerable. One interviewee, Tsutamori Tatsuru, however, pointed out that I was being paternalistic and should not think for others. Eventually I decided to engage in any kind of relationship I wished, while trying to be honest about my feelings. I even ended up picking up a young man in a gay bar, which I do not usually do. In total I had amorous relationships with ten men, ranging from 19 to 40 years old from various walks of life, during my research period.

Western ethics are very constrictive about sex and I am not the first fieldworker to get tangled up in them. I have come to understand that in fieldwork situations it pays to adapt to local values (Cesara 1982: 148), which in my context meant freedom from values concerning constrictions on sexual activity. The only ethic I maintained in this respect was honesty, which was not and did not need to be reciprocated by all lovers. Contrary to people who think that sex in fieldwork needs nothing but the same morals one usually follows (Abramson 1993), I believe that there is an essential difference in relationships outside fieldwork and those inside. Outside fieldwork anything goes: people lie, betray and cheat all the time. When relationships are part of research more overtness and honesty on the side of the researcher are ethically required.

Another line of reasoning that having love relationships in fieldwork is unethical seems to stem from a comparison of the position of the fieldworker with physicians or psychologists. The idea is that a fieldworker has power over her or his informants (Abramson 1993). This may be a problem in some settings, especially when economic inequality comes into play, but in my research setting I am quite confident that it was not. If money played a role, it was because some lovers paid expenses for me.

Sometimes people tried to force sex on me. Especially in the beginning I encountered sexual harassment a number of times. Such experiences were, like more pleasant sexual experiences, valuable sources of information about sex in Japan and helped me to understand informants' experiences. Having experienced sexual harassment was helpful when informants talked about harassment and rape. I could communicate that I knew how it feels when a man stronger then you with alcohol on his breath in smelly clothes restrains your movements and fondles your crotch in a train where everyone tries not to notice. Like sexual harassment, love relationships are part of my life in Japan and thereby part of participant observation. They provided information on areas that are difficult to investigate otherwise.

## Inside the Outside: A Fieldworker's Personae

Dorinne Kondo, an American with a Japanese background, wrote that Japanese have an 'eminently biological definition of Japaneseness' and that this made her, being an American of Japanese origin, 'a living oxymoron'. She devoted her first nine months of fieldwork in Japan to an attempt to become 'Japanese' and eventually people ended up putting her in 'a meaningful cultural role'. Eventually she was treated by her environment as 'Japanese', albeit one that was somewhat strange. She uses the word 'war' when describing the fragmentation of her self and the collapse of her identity that 'naturally' resulted from this (Kondo 1990: 11–13).

What is a meaningful cultural role? Unlike Kondo, I set out for Japan with the intention of not becoming 'Japanese' any more than I was already. I am not used to having 'a meaningful cultural role' other than questioning roles cultures provide, in the Netherlands, in Japan and in England. Being 'a living oxymoron' is perhaps a role that fits me. This is not necessarily anomalous in my research context in Japan. My character and personality fit in quite well and it is not hard to find Japanese who act and react in ways similar to me. As stated in the introduction, in general I feel quite at home in Japan and Japanese seem to agree that I fit in quite well. Not looking like a Japanese to most people makes my position different from Kondo's, who is of Japanese descent, and possibly gave me more latitude in what behaviour was allowed. On the other hand, informants often said that I was more Japanese than they were, which may partly be a result of the fact that they see themselves often as uncharacteristic of Japanese. Strangers asked me the way, especially when my eyes were behind reflecting sunglasses, and some asked me whether I was *hāfu* (lit. half), i.e. whether one of my parents was Japanese, or even whether I was Japanese. To me, the field 'Japan' is not a 'negative category, the place that is not ours' (Killick 1995: 103), but rather the place where I feel more at home than in most places.

Hamabata (1990: 10–20) describes the anomaly of his position in Japan as an unmarried man, something that is also discussed by researchers in various other contexts (Angrosino 1986, Back 1993, Killick 1995, Wade 1993, Whitehead 1986). This anomaly was an integral part of all my personae in Japan. There are Japanese unmarried men and therefore there is nothing un-

Japanese about being anomalous in this sense. In the contexts in which Kondo and Hamabata worked, a traditional sweets bakery and a wealthy business family respectively, being anomalous may be contrary to one's goals but in my case it often was quite beneficial to be outright queer: it got people talking. I do not see my own identity as of much importance to all this. I experience no sense of breakdown of identity if people do not place me in a 'meaningful cultural role', like Kondo, or if my sexuality is not recognized, as Evelyn Blackwood experienced among the Minangkabau in Indonesia (Blackwood 1995). This may all be related to my particular personal background, in which sexuality is not as much a matter of identity as it is a matter of pleasure. As I suggested in the introduction, I feel that presenting oneself in a variety of ways is more interesting than having some set identity. I like people to be confused about what I am.

There were contexts where my persona was that of a heterosexual single man. I learned ways of dealing with those contexts, ranging from saying that in my country many people do not marry, that leading my life, moving from country to country, I could not possibly settle down and start a family, to that I did not wish to marry because I was gay and even if I were not I would not marry because I considered marriage to be a ridiculous institution. The last explanation is unheard of for most Japanese, although many informants agreed. It would end further discussion on the subject or lead to more interesting discussion on the topic of marriage in Japan or in their personal case, instead of my particular case. Some heterosexuals, on the other hand, were adamantly trying to find a bride for this young unmarried foreign man, which led to some complications, discussed in chapter six. In some of the families I visited, my being single was accepted for the moment but especially the matrons of the houses tended to keep insisting that one day I would meet the right person. In these contexts I deliberately did not say that I was gay, in order to experience to some extent what gay people in Japan experience when they hide their sexuality from their relatives.

I played many roles, ranging from what an informant called *burikkoburi* (acting the *ingénue*), of which singer Matsuda Seiko, who continues acting like a naive girl even though she is well past that age, is perhaps a prototype (Ogura 1989), to someone who is very knowledgeable and has much to tell, especially where it concerns personal relationships, sexuality and gender. The roles I played and the ways I presented myself were not so much thought out in advance but rather invented on the spot, influenced by whatever happened, as everybody does always to some extent (Goffman 1987). I adapted to different situations continuously. This was not alienating because, while I am an outsider as a white Western European in Japan and in some of the contexts I conducted research, I am an insider in most research groups as a feminist gay lesbian single person.[13] This made it easy to overcome the distrust of academics prevalent among informants. I was more queer than academic and agreed with informants that what scholars produce was often homophobic or otherwise unacceptable.

Often I was taken for an English language teacher, a profession that in Osaka seems to be occupied by the majority of white people. On other occasions I was thought to be a professional ice-skater or a dancer or singer. Most people at the time estimated my age at 26 or 28 years, with extremes of 22 and 30. Gay men and lesbian women were quick to recognize me as gay, which usually posed no problem because they were aware that, while they recognized me as gay, the majority of Japanese did not because they did not have a realistic concept of how gay men look and even if they would have, being with someone who is recognized as gay was not usually related to the possiblity that they might be seen as gay or lesbian by implication. It was interesting to notice later in Singapore that there fear of being seen with me, unless I dressed very neutrally, was much greater. Before leaving for Japan I bought clothes to achieve the looks that made many informants see me as *suteki* or *kakkō ii* (stylish or handsome)[14] because I expected people to be more eager to talk with me if I fitted their aesthetics. I also had regular haircuts[15] and kept myself clean for the same reason.

Playing different roles eventually led to some awkward situations, especially in Umeda, the entertainment and shopping area in the north of Osaka, which many informants regularly visited because it is the most important centre for railway connections in the area, has a large concentration of shops and the highest concentration of gay bars in Japan outside Tokyo. It happened that I ran into someone I knew from one group while setting out with someone else to find a coffee shop to do an interview. We had to get rid of the person, who looked terribly disappointed at being excluded by us. Other occasions are discussed in chapter six. These experiences taught me the complexity of a compartmentalized life through experiencing it myself. This method, which is similar to learning from experiencing sexual harassment or having sex, is what I, bending Reinharz's concept of 'experiential analysis' (1983), call experiential research: learning to understand mechanisms by experiencing them oneself. One becomes a subject in one's own research.

Part of this was coming out in the media as a gay man, invited by my lover Onitsuka Tetsurō, about which more in chapter six. This changed my persona in certain parts of the field, especially in gay bars and in some clubs, where it seemed that everyone knew me all of a sudden. A result was that people came up to me to ask for information about lesbian and gay circles, which brought some new contacts. In the gay and lesbian circles I participated in, little changed because they knew me before and coming out in the national media was becoming increasingly common by then. The exposure of my relationship with Onitsuka served to further discussion on having multiple relationships and sex because I acquired an explicitly sexual persona. Some informants, however, never found out or if they did, preferred not to discuss it with me.

In feminist circles much is made of the special position of the female researcher, who is supposed to have better access to women in particular and to be better at discussing sensitive subjects (e.g. Warren 1988). This may of course be true in large-scale fieldwork in which time to establish rapport with informants is limited, which in turn causes them to judge the researcher on directly visible features (Whitehead and Brown 1986), or in more traditional contexts (Schrijvers 1985, 1993), where men may be seen as threatening to women (Angrosino 1986, Wade 1993). The idea that women have easier access to discussing sensitive themes is based on the assumption that women have certain qualities men do not have. I believe this to be a very rough generalization.

When interviewing women I found them to be very obliging in answering the most personal questions and some said that they did not have such open discussions with their best female friends. Sometimes I stressed that they did not have to give answers to everything if they did not feel like it but except for two instances – a woman who refused to give her age and a woman who refused to give the direct incentives for her divorce because she did not wish to talk about it at that time – women answered whatever I asked and often more than that, regardless of whether they were heterosexual or lesbian. This may have been the same if I had been a woman, but many women would have difficulty asking men the questions I asked. According to a female colleague, men did not see her as a suitable person to discuss their sexual activities with. This may have to do with her personality, which is precisely my point: in intensive in-depth and personal research personal qualities far outweigh the influence of one's sex.[16]

## Conclusion

Throughout my research the topics I wished to investigate turned out to be important topics to informants who fell within the research categories but less so for those who remained outside them. This suggests that I happened to start out with the right questions, to hit the right tone with the right people. Possibilities for living in Japan that are generally glossed over because the number of people involved is too low to be statistically significant, are relevant as extremes on various continua. They provide insight into how loose boundaries can be for those who wish to avoid being moulded by their environment.

Apart from being representative in scope, or qualitatively, the findings can also be used in order to achieve a representation of not only the categories this research is concerned with but also of Japanese society as a whole in relation to them. It is possible to reach judgements on how Japanese society is structured in relation to the research categories because all people who were interviewed had to deal with Japanese society and ways of dealing with it were a focus of the interviews, of many discussions and of the examination of myself. Quantitative analysis is limited but nevertheless judgements can be made as to which patterns of thinking and behaviour are more widespread and which are more limited.

## Notes

1 To give an example, in England I was asked to fill out a questionnaire about attitudes towards AIDS prevention. Gradually it dawned on me that the questionnaire assumed that I was heterosexual, had one steady partner and possibly occasional sex with other people and that sex was vaginal sex. I had to think very hard about how to cope with questions like: 'If you have sex with your partner do you use a condom?' that I ended up circling 'Don't know' most of the time, although I have a clear safe sex policy.

2 Five gay magazines existed in Japan at the time, of which I read four throughout my fieldwork period: *Adon*, *Barazoku*, *Sabu* and *Za Gei*. The fifth, *Samuson*, was not read regularly because it was not particularly different from the others and included less journalistic material and reader's pages. Two new magazines, *Badi* and *G-men*, have since appeared.

3 Occur or Akā, as they call themselves in Japanese, is a group at the time numbering about 200 gay men and lesbian women (in this order, as it is theirs) who are relatively widely known for suing the Tokyo metropolitan government for having been denied the use of a youth hostel-type facility in Fuchū, a town on the outskirts of Tokyo.

4 ILGA is an international network of gay and lesbian groups, that tries to promote the liberation of homosexuality worldwide. Its main base is Western Europe (at first especially the Netherlands) but the late 1980s brought major inroads into Latin America, Asia and Eastern Europe. Minami

Teishirō headed JILGA, fashioned as the Japanese chapter of ILGA, which was building a network in Asia. I met Minami at the second Asian Regional Conference in Tokyo in 1986 and again at the ILGA World Conference in Vienna in 1988, where I interpreted and translated for him. Contacts were thus well established before I started my fieldwork.

5 'Transgender' is a literal translation of the Anglo-Japanese term *toransu jendā*, which comprises everything that crosses gender boundaries. The term is further discussed in chapter seven. See also Tsutamori ed. (1990a).

6 This tour of Japan, held in order to raise interest in the proceedings of Occur's court case, comprised visits to Sapporo, Sendai, Nagoya and Osaka. The visit to Osaka was boosted by the presence of some members of GAPA, Gay Asian Pacific Alliance, an organization based in San Francisco.

7 One interviewee drew my attention to a magazine called *Gekkō Bunka* (Moonlight culture), with articles ranging in subject from witchcraft to ghost stories, sadomasochism and lesbianism and suggested that I reply to advertisements placed by lesbian women. This produced no result. Replying to advertisements in gay magazines, however, produced some interesting results.

8 See also Ueno and Dentsū Nettowāku Kenkyūkai (1989), which is an investigation into women's networking in this very area and was criticized by Yamashita Etsuko (1991) for being too positive about the progress of women's liberation because the sample Ueno used were housewives who were in the minority position of having a husband who earned enough for them to be able to freewheel in whatever activities they wished.

9 Some of these groups do not have a 'membership system' and in most everyone could join activities at any time, hence my use of 'participants'. The people at the centre of these groups can nevertheless be described as 'members' and one of these groups was more or less closed to new participants for a particular period, making members a good description of its participants.

10 At a seminar I presented my interviewees in four categories of gay men, lesbian women, straight men and straight women, superimposing on them the numbers who were familiar with feminist ideas. Most straight men were familiar with feminist ideas and most gay men were not. Ueno Chizuko drew the conclusion that gay men were less informed about feminism because they had less contact with women, which agrees with her earlier writing (Ueno 1991a), but it is nonsense. The reason that in my sample straight men were more informed was that they were chosen as interviewees because they had lifestyles or were involved in activities that made it likely for them to be familiar with feminist ideas, whereas gay men were chosen because they were gay, regardless of their views of feminism. In order to pre-empt such false deductions, I prefer to avoid quantifications.

11 Informants include Koreans living in Japan (*Zainichi Kankoku-/Chōsen-jin*), South East Asians, Chinese, Europeans, North Americans and Latin Americans, the last mostly of Japanese origin. Of these groups, only some Koreans were extensively interviewed. In one case I was unaware of my informant being Korean until halfway through the interview.

12 When I met people from the same circle in 1995, they did not use *kowai* any more: it had largely been replaced by *jān*, which has no particular meaning but in this context is used to express shock or surprise.

13 The attributes are in alphabetic order. The idea that men can be lesbian is proposed by Hashimoto (1992a) and I instantly recognized it because on the rare occasions I had sex with women I felt more feminine than in any other situation.

14 Clothes I bought before setting out for Japan included a leather jacket, some shirts and shoes. Other clothes were sent later. Apart from the fact that Japanese sizes may not fit very well, I picked clothes to coincide with what I expected my informants to like. I appeared to have chosen correctly.

15 It was interesting to note that when I lived in Japan with long wild hair in 1996, people also thought I might be a professional dancer, only now of classical ballet rather than modern dance. This time I thought that more extraordinary looks would be conducive to my research purposes.

16 My positions in the field, including love and sex relationships and ethical matters concerning them, are more thoroughly investigated in Lunsing (1999a).

# 3 Discourses and Politics of Marriage

What is marriage supposed to be? Why are those who do not marry seen as problematic? And how do they feel about marriage? This chapter investigates various constructions of marriage. It starts by discussing mainstream discourses, or *jōshiki*, of marriage as they exist today in Japan. The reasons why marriage is thought to be an important part of people's lives and implicitly a fundamental organizing feature of society are presented. It goes on to describe socio-political and legal dynamics which are the focus of several movements that try to change marriage, in content or outward appearance. Finally, some examples of discrimination related to marriage are investigated.

## *Kekkon*: Common-Sense Notions of Marriage

As proposed in the introduction, the only fully adult person is a married man (p.14, Hashimoto 1988: 20–8, 62, Kawashima 1974: 36, Ueno 1990a: 65, 103–6). Indeed, in Japan one of the most widely held *jōshiki* related to marriage is that in order to become *ichininmae no shakaijin* (a fully adult social being) one has to marry (Edwards 1989: 124–9, Hamabata 1990: 129, Hendry 1986b: 115, 206–7). In this line of thinking men who do not take upon themselves the responsibility of supporting a household are not considered to be fully mature and thus can not be given responsibility for the most independent or powerful types of work. Women can, in relation to the concept of *ichininmae*, at most become *ichininmae no onna* (fully adult women), which is a fully adult but gendered being (Kondo 1992), derived from the male norm, a position that is obtained by marriage and having children (Hendry 1986b: 100, Lebra 1984: 87–100), often preferably a son (Higuchi 1986, Lunsing 1989).

One married couple amongst my informants whose sympathies lie with the left-wing in the spectrum of Japanese politics, said that marriage is more than a man and a woman pledging to share their lives together. While the man's brother, who had remained single, looked increasingly displeased, they continued to explain that man and wife are in fact physically combined into one entity; they become one person and this person, that is represented by a married couple, is the *ichininmae*. In this line of thinking unmarried people are *hanninmae*, they are but half of a couple, which means half of a person. Those who are not married are not independent individuals but like children waiting to grow up, no matter what their age is. This idea of the oneness of the married couple has been traced back by Idota to the situation of peasants and townspeople as opposed to the *samurai* class in the Edo period:

> one can say that a united (*ittaiteki*) couple-family cooperative was the basis of society. This united couple-family cooperative can be divided into two types: 1) the non-patriarchal, which is a relative qualification, based on equality and 2) the patriarchal, a union in which the woman is subordinate to and absorbed by the man and his family. (Idota 1993: 81)

Both types are based on the idea of the physical unity (*ittaika*) of husband and wife. The first type is a blending of the male and the female and in the second the male and his family absorb the female, which denies the possibility that the female might make any significant contribution as a person in her own right to the outcome of the union. This second form also stresses that the woman enters her husband's *ie* (household), where she becomes subordinate not only to her husband but to his entire family. The *ie seido* (household system), which was continued by way of marriage and having children, has even been used, with considerable popularity, as a metaphor to describe the social structure of Japanese society (Nakane 1973).

The *ie* system is usually described as a household organization in which the members of a household share an economic activity and in which ideally the eldest son brings in a wife to continue the essentially vertical line, a line of continuity through generations, from ancestors to generations yet to be born (Hendry 1986b: 15–17, Lebra 1984: 20–1, 1993: 108–11). If no suitable son is available other possibilities exist, such as the eldest daughter bringing in a husband (*muko yōshi*; Hendry 1986b: 99–100, Lebra 1984: 20, 1993: 112–15) or even the adoption of a couple (*fūfu yōshi*; Bachnik 1983, Lebra 1993: 111–12). Thus, although ideally the blood lineage is continued, in practice economic reasons and the continuity of the *ie* are considered of such importance that they may override the blood links (Bachnik 1983, Hendry 1986b: 101, Lebra 1984: 20, 1993: 109–10). From this it follows that, within the *ie*, positions or roles that must be filled by members are considered of more importance than individual proclivities.

Both of Idota's types can still be discerned in Japan, although the extended family moved somewhat to the background of academic discourse as a result of the legal demise of the *ie seido* after the Second World War and the subsequent nuclearization of the family. The low incidence of women whose name a couple chooses after marriage[1] suggests, perhaps, that *muko yōshi kekkon* is no longer as widespread as it may have been, which in turn suggests a decline in the influence of the *ie seido*. Present-day rhetoric is strongly based on the concept of equality in difference: husband and wife have different capabilities that are complementary to each other (Edwards 1989: 120–9). On their own they would be hopelessly helpless, they need each other to stay alive (Lebra 1984: 132), which is explained, as by my informant couple, with the concepts of *ittaika* and *ichininmae*. The idea of the physical union as a method of explaining the importance of marriage is popular and endorsed by, for instance, Lebra when she described the impossibility of talking with women when their husbands were present (ibid.: 27). The closeness of husband and wife makes it unnecessary for them to display intimacy and even conversation beyond the indispensable may be seen as superfluous (Lebra ibid.: 124–5).

Historical evidence indicates that the ideal type of marriage of two spouses who share their lives and love as it exists today, developed quite recently (Kawashima 1974: 167, Takamure 1991). Different from the expectation, common among my informants, that husband and wife should be true to each other, only a hundred years ago it was considered to be 'normal' for a man to have more than one wife, if he could afford it. This was called *ippu tasai sei* (one-man–several-women system; Kawashima 1974: 143). The Smith and Wiswell (1982) book on a poor village in Kyushu based on research in the 1930s, showed that extra-marital relationships were common, although it seemed to be preferable to keep things quiet and discreet in order to avoid gossip which, nonetheless, was widespread.

While on the surface people may act out their roles as spouses and pretend they are true to each other, in reality having affairs (*furin*) and sex outside marriage is not uncommon for both men and women – almost as common as in America[2] – and it seems that whatever the husband or the wife does, does not matter much as long as it remains discreet (Condon 1986, Ishikawa 1984, Maruyama 1988, Murata 1992). According to Lebra, structured promiscuity, that is a husband who keeps his involvement outside the house strictly separated from his wife, is less problematic than unstructured, in which case the other woman can become a nuisance to the man's family (Lebra 1984: 138–41). As long as the shape or the illusion of a one-man–one-woman relationship (*ippu ippu sei*) is upheld, there is no problem. Outward appearance matters more than contents: as long as the wrapping (Hendry 1993a), or *sekentei* (public face; Inoue 1971), remains intact, the contents matter less.

The most general term for love nowadays, *renai*, can, according to *Kenkyūsha's New Japanese–English Dictionary*, be translated as 'love, tender passion, *amour* or romantic attachment' (Masuda ed. 1988). It was introduced in the Meiji period to translate the Western concept of love (Inoue 1995).[3] *Renai* combines *renjō* and *aijō*, respectively the feelings of *koi* and *ai*, whereby *koi* is the passionate, romantic emotion and *ai* the stable affection or tender feeling. According to informants, the difference between *koibito* (with the character for *koi*) and *aijin* (with *ai*), both of which may be translated as 'lover', consists of *koibito* being the one and only love, whereas *aijin* could be translated as mistress or its male counterpart. As elsewhere, both words for lover are seldom, if ever, used to refer to spouses. While the ideal of romantic love leading to a marriage with a *koibito* exists, in general marriage in Japan can be said to be less bound by love than by a felt necessity either to comply with general standards about how one should live or to achieve enough economic power to afford what one thinks is necessary for leading an agreeable lifestyle. Love in association with marriage is in the first place expressed by the term *aijō*, which stresses not the romantic or passionate but a stable emotional affection which is supposed to grow between spouses over time. A romantic attachment may not be regarded as conducive to a good marriage because such feelings are thought to be unstable (Lebra 1984, Hendry 1986b).

The type of marriage that is discussed by many Western scholars in the field is the type in which the husband works outside the house and the wife inside (e.g. Imamura 1987, Lebra 1984). The husband makes the money and the wife holds the purse strings. According to many informants it is a generally accepted *jōshiki* that this marriage is what happiness for women (*onna no shiawase*) consists of. The description of the housewife's position as lifetime employment with three meals a day and an afternoon nap (Higuchi 1984: 57) also suggests that housewives lead easy lives. When asked explicitly, older married informants often presented reasons why it is important to marry in seemingly rational materialist ways. They said, for instance, that because Japan lacks a good system of care for the elderly and the ill, one needs to have a partner or children to take care of one in old age or when one becomes ill.

From at least the Heian period (794–1185), in which women's positions have been described as quite independent because high-class women remained in their parents' houses and their suitors or husbands visited them there (Takamure 1991), women have been seen as dependent on male family members, which culminated in the three obediences to the father, the husband and the son, of neo-Confucianist thought in the Edo period (1603–868; DeVos 1985, Hendry 1986b: 20–1). There is, however, a difference between the influence of Confucianism in Korea and Japan. In Japan it was much more limited to the upper classes, especially the *samurai*, and never really filtered down completely to the farmers, who comprised the largest part of the Japanese population. In Korea Confucianism arrived earlier and spread among the farmers, so that the position of Korean women was affected more by the low position women are accorded by Confucianism (Moon 1992).

This agrees with the view of Minamoto (1991) that the influence of Buddhism is of vital importance for the understanding of the difference between the sexes in Japan. Both intellectual traditions and folk traditions were strongly influenced by the Buddhist notion of women as less than people, as persons who were a danger to the purity of men and who could not attain enlightenment in this life. The best they could hope for was to be reborn as men (Marra 1993, Minamoto 1991, Wōss 1981). This argument offers an explanation for the general decline in the status of women starting with the arrival of Buddhism in Japan in the Nara period and the easy acceptance of the Confucian depreciation of women (Imai 1994, Minamoto 1991). It further offers an explanation for the discrepancy in marriage mores between the *samurai* class and the lower classes. However, while the women of farmer, trader and craftsman origin may have had more freedom as to choosing partners for marriage, their role in the household was also subordinate. Already in the eighteenth century 'women working outside the home were not perceived to be "real women" ' (Imai 1994: 49).

A male interviewee, who was married to a feminist woman, said that many people think that the marriage system is there to protect women, which is a traditional stance based on the idea that if a man is not married legally he may always desert his wife who then must take care of the children on her own. According to this line of thinking, marriage provides the woman with the security that the man is legally bound to his responsibilities as a husband and father. In this construction, that stems from post-war rhetoric, the husband is a provider for and protector of his wife, who is a weaker caring creature (Ortmanns 1993). My interviewee seemed to be afraid to identify with this idea personally, possibly because his wife might not endorse it. When I asked him what he himself thought, not what many people think, he said this was not his opinion. He apparently preferred to keep his opinion secret: he failed to give any, and became very defensive when I asked him what he saw as the reason for his marriage. I suspect that the answer was one that according to a government survey in 1974 was the answer 42 per cent saw as the reason for their marriage: because all marry, because the surroundings press one to marry, or because it is 'normal' (Herold 1980). It is common sense (*jōshiki*), natural (*shizen*) or a matter of course (*atarimae*).

## Dealing with Marital Roles

*Jōshiki* concerning femininity prescribed that a woman's job is essentially of an assisting nature, which is expressed by the content of the job, ranging from nursing to private secretaries, and in the reasons why the job is held, ranging from the need to save before marriage to the need to boost the household budget (Fuse 1984, Higuchi 1984, Imamura 1987, Lunsing 1989). For a married woman to work in this context means to work for her family (Higuchi 1984: 182–4). Even in cases of women who work in traditional fields and appear to be independent, such as the *ama*, female divers, it appears that the allocation of the work to them came about because of its low status and that their outward independent look has no relation to their status within their families or communities (Martinez 1993). Women who work because they like their jobs or because they wish to have an independent income cross the boundary of their assigned gender role into the realm of masculinity. Women are not supposed to be independent. In the case of men a reverse picture can be discerned. Men are supposed to go out of the house and work for an income to provide for the financial needs of the family (Lunsing 1989, Linhart 1984).

The freedom of Japanese 'professional' housewives whose husbands earn enough for them not to have to work outside the house and can thus provide their families with a home that is well cared for to come home to (Hendry 1993b), may be a debatable sort of freedom. For example, an informant quoted in Rosenberger (1992: 79) says: 'We would rather be out making good money than doing hobbies', but since she has no hope of getting a reasonable job she does *ikebana* (flower arranging). This case indicates that women are coerced into a particular lifestyle, which qualifies the fact that many women think that they like what they are doing. What matters more than the question of whether some women are happy as housewives is the question of whether they feel that they have a choice not to be a housewife and many women feel that they lack such a choice (Higuchi 1984, Lunsing 1989).

Research by McKinstry and McKinstry (1991) on the 'life advice column' in the newspaper *Yomiuri Shinbun* indicates that dissatisfaction with the role of the housewife is a main focus of the complaints and in a column in the women's magazine *Fujin Kōron* it is likewise the main focus of complaints sent in by women (Lunsing 1989). The prize-winning investigative journalistic *Tsumatachi no Shishūki* (Housewives' autumn) by Saitō Shigeo (1983) discusses some of the problems the dissatisfaction of housewives can lead to, such as alcoholism, loneliness and feelings of uselessness. Higuchi (1984) also gives a number of examples of dissatisfied housewives. Abundant material can further be found in, for instance, *Waifu*, a magazine in which women write about their personal concerns. For instance Yamada (1993), who writes on the relation with her husband's family, shows clearly her feelings of being trapped in an undesired situation.

Lebra (1984: 78–9) discussed essays she asked schoolgirls to write about their future. They tended to stop on the wedding day, the day when life ends in a way. One girl even thought it might be better to commit suicide before she had to marry and indeed, as Cecchini (1977) showed, there is a peak in suicides among women of marriageable age. This issue is also discussed in Ogura (1988: 107–8), who also relates it to the confrontation with a society that, different from schools and universities, discriminates against women. Wōss (1990), on investigating reasons for suicides among young women in Japan, found that financial problems are the most often cited reason. Many are unemployed. Official unemployment figures in Japan are low because the category is very narrowly defined. If one only works for one hour in a month one is not counted as unemployed in that month (Bosse 1994). An alternative solution for their problems would be to marry someone with a good income, which they obviously either see as not feasible or as not desirable.

In the households I visited, that can be described as being more or less in accordance with *jōshiki*, the role of the housewife was invariably subordinate. As is described elsewhere at more length, the role of the housewife demands that she is present whenever the husband or the children are at home, to have the food on the table when they want to eat, to keep things clean and to provide whatever else may be demanded. This greatly limits the freedom the housewife has to engage in activities of her own, in or outside the house, including paid work (Higuchi 1984: 23–4, 61–2, Imamura 1987: 14–30, Lock 1987). Marriage may be a matter of practical choice for women who cannot hope to obtain a position in the main career track and, by marriage, have more chance of a relatively comfortable lifestyle.

Older married male informants usually had little difficulty with seeing the virtues of marriage as far as they themselves were concerned. They may see marriage as desirable because they want a warm (*atatakai*) home to return to after a day's work. The day of marriage for them is a transition to an easier life in which they may actually gain in freedom because, if they were living alone and taking care of themselves, they no longer have to do their own shopping, cooking and cleaning. This gives them more time to spend as they please. If they were living with their parents, marriage provides the idea of security in being taken care of in the future, when the mother may become too old and physically weak. Their main role is in the workplace and when they marry they receive spouse benefits. Their position is enhanced by having become *ichininmae* because they have taken upon themselves the responsibility of supporting a household, which makes them more trustworthy in the eyes of their superiors at work. Although the above reasons surfaced, in general married men seemed not to have thought much about the question of why they married. *Jōshiki* holds that marriage is what you do and they had no reason to question that, as was the case for many female informants, who only after marriage started to wonder whether they took the right step, as will be discussed in the following chapter.

## Some Alternative Views

The prolific gay writer Hashimoto Osamu turns the *ichininmae* argument around and makes something positive of not being *ichininmae*. Being adult in his context is related to being dishonest and to the corruption of one's truer self, leading to its pollution. Therefore it is better to remain pure and a child, to remain unmarried (Hashimoto 1988). Such ideas exist among Japanese who oppose marriage but are not widespread. The imperfectness of being unmarried is expressed by the Japanese term *mikon*, which means not yet married. Only recently new inventions like *shinguru* (single; Ebisaka 1986) and *hikon* (unmarried; Yoshihiro 1987, 1988) have come into use, especially among those who take a positive political stance in this field, as will be discussed in chapter five.

Ideas about the physical union of marriage as being the only way to attain the status of *ichininmae* are under attack by feminists, men's liberationists and people from singles' networks. It is not very hard to undermine such ideas by making use of logical argument, such as that it is more *ichinimae* to be able to live on one's own and take care of oneself than to depend on a partner, but rationality is not very effective. Logic does not impinge on people who have believed all their life that marriage is the natural way of living for everybody and anybody who is not in a marriage must surely want to be. In their view, people who say they do not wish to marry are absurd and hence not worthy of serious attention.

Many informants said that the materialist arguments mentioned above, such as that marriage is necessary in order to have a spouse or children take care of one in case of illness, are outdated because many parents do not wish to live with their children and increasingly children do not want to or, due to their occupations, cannot live with their parents. Furthermore, it was argued that the idea that a spouse will take care of one in case of illness and old age does not stand up for women, who more often than not outlive their husbands and, even while they are younger, may not be looked after by their husbands in the case of illness. Common sense is, however, strong, resulting in many people 'knowing' that if you do not marry and have children you will end up lonely and sad. Similarly, the idea that housewives have power because they hold the purse strings is also debatable because it does not mean that they have the power to spend the money any way they like. Housewives are often bound by such tight budgets that they have no money to spend on themselves, while the pocket money men receive can be used by them at their own discretion (Higuchi 1984: 80–8, Imamura 1987, Lunsing 1989).[4]

It seems that people who believe marriage is the right way of living and are married themselves, are reluctant to give up this belief, which forms a secure base for sustaining their worldview that the life they live is 'normal' or 'natural'. The idea that other ways of living might be equally feasible appears to undermine their whole philosophy of life. People who criticize ideas that say that marriage is the natural thing to do, are fobbed off with the expression *rikutsuppoi* (argumentative), which has the derogative connotation of 'know-all', a very convenient word to use when one is confronted with an unwelcome argument to which one does not want to give proper attention. How people may deal with this lack of possibilities to discuss their opinions is investigated further in chapter six.

Japanese scholars rarely discuss lifestyles other than marriage. Ueno gives a clue as to why this might be so. In the introduction to an article on alternative lifestyles she discusses the fear that conservative people have of what they perceive as the disintegration or destruction of the family. She counters this by arguing that the family is not being destroyed but changing into a variety of different shapes, such as the single-person family or the same-sex couple family (1991b: 2). Precisely these changes, however, make the people in question feel unsettled. The idea that marriage may be something different than a union between man and wife has implications they are most likely to find unsettling. A variety of different shapes suggests that one has to choose. Placing for instance lesbian couples on the same level as heterosexual couples is felt as a threat by heterosexuals who are used to thinking that their way of life at least is more 'normal' than that of lesbian couples. Due to these dynamics Ueno appears to have felt the need to defend her writing on lifestyles that are at variance with marriage and to appease those who might feel cornered, who are likely to be the majority that upholds common sense.

Japanese scholars discussing anything different from some standard lifestyle use terms like *shakai byōri* (social pathology) or *shōkōgun* (syndrome). Many *shōkōgun* concern married women who are not happy with their lives or problems children have, both of which are generally blamed on the housewife or mother (Lock 1992b). The term *shōkōgun* also permeates discussions on the increase in numbers of single women, resulting for instance in a book entitled *Kurowassan Shōkōgun* (The Croissant syndrome), the author of which concludes that positive articles on independent single women in the popular women's magazine *Kurowassan* (Croissant) have led to a large number of women who did not marry, although it would have been better for them if they had (Matsubara 1988). Countering this argument, feminists have written a book called *Anchi Kurowassan Shōkōgun* (Against the Croissant syndrome; Waifu Henshūbu ed. 1989), in which Matsubara's argument is undermined. Nevertheless, Matsubara's line of thinking probably remains more widespread. A book along the same lines called *Kekkon shinai ka mo shirenai Shōkōgun* (The maybe-I-will-not-marry syndrome; Tanimura 1990) has seen the light of day since. This is reminiscent of the use of the term 'deviance'. As earlier work of Western scholars discusses, people who do not observe *jōshiki* regarding the roles of husband and wife, or any other *jōshiki*, may be stigmatized as deviant or mentally ill (Lebra 1976: 169, DeVos 1986a, b).

Among gay men and lesbian women many believe that marrying is the proper thing to do. Like most people, lesbian and gay informants often thought that remaining single would make them rather sad people and they also feared the loneliness old age might bring them. While they recognize the fact that their sexual preference poses a problem in relation to marriage, some think that they can become heterosexual upon marriage and others are confident that they can put on a show of heterosexual affection. Some are resigned to the idea that they cannot marry, although they find this a sad fate, a *nayami* (worry). In general, being lesbian or gay does not mean that people's ideas are different with regard to the pervasive importance attached to marriage. As the next chapter discusses, many do not escape the *jōshiki* presented in this chapter, which confirms their pervasiveness.

Single people, whether they are single by choice or because they just happened not to marry, do not have much trouble with countering economic arguments. The problem is again, however, that it is not so much rationality that counts but rather what the base of the argument is. The argument that one must marry and have children in order to have a comfortable old age is based on established *jōshiki* and backed up by a bureaucracy that still proposes that the old and the needy should be taken care of by their offspring (Lock 1987, 1988), especially by housewives, i.e. the wives of their sons or, according to Ueno Chizuko (verbal communication), lately increasingly their daughters, who are expected to put aside their personal interests whenever their assistance is needed. As discussed in the introduction, Japanese society still features systematic discrimination against women in the labour market (Lam 1993, Tsumura and Kita 1994). Marriage may be a mainly economic event and if women could have had the money without the husband, they might very well have preferred that (Lunsing forthcoming).

Feminists in Japan have been struggling with the problematics of marriage ever since they came into existence. In the magazine *Seitō* (Blue Stockings) at the beginning of this century, for instance, Ibsen's play *A Doll's House* was much discussed. The 1950s saw the *shufu ronsō*, the discussions about the position of the housewife and mother, and one of the major recent discussions centred around the question of whether housewives are enemies of women's liberation or victims of patriarchy (Ueno *et al.* 1992). The more radical, such as Ogura, hold that married women are enemies and feminists who are married have no credibility, which she sees evidenced by early feminists who started out demanding change in marriage and sexual relationships only to eventually change into a movement for obtaining the vote for women (1988: 199–201). Others criticize housewives while showing understanding, like Ueno (Ueno *et al.* 1992) or, and this is probably the majority, work themselves from the position of housewife and often mother, of which Hiratsuka Raichō was a proponent from the *Seitō* days to the 1950s (Takamure 1991: 250–1).

Feminist women do not usually endorse marriage as it is in Japan. They want to change its contents, which means in particular the husband playing a larger role in the household, more equality and the possibility for women to have a career besides being a mother. Otherwise they are usually quite in line with the idea that marriage as such is 'normal'. It should only be arranged differently, so that women have more freedom and relationships between husband and wife are more equal. This last position was ridiculed by two female interviewees, who found it rather useless to devote one's energy to changing something you do not like and therefore did not understand much of the feminist movement. Their solution: 'Why, instead of complaining that this or that should be changed, don't they just quit marriage?'

## Courting for Marriage

Methods of courting, as discussed by Hendry (1986b: 116–49), Lebra (1984: 79–105) and Edwards (1989: 53–63), vary according to period, region, class and the individual. In explaining Japanese ways of recruiting marriage partners, usually a division is made between *miai* (arranged) or *renai* (love) marriage. *Miai* means literally 'see each other'. Ideally, a *nakōdo* (go-between) arranges a meeting between a woman and a man so that they can meet and decide whether they want to continue meeting each other and eventually marry. Whereas there are people specializing in match-making, anyone can act as a *nakōdo*. Apart from very explicit cases of *miai* marriage, the distinction between *miai* and *renai* is mystifying rather than clarifying. Most marriages are a combination of the two (Lebra 1984: 87–100, Hendry 1986b: 147–9). Partners may have a *miai* arranged after they have fallen in love or they may fall in love after a *miai*. Love marriage does not preclude the possibility of coercion. A woman may feel forced to marry a man against her will, for instance because he made their colleagues think that she would marry him (Saitō 1983: 169–78) or because the man emotionally blackmails her (ibid.: 221–7). For men it may be considered impolite to refuse a proposed marriage because 'women are thought to be delicate and easily hurt by outright rejection' (Edwards 1989: 60).

Notwithstanding the vagueness of the difference, Japanese statistics categorize marriage as *miai* or *renai*. They show a steep decline in *miai* marriages, from 36.9 per cent in 1973 to 12.7 per cent in 1991 (Keizai Kikakuchō ed. 1992: 40), in favour of *renai* marriages, a decline that may very well be a mere result of the fact that the idea of love marriage has gained in popularity, something that can be related to the growing stress in the media on the supposed virtue of individual choice. This makes *miai* less appealing because the influence of third parties in determining one's life is so evident. Remarkably, in the statistics of 1991 a new category of what is called *renai kekkon* (love marriage) is introduced. It is the category in which partners met through the introduction of friends, which comprises 25.7 per cent of the total. Since the other major way of getting to know each other is meeting at the workplace (ibid.), where the influence of colleagues or superiors may be present, the stress on a change from *miai* to *renai* is not very convincing. It rather seems that *miai* has become less rigidly structured.

Love marriages are often based on calculations that take into account the other's status and capacities and one's own age and chances of finding a good match, more than the question of whether one is actually in love with someone (Lunsing forthcoming). Although romantic love is the incentive for marriage according to what is presented to the outside world, or *seken*, in many cases other considerations may play important roles, regardless of whether it concerns *miai* or *renai* (Lebra 1984: 90–7). As a female interviewee said: 'As long as he loves me, any man will do.' Apparently, she did not consider her feelings towards him to be of much relevance. This may be wise because, as she argued, while the love of the other for oneself is not a guarantee that everything will work out well, one's own love for the other is even less so.

The choice of marriage partners is influenced by many factors. Great influence is exerted by the *jōshiki* that one of course marries (*kekkon suru koto ga atarimae;* Tsuji 1989: 82). The basic question of whether one wants to marry or not is not really asked, because it is taken for granted that one will, which shifts the focus directly to the question of with whom. This of course limits one's freedom in relation to the choice of partners (Lunsing 1989). Another factor is ideas concerning the proper age to marry, *kekkon tekireiki*. Once past this age, which is not wholly stable, women may be written off as *Kurisumasu kēki* (Christmas cakes), which lose their value after 25 December, a reference to the age of 25 years (Brinton 1992). This plays a greater role in the case of women than in that of men, as having children is inevitably connected to marriage and a woman's fertility is thought to decline after 30 years of age. For men this is hardly a problem but they are, as many informants indicated, also increasingly seen as weird and confronted with proposals for *miai* when they reach their 30s and are still single.

Young people interviewed on radio and television programmes about their future plans often come up with the exact age at which they expect to marry. The idea that a partner might not be available at that precise moment is not considered. A woman on the radio made a whole speech about what sort of man she wished to marry: 'Tall and handsome, with a good salary and a taste for outdoor sports, someone who would like to travel together.' While it is of course a good thing to know what one is looking for, this also indicates that the individual one marries matters less than certain attributes he or she possesses. In this context there is the much discussed phenomenon of *san K*, the three highs, which a man, according to the mass media, is expected to possess if he wants to stand a chance with many women: he must be tall, be highly educated and have a high-status occupation. Glossy women's magazine *SAY* even ran an article featuring the average lifetime earning expectation of men according to their education, apparently intended to make it easier for women to make up their minds about what sort of man they wish to marry.

Before anyone is actually encountered, a strong ideal is developed of what kind of person they should be and when men found it increasingly hard to find a spouse in the early 1990s, the media were quick to develop surveys and reports to show that the demands of the women had become too great, resulting in a decline in the overall percentage of marriages and especially in an increase in the number of men who remain unmarried. While the media first pointed at the women for being haughty, this attitude has changed to young men's magazines now describing what are good strategies for a young man who wants to hook a woman (*Tarzan*, *Men's Nonno*, *Popeye*, etc): giving expensive presents, taking dates to dine in the right restaurants and making good conversation (Lunsing forthcoming). The mass media increasingly present a picture of men who have difficulty finding a woman (Ueno 1990b). For desperate cases, there are even *hanamuko gakkō*, bridal schools for men, where they can learn how to be interesting and witty when taking a woman on a date (Higuchi *et al.* eds 1990, Itamoto 1992b, Kawauchi 1992).

As table 3.1 shows, recently the numbers, particularly of men, who pass the proper age for marriage has grown considerably. Of men between the ages of 35 and 40 years 22.6 per cent had not married in 1995, compared to 19.0 per cent in

*Table 3.1*: Percentages of people who remain unmarried, by sex and age

| | Men | | | Women | | |
|---|---|---|---|---|---|---|
| | 30-34 | 35-39 | 45-49 | 30-34 | 35-39 | 45-49 |
| 1970 | 11.6 | 4.7 | 1.9 | 7.2 | 5.8 | 4.0 |
| 1980 | 21.5 | 8.5 | 3.1 | 9.1 | 5.5 | 4.4 |
| 1985 | 28.1 | 14.2 | 4.7 | 10.4 | 6.6 | 4.3 |
| 1990 | 32.6 | 19.0 | 6.7 | 13.4 | 7.5 | 4.6 |
| 1995 | 37.3 | 22.6 | 11.4 | 19.9 | 9.7 | 5.7 |

Source: Keizai Kikakuchō ed. (1992: 26, 409) and Sōmuchō Tōkeikyoku ed. (1996: 49).

1990, 14.2 per cent in 1985 and 8.5 per cent in 1980. This rise set in 1955, when the figure was 3.1 per cent and is accompanied by a rise of unmarried men in all age cohorts as the table above indicates. In the case of women the same tendency exists, albeit less marked, with a rise from 6.6 per cent in 1985 to 7.5 per cent in 1990 and 9.7 per cent in the age range 35–9 years in 1995 (Keizai Kikakuchō ed. 1992: 26–409, Sōmuchō Tōkeikyoku ed. 1996: 49). Hitherto this appears, however, to have had little influence on the idea that marrying is the only proper thing to do.

While the numbers of unmarried men have increased, the media until recently stressed the growing numbers of unmarried women, though they are much smaller. This is likely to be related to the fact that relatively more women in high positions (*kyariā ūman*: career woman) remain unmarried, as opposed to unmarried men who tend to be in lower social positions. In general, it is believed that the husband should have 'natural authority' over the wife, be taller, older and have had more education, which makes it very plausible that men with a low education and women with a high level of education have difficulty finding suitable partners and thus a relatively good chance of remaining unmarried.

Two interviewees who married a partner who was not suitable in this sense had great difficulty in convincing parents and superiors of the viability of their matches; one was a feminist woman who had a much higher level of education than her husband and the other a gay man who was ten years younger than his wife, who was well past the age of childbearing. These two are types of marriage that have recently come to be discussed as possibilities. Terms for marriages in which the woman is older or has a higher level of education have already been developed, such as *akiramegata* (give-up type), which refers to people who decide to look no longer for the love of their lives, but settle for less, or *chōkōgakurekigata* (extremely-high-educational-record type), which refers to people whose marriage was postponed by long years of education, both of which are types of marriage that bind couples who are both in their 30s, and *otoko pettogata* (man-as-pet type), for couples where the man is younger and economically less powerful than the wife (Tamura 1989).

The decline in marriage can partly be attributed to the phenomenon of *bankonka* (marrying later in life) but at the same time people who reached their 30s without having married are more likely to decide not to marry at all. They may have seen dreariness in the life of married friends and they may believe that they have discovered the joys of being single. The contradictory phenomena of Japan having a high marriage rate and at the same time a high average age of marriage,[5] suggest that many people tend to postpone marriage rather than rushing into it. People may wish 'to have some fun' (*asobu*) before they take the supposed social burdens of being married on their shoulders and become *ichininmae*. Two informants married but decided to postpone having children, so that the wife in particular could enjoy working life and the freedom to go out at night a bit longer. They presented themselves as very alternative compared to *jōshiki* that, in their interpretation, dictate that one has children straight after marriage. Indeed, they pointed out that their parents showed little understanding for their decision.

## Law and Politics

The Japanese language possesses a number of terms for marriage, the meanings of which are varied. There are fully Japanese words like *enmusubi* (tying a bond), which is not much used any more, and the viricentric[6] *yome o morau* (receiving a bride), still much in use, the Sino-Japanese words *kekkon* and the legal term *konin* and modern words like the Anglo-Japanese *marijji* (marriage, often combined with 'in the chapel'). The most commonly used word *kekkon* may be used to refer to legal marriage, to common-law marriage and even to same-sex unions, depending on the context. For this reason the word *kekkon* proved to be rather confusing in relation to the questions my research was concerned with.

Marriage as expressed by the word *kekkon* does not necessarily mean anything more than two persons whose involvement with each other has an element of permanence in intention or reality. They do not even have to live together, as there are types of *kekkon* like *bekkyo kekkon* (living apart marriage) and *kayoi kekkon*, in which partners commute to be together, for instance at weekends. The system of *tanshin funin*, whereby usually the husband is temporarily located elsewhere on his own for the sake of his job,[7] is widespread and much discussed (Tanaka 1992, Shiina 1994). Even if people live together they may not share much of their lives, which may amount to what is nowadays called *kateinai rikon* (divorce within the household; Kanda 1992).

People may claim that they are married when they are not married legally. At the same time people may be considered as married, when they wish not to be seen as such. According to law, *kekkon* is supposed to consist of a relationship of a male and a female bound by a legal document, the *koseki* (household register), which is supposed to be set up when a couple marries. As the following discussion intends to clarify, the actual connotations of the way the word *kekkon* may be used can be at great variance with this view.

Before my fieldwork started, rumour reached me that a friend had married. This friend, however, was known to be the kind of person that I expected to have political objections to marriage, something which in Japan is an issue that has lately become a matter of growing public interest (Fukushima 1991b, Ninomiya 1992a, Idota 1993). The fact that when one legally marries one of the partners has to adopt the name of the other, which usually means that the woman adopts the name of the man (see note 1), is a focus for movements concentrating on the law that does not legally permit married couples to retain both their own names.[8] The Japanese bureaucracy even started to discuss seriously the option of changing the marriage laws, in order to make it possible for spouses to keep their own names.[9]

As it turned out, my friend had married in one sense while in another he had not. He and his wife held a marriage ceremony for their families and she transferred her official home address (*jūminhyō*) to his. They did not set up a shared *koseki* (household register) or, in other words, they did not do *nyūseki* (entering the register, which is a rudimentary term, left over from the *ie seido,* but still much in use)[10] or *kekkon todoke* (marriage registration), which made their marriage not a legal one. Technically they had a common-law marriage because she changed her *jūmin todoke* (official address) to his house. I write technically because in practice they did not live together. Living together was practically impossible because the workplaces of the woman and the man were separated by 600 kilometres. Thus, in practice, they were in what one could call *bekkyo jijitsukon* (living-apart common-law marriage) or *kayoi jijitsukon* (commuting common-law marriage), terms I invented by analogy to existing terms but that did not exist in Japan at the time.

At his work, superiors of the man think he is married and according to Japanese law he or his partner might even receive spouse benefits, if the income of the partner remains below the 1 million yen a spouse can earn per year before this benefit is lost. According to law, she or he could be included on his or her health insurance and they are entitled to almost all benefits that married partners have, such as pensions, the right for the partner to stay on in the rented house when the one whose name it is in dies and even compensation money (*isharyō*) in the case of divorce (Ninomiya 1991: 123–43). In practice, however, informants living in *jijitsukon* seem not to expect most of these rights to be granted, although Ninomiya writes about people who received, for instance, time off for a wedding, for childbirth and for taking care of a partner who falls ill (ibid.: 132). A condition for the granting of such rights is often that the couple have the same official address (*jūminhyō*; ibid.: 133). Although such rights exist, many people are not aware of it and those who are may not wish to make use of them, especially in the case of a divorce. Informants who live in *jijitsukon* usually do not want the state (*kokka*) to interfere (*kanshō suru*) in their personal lives.

The *naien* laws, that give common-law couples equal rights to married couples, are based on the situation before the Second World War, when many people did not marry legally for various reasons. *Naien* is expected to be a temporary state of living together with the goal of marriage but there is no limit to the period of *naien*. The laws made for *naien* had different goals from what they may be used for nowadays (Hendry 1987a, Ninomiya 1991). The *naien* these laws were made for were in many cases born out of necessity. For example, the partners could not marry legally because one of the partners was married and could not get a divorce, or because parents failed to give their consent (before the war consent of parents was needed for men until 30 years of age and for women until 25 years of age), or because both partners were the main inheritors of their parents' *ie*, which made it undesirable for one to enter the *koseki* of the partner's *ie* because that would mean there would be no successor to their own *ie* (Ninomiya 1991: 29).

More common reasons for *naien* were that the bride was not officially accepted into the new house until she had proved to be able to adjust to the culture of the house (*kafū*), or to have children. If she could not adjust she could be sent back without having to go through a divorce procedure, something that would pollute the *koseki* (ibid.: 28). For many of the working class the bureaucratic procedure was difficult to fulfil. They had to take leave of their jobs to go to the town hall where their *koseki* was kept, which was often far away because most factory labourers were registered in the village they had left to go and work in the city. They also had to write their own declaration of marriage because there were no pre-printed forms as there are today (ibid.: 30–1).

Tsunoda (1992) and Ninomiya (1991) suggest that the *naien* laws technically might even apply to same-sex relationships because they do not specify the sex of the partners but use the neutral term *haigūsha* (spouse). Tsunoda said at a meeting in Tokyo that even the law of marriage itself does not necessarily exclude same-sex marriages because although it is stated explicitly that marriage is based on the mutual consent of both sexes, this merely reflects the fact that those who drew up the law could not imagine the possibility of same-sex marriage. Examples of gay or lesbian couples using these laws are not known to me and it would not be likely for the Japanese bureaucracy to grant gay and lesbian couples these rights. If demanded, though, they might produce interesting law-suits.

A possibility of casting a legal bond between same-sex partners that is being used to a small extent is the adoption law. In Japan it is perfectly acceptable to adopt an adult, who is entered into one's *koseki* as a legal child. A remnant of the *ie seido,* this possibility was used to safeguard the continuity of the *ie* when a suitable successor was not present (see pp. 76-77). This law makes it possible for anyone to adopt someone who is younger. Usually even couples of the same age are not born the same minute, which makes the use of this law a viable possibility for those who wish to have a legal tie to support their relationship (Tsunoda 1992). As an informant who lived in such an arrangement pointed out, sexual activities with his partner would legally count as incest.

The couple living in *jijitsukon,* mentioned above, live in an area in Osaka where many people refuse to marry. Further, there are relatively many Koreans and disabled, and anti-discrimination activities are a strong binding factor. Many parties are arranged with what at times seems to be the excuse of discussing particular cases of discrimination, for instance the case of a Korean Japanese man who sued Osaka city for not allowing people of other than Japanese nationality to rent newly built public housing.[11] In these circles it is almost inconceivable to marry legally and set up a shared *koseki.* It is more or less *jōshiki* that one does not set up a joint *koseki* but defies the *koseki seido,* which is the legal side of what is left of the pre-war *ie seido,* and supports a popular understanding of marriage that finds its roots in the *kafuchōsei* (patriarchate) of the pre-war period. It is felt that this must be opposed. How strongly this opposition operates in some circles is shown by the case of a couple who married secretly. This was only found out by a friend when he called the woman at her workplace and there was no person of her former name working there anymore. Two informants living in a similar context married abroad in order to have a legal tie that would make the employer of the man pay spouse benefits, so that he could support the woman, while avoiding setting up a *koseki.*

An example of a couple at variance with the idea that living in a *jijitsukon* is a good way to show disagreement with the position of women in marriage concerns an interviewee in her 40s who works full-time while engaging in various political activities. She lives together with a male lover but does not want anyone to know this because she fears people would start treating her as the *yome-san* (bride) of her partner. To avoid discovery by friends, family, colleagues and fellow activists, they have separate phone lines. While in practice they live together, the man still officially lives in the apartment where he lived before he moved in with her. Without living together, this couple could not have much of a relationship because they both work extremely long hours which do not coincide most of the time, so there would hardly be any chance for them to meet if they did not see each other when they both happen to be home. Having separate telephone lines is a way of coping with the idea that the outside world must not know about one's relationship that I also found to be employed by several lesbian couples who live together.

The riddle of the marriage of the couple that is the main example of this section is not solved by political opposition against the *koseki seido* only. Could they not have continued the way they did, after all they had had a more or less stable relationship for over most of the past ten years? The reason for this change of heart is not to be found in financial benefits, for they are few. The parents were not happy with the fact that they did not follow what they saw as *jōshiki* and set up a *koseki* but they still had the *kekkonshiki* (marriage ceremony) in which they witnessed their son and daughter pledge fidelity to each other. To make the parents happy was, however, hardly the major motive. More important were the feelings on the side of the spouses themselves. By having a marriage ceremony they pledged their intention to share the rest of their lives and by transferring her official residential registration to his house, they pledged their intention of living together as soon as economic circumstances, i.e. their job situations, allowed it. In fact they pledged that they would be husband and wife, and socially their position changed accordingly.

It is important to note that *jijitsukon* is typically based on the wish to share each other's lives, more than on the wish to improve one's status by marriage or to follow *jōshiki*. Partners living in *jijitsukon* are, unlike those in legal marriage, necessarily interested in each other as people, otherwise they would not have started to live together. This is linked to a distinct ideology which counters the position of marriage in the Japanese social structure. People in *jijitsukon*, as opposed to those in *hōritsukon* (legal marriage), are opposed to the *ie seido*, to the *koseki seido* and, at least in name, to the oppression of women they feel is reinforced by it.

## Children: *Shiseiji, Rabu Chairudo, Hichakushutsushi*

Closely related to the *bessei undō*, the movements striving for the right to keep different names in marriage, Japan has a number of groups that oppose discrimination against illegitimate children.[12] According to progressive authors in Japan, one of the major problems of discrimination the *koseki seido* brings with it is that of the illegitimate child, rendered by the terms *shiseiji* (illegitimate child), *kongaishi* (extra-marital child), the legal term *hichakushutsushi* (illegitimate child), or the more positive term *rabu chairudo* (love child; Fukushima 1991a, Hino 1991, Ninomiya 1991, 1992a, b, Shigekawa 1990, Satō and Kaibara 1990). Legal discrimination consists of a different way of describing illegitimate children in the *koseki* – 'only' son or daughter instead of the first, second, etc son or daughter – and fewer rights of inheritance than legitimate children (Ninomiya 1991: 154–5, Satō and Kaibara 1990: 97–8). Since this illegitimate status is explicitly reflected in the *koseki*, the *koseki* has become the focus of attention of these movements.

Illegitimately born interviewees drew a picture of social discrimination in the fields of education, marriage and employment. A young interviewee related this to a suicide attempt. Another interviewee, who was born before the Second World War, related his lack of a career and the fact that he had not been admitted to a good university to study medicine directly to the fact that he was an illegitimate child, born to his father's second wife, or mistress, instead of his legitimate wife. While his father was a surgeon at one of Japan's top hospitals, he spent much of his life as a cleaner. Even today, being born as a love child appears to have repercussions on career opportunities and marriage possibilities, that is for those who want to marry into 'good' families, where conservative ideas may dictate that having somebody who was born illegitimately marry into the family might defile the purity that is strived for – 'if I let my child marry someone whose father is not known, the *koseki* will become polluted' (quoted in Fukushima 1991b: 100) – and for those who wish to work at companies that treat illegitimacy as a fault in character.

According to Hendry (1987a: 16), referring to Seward, little stigma is attached to being born illegitimately.[13] While in everyday life not much stigmatization may occur, I found all informants who were born outside a legal marriage had felt some sort of stigmatization, which would become most evident when they had to deal with the bureaucracy or with anything for which they needed to reproduce their *koseki*. Feminist novelist Ochiai Keiko, who was a love child herself, felt a strong stigma attached to being illegitimate (Fukushima 1991a, Kawachi 1992: 121), which can be found reflected in some of her novels (e.g. Ochiai 1990) and her answers in *Yomiuri Shinbun*'s 'Jinsei Annai' (Life's guide) column, where she advises a woman not to have an illegitimate child because that child will 'suffer the consequences' (McKinstry and McKinstry 1991: 152, quoting Ochiai).

According to Mouer and Sugimoto (1990: 259), children of single mother (*boshi katei*) or father households (*fushi katei*) have been systematically singled out at school as probable trouble children, something that may not always be true because many school teachers I know said that they think this is undue discrimination. What this suggests, however, is that not having a father or mother at home is of more importance than the question of whether one was born illegitimately. Children with an absent father or mother are widely expected to become troublesome and until they do they are regarded as *kawaisō* (pathetic) and may become the victim of harassment by classmates calling them *chichinashi ko* (fatherless child). In 1990 there were over 2.7 million single-parent households (Sōmuchō Tōkeikyoku ed. 1992: 19) and such problems may thus affect several millions of children.

As Marumo (1993) wrote, people frequently ask children who are out with their mother where their father is and what he is doing. While such questions do not need to be taken seriously, the simple fact of being asked time and again is likely to have a stigmatizing effect on the child because she or he is confronted with the fact that she or he does not have a father, something that apparently is thought to be strange. Fathers' days in schools do not do much good either because they confront children with the fact that they do not have one. Marumo's (1993) son found the solution in letting a friend of the family take on this role, as did the little boy in a novel of Ochiai Keiko (1990), a solution that indicates in itself how strongly the difference is felt. Children are taught at school not to 'stick out' but to appear to be the same as everybody else (Hendry 1987b), which obviously makes not having a father unpleasant.

In accordance with the position of the child of a single mother, unmarried pregnant women are treated badly. In 1991 a woman who worked at a nursery school in Fukui was dismissed when she became pregnant because 'she represented bad morals' (Ōta 1992: 117–19) and the bureaucracy in general appears to put much effort into making pregnant unmarried women feel that they are immoral and a nuisance to society (Yoshizumi 1992: 141–2). For those in financially difficult situations, it is possible to get assistance for buying the many goods needed in connection with the birth of a child and, when one cannot work during pregnancy and after giving birth, it is possible to receive social security payments. Many single women, however, make as little use of this as possible because they prefer to avoid having to deal with the bureaucracy. Single mother Satō Fumiko was in hospital to have her baby. To her pleasure, she was placed on a ward with single mothers only. There she learned that all the other single mothers were so not by choice and that all of them were anxious to start working again as soon as possible in order to avoid further harassment by the bureaucracy (Satō 1982: 75–8). Women who become pregnant and are abandoned by the father of their child, that is those who did not positively choose to become a single mother, have most difficulty with the treatment they receive. Fathers can walk away just like that: if they do not care to recognize a child, they cannot be made to (Shimazu 1992: 211–12, 1994: 85).

An informant couple that was living in a common-law marriage had a child and for reasons such as access to the man's health insurance they decided to enter the child in the *koseki* of the mother, while the father would recognize the child (*ninchi suru*) as his own. The reaction of the civil servant on duty when they went to register it was that once the couple set up a shared *koseki*, the child would become legitimate, which was supposed to be a reassuring remark for the parents: even though they were at the moment living somewhat messily in a non-legal marriage, once they married legally, their child would become legitimate as well. Clearly, according to my interviewee, the civil servant in question did not begin to understand the reasons why this couple was not legally married. The civil servant assumed that it was a matter of fact that everyone wants to marry legally.

A problem related to this is that encountered by children with a gay or lesbian parent. Usually gay or lesbian parents will not let their sexuality be known to a child, or they will keep it from becoming known at the child's school. Not so Tōgō Ken, who came out as gay in the mass media in the late 1960s, while his children were attending elementary and high school. His daughter described the terrible times she had being told by her classmates that her father was an *okama*, a term for homosexual that generally has a strongly effeminate and derogatory connotation. As a result, she refused to go to school for years. The children of some lesbian couples I interviewed until then had not encountered any major problems, although their mothers found it extremely difficult to engage in activities related to their child's school, such as the Parents' and Teachers' Association (PTA). The subjects the other children's mothers talked about were simply too remote from their interests.

The movements against the discrimination of *hichakushutsushi* are closely related to the movements advocating free choice to keep one's name for both partners in marriage.

They claim that children are used by 'the state' in order to pressure people to marry (Fukae 1988, Ninomiya 1992b: 219). If they do not, their child will be the object of discrimination. As the discussion of divorce below shows, this is but one way the bureaucracy influences people's choices, be it one that is an easy target for movements because those concerned are 'innocent' children who have done nothing apart from being born to parents who are not married. In this sense one might also take the view that the movements, by focusing on the discrimination of children through the registration system, also use children as a means of gathering support for their ultimate goal: i.e. individualization of the registration system, using *koseki* with *ko* written with the character of *ko* in *kojin* (individual), which would mean personal register instead of the character for *ko* used in the present *koseki*, which literally means door and refers to the household. As Satō Bunmei, author of a number of books about *koseki* explained, it is not feasible to start a movement to abolish the *koseki seido* as such but it is much easier to organize people to oppose particular effects and results of it.

## *Rikon*: Divorce

Legally, divorce is possible either if both partners agree to have a divorce or if the partner applying for divorce has been wronged by the other in a number of clearly determined ways (Tsunoda 1992). Among some informants this led to a problem when the spouse would not consent, while they themselves were legally in the wrong by having another lover or by neglecting their spouse. Tōgō Ken, mentioned above, is such a case. He deserted his wife to pursue a gay lifestyle but his wife refused a divorce. In a similar situation were several heterosexual women who were legally bound to a man who refused a divorce. While this deadlock situation continues, they may share their lives with another lover, whom they would rather not marry, even if they could. Such situations can continue for extended periods.

According to *jōshiki*, divorce is seen very negatively. Many people believe that traces remain in the *koseki*, which as a result is 'polluted', but it is possible to return to the pre-marital *koseki* or to set up a new one, in which case no trace of the marriage remains (Satō and Kaibara 1990: 140). Further, divorce is still widely held to be the fault of the woman. Even though husbands can be brutes and this is acknowledged, the wife is expected to endure (*gaman suru*) and try to make the best of it with all the powers in her might. This leads to surprising autobiographical material, like a book by Ōhayashi Masako (1991), a singer and *tarento* (mass media personality with no apparent talents), who was more or less forced into a marriage with a famous singer who was thirty-seven years her elder. From the beginning this marriage was problem-ridden and it did not improve: her step-children regarded her as a gold-digger and worried about their inheritance, her husband forced her to have abortions and scolded her for being too fertile while he had sexual affairs with other women. It made me wonder why she did not try to escape this situation sooner. Part of the answer is provided by the title of the book: *Warui Onna ka Shira?* (Does this make me a bad woman?).

Yamashita Noriko, ex-wife of the famous singer James Miki, also felt the need to justify her divorce with an autobiographical explanation under the ominous title *Kamen Fūfu* (Masked married couple, Yamashita 1992), and many are the reports on what is called *kateinai rikon* (divorce within the household), which refers to a couple whose relationship is emotionally finished but for the sake of *seken* (the public world, the surrounding people), or children, continue to live together

(Kanda 1992). Hayashi (1990) wrote a much acclaimed book discussing this phenomenon. The shape is that of marriage, the contents are not, the wrapping counts more than the contents (Hendry 1993a). An interviewee thus shared a house with a legal husband and children and husband and wife paid half of the bills and the rent. She had lovers outside the house, something she made no effort to hide from her family. In this case most friends were aware of the situation, but neighbours were probably not.

In line with the idea that women are the ones at fault in cases of divorce, the first divorced woman I met in Japan burst into tears when I asked her how people saw her after her divorce. Although parents increasingly seem to enjoy having their daughter return, so that she can take care of them in their old age, prejudice against divorced women remains. An interviewee, who was divorced after he had come to use violence against his wife, commented on the pending divorce of a couple who were in a *jijitsukon*: 'It's terrible isn't it. And there are children.' It did not occur to him that divorce might be good for both partners and for the children. Divorce is seen as a problem rather than a solution.

There is some rationality in this because in Japan women usually feel or are made to feel that they must be able to be economically independent of their husbands after their divorce and, unless they either have large savings or special skills, they will usually have to lower their living standards considerably, if not live in what they are likely to perceive as poverty. This incentive is used very much in official divorce counselling. An informant who worked as a divorce counsellor said that if the woman in question cannot be sure that she will find a good job, divorce is usually advised against. Nevertheless, most divorced women I spoke with in Japan are happy to have made this decision, even if it meant that they had extreme financial hardship and were living from day to day: at least they were living their own lives and not having them lived by a husband they did not care to be with.

Lately some groups have started to give advice on divorce that is more directed at supporting women to brace themselves to enter the labour market, or in assisting them to find ways of having husbands pay alimony, usually in a lump sum, something that is perfectly possible in the case of husbands who became violent or committed adultery. Such assistance is still scarce and only provided by some more radical women's organizations, for instance Nikoniko Rikon Kōza (Divorce with a Smile Course), a course teaching women how to get the best deal out of a divorce and how to brace themselves for economic independence. Most women, however, do not have access to such organizations because they are not aware of their existence. As the divorce counsellor mentioned above suggested, divorce counselling as it exists in Japan at the moment seems mostly directed at keeping the divorce rate down, without much consideration as to what the costs, in terms of personal emotions, are.

## Marriage and Discrimination

While, as discussed, in some circles it is considered wrong to marry, in most of Japanese society today and in most of that of the recent past,[14] marriage is and was considered to be the right thing to do: couples living together without setting up their *koseki* are frowned upon by the bureaucracy and often also by family members. Although Japanese laws related to *naien* do not recognize discrimination against those who are not legally married in most fields – they stipulate for instance that those in a *naien* relationship have the same rights as those who are legally married when it comes to the right of housing (Ninomiya 1991) – many landlords will not accept people who are not legally registered. The rights exerted by landlords supersede any rights of renters, not legally but in practice.

Apart from this, functionaries at the town hall or any other place may be *urusai* (troublesome): they may ask again and again why you do not put things right and make the marriage 'properly (*chan to, kichin to*)' legal. This is something people of course may become tired of. Also because setting up a register takes hardly any effort at all – it can be carried out in a few minutes – the merits of not having to answer the *urusai* civil servants about one's personal choices may make it increasingly appealing. A number of married informants, indeed, gave the insistence of civil servants as the reason why they finally gave in and set up a shared *koseki*, even though they were against it for political reasons.

A young female informant said that she and her husband set up their *koseki* because of their landlord. They were adamant that in the 'conservative town (*hoshuteki na machi*)' where they lived, Kyoto, it would be terribly difficult to find agreeable living quarters for themselves unless they set up a *koseki*. The landlord let them rent his apartment only on the condition that they would make their marriage legal. As he kept asking about their civil status after they moved in, they decided to silence this nuisance and set up a *koseki*, even though they were ideologically opposed to the *koseki seido*.

Gay men who do not wish to marry may have obvious reasons but that does not mean that they feel they can relate them or that they are accepted by those who wish to see them married. A gay informant wanted to live straightforwardly and therefore did not want to deceive a woman and marry her. His boss introduced him to a woman but he refused to marry her, after which his boss dismissed him. Of course refusal to marry is not a legal ground for dismissal but trials in Japan tend to last for many years and cost large sums of money. In general, trials about having been dismissed unjustly are a sort of race of exhaustion between the two parties concerned. Financial means and perseverance are paramount. One woman and her lawyer said that they spent six years fighting her case after she lost her job because of illness which was caused by the labour circumstances in the first place. She could only proceed because she had the support of women's networks that brought together much of the needed money. An interviewee gave up after five years of fighting her dismissal caused by her protest against wage discrimination of women, in order to sort out her life and go to university. If the man in the case above had had the financial means and perseverance, he might have been able to win compensation money.

The oldest never-married man I met was Hase *san* (Mr Hase), aged 60 years, who spent his life changing from one job to another and knew very well that the fact that he was not married increasingly restricted his job opportunities. Nevertheless he always thought that it was wrong for a gay man to marry and persisted in his principles. He never had a lover because he would not start an affair with someone who wanted him if he did not love them, and, similarly, the men he fell in love with rejected his advances. Hase *san* spent many years of his life working as an office cleaner, which was one of the few jobs he could obtain once he was 40 years old and was made redundant at the publishing company where he worked until then.

Hase *san* discovered that many gay men worked in the cleaning business. Among his colleagues at least 50 per cent were gay men. Likewise, gay men are over-represented among the day labourers (*hiyatoi rōdōsha*) who are concentrated around Kamagasaki in Osaka and in smaller numbers in Sanya in Tokyo, Kotobuki in Yokohama, and elsewhere. In Kamagasaki I intuitively recognized many men as gay. When I checked the validity of my intuition it usually turned out to be right. Among men who sexually harassed me in public situations, homeless and *hiyatoi rōdōsha* were over-represented. Discussions with people involved in voluntary work or living in Kamagasaki supported my hypothesis. One of the major reasons for men to end up living in Kamagasaki is the breakdown of their social networks. Gay informants whose wives, or other relatives, found out about their homosexuality sometimes felt compelled to leave their village or neighbourhood and, if they had no friends or understanding relatives to go to, one of the places they could go was Kamagasaki. Kamagasaki figures often in fantasies of homosexuality, especially in the gay magazine *Sabu*, which even runs a *manga* (comic) series based on men from Kamagasaki, as well as in real-life accounts by readers in gay magazines.[15]

Job discrimination also applies to single foreign men. An English teacher with the best of references found that he was turned down for a number of jobs because there was no Mrs, while his age was one at which people are expected to be married. Likewise, the general difficulty for foreigners in finding housing is exacerbated when they are single and past a certain age. I personally experienced people in Tokyo who would not let me stay at their house, after having been asked by a mutual friend, giving as the reason that I might be gay because I was unmarried and over 30. Many people 'know' that many foreign single men in Japan are gay and many think that they also know that many foreign gay men have AIDS.

Another problem related to marriage is discrimination against the dead. In Japan most graves are family graves and many temples refuse to house the graves of people without a family to pay for their upkeep and for occasional prayers. Funerals are big business but if there is no family there appears not to be much trust that other relations will be interested enough in the deceased to fulfil the duties of piety. Onnatachi no Ishibumi no Kai (The Group of the Women's Memorial Stone) is a group that erected a memorial stone to commemorate the loss of life the Second World War brought, consisting mostly of single women who claim that they could not marry because so many men died during the war. Their president, Tani Kayoko, related in her speech at the yearly meeting in December 1992 that she had given a younger friend money to bring her ashes to Hawaii after her death. In the meantime, however, Onnatachi no Ishibumi no Kai had founded a grave for single women at the Jōjakukōji, a temple in Kyoto. For 100,000 yen a single woman can have her ashes set in the grave, which consists of a deep round hole inside a tomb beneath a monument, and she can expect yearly ceremonies to be held by the members of the group that in 1992 numbered about 400 members and is growing faster than members die (Tani 1993). Gay activist Tōgō Ken said that he wishes to found a temple where gay men can have their ashes buried.

However, even when one is a member of Onnatachi no Ishibumi no Kai one is not sure that one's ashes will rest in the desired spot. The year I visited the annual meeting there was talk of a woman who had died in the previous year and whose ashes had been placed in a municipal grave by the city of Kyoto. When another member found out about this she went to the responsible bureaucratic body and asked for the ashes to be moved, but this could only be done with the consent of the family of the deceased. When calling on them, she found that they were not at all interested in the deceased and did not care what happened to her wish to have her ashes placed at the Jōjakukōji. Although all they needed to do was to put their seal on a document, they refused. Likewise, an interviewee related the story of an unmarried friend who was highly regarded in the community where he lived and wished to be buried there by his friends. In this case too, the family moved in and put him in the family grave without even consulting his closest friends. This dominance of blood ties and legal ties over actual social ties is supported by the *koseki seido*.

## Conclusion

This chapter has sought to provide a basis from which to understand the next one, which is concerned with marriages of gay men, lesbian women and feminist women. Whether one is legally married or not may make great differences socially, politically, legally and economically, but not always. Socially, i.e. in neighbourhoods, the difference between legal and common-law marriage can be marginal and the law provides loopholes in other fields. The ways people devise to overcome problems caused by the omnipresence of the *konin seido* are a focus of investigation in chapter six. Here one example was given: founding grave monuments for particular groups. Reasons why people within the various research categories wish to marry or think they cannot avoid marriage, should be clear: *jōshiki* have it that the only proper way to live is to marry. Most people think that it is important to live 'the proper way'.

# Notes

1 According to Toshitani, in 1987 97.8 per cent of all marrying couples chose the husband's name, and presumably 2.2 per cent the wife's (1994: 79). Idota gives the figure of 98 per cent (1993: 98) and Fukae writes almost all (1988: 116).

2 Condon, Murata and Ishikawa all write that about 20 per cent of male respondents said that they had extra-marital sex in the last one or two years. For women these figures are much lower, about 4 per cent, but this still could lead to quite an accumulation over a lifetime (Condon 1986, Murata 1992: 76, Ishikawa 1984: 141–2). Maruyama (1988: 24–9) presents a figure of 30 per cent of married women who have had the experience of extra-marital sex, based on a questionnaire conducted by a newspaper with 2,000 women in a *danchi* (a housing estate) in Tokyo in 1978. Comparable figures presented in Ishikawa (1984) show, however, that extra-marital sex was slightly more common in America than in Japan.

3 I am indebted to Andrea Germer for making me aware of this fact.

4 The power Japanese housewives yield in the household is often discussed (e.g. Lebra 1984: 129–38, Vogel 1978). This power clearly has nothing to do with autonomy. Dependence on the income of the husband excludes this idea. Further, the activities of the housewife can be restricted by the husband or his father or mother. Lebra (1984: 294–300) presented a totally incomparable (because highly educated and highly mobile) American group for comparison, who she refers to as having declared that 'women are better off in other societies including Japan' (ibid.: 315) in what seems an attempt to say that Japanese women are possibly better off than American. I

think that the problem here lies with the idea that American women are relatively liberated, which recently has been refuted by books like *Backlash* (Faludi 1992) and *The War against Women* (French 1992), rather than saying much about Japan. Just as Japanese women cannot be represented by contented housewives, American women cannot be represented by independent women.

5 In 1991 the average age for women to marry was 25.9 years and for men 28.4 years (Keizai Kikakuchō ed. 1992: 23–4, 408).

6 Viricentric is a term proposed by Schrijvers (1985) and others, who think that the term androcentric, prevalent in America, is vague because the Greek term *andros* means human as well as man. The Latin term *vir*, from which viricentric is derived, means only man, and is therefore clearer. I write viricentric rather than *ie*-centric here because that is the way I was confronted with the term. Informants who mentioned it, referred mostly to colleagues and friends who said things like: 'Isn't it time for you to receive a bride?', without any reference whatsoever to the *ie*. Although the character for *yome* is a combination of the characters for *ie* and *onna* (woman), which suggests the centrality of the *ie*, people may not realize this when they are using the word.

7 This is usually the husband but I found one case of the wife having started a successful career and leaving her husband and children to live temporarily elsewhere for the sake of her work.

8 Two of these groups are Fūfu Besshi no Hōseika o Jitsugen suru Kai (Group for the Realization of Separate Names for Spouses) and Fūfu Bessei Sentakusei o Susumeru Kai (Group for the Promotion of Free Choice of Separate Names for Spouses), both in Tokyo (Josei no Jōhō o Hirogeru Kai ed. 1991: 234).

9 Idota (1993: 72–88) points out that the practice of husband and wife sharing the same name is a relatively recent development in Japan, established no earlier than the late nineteenth century. The only other countries that have *koseki* rather than individual registration are Taiwan and Korea, which suggests a relation to Confucianism. In Korea the wife is still not included in the *koseki* of the husband's family but remains an outsider, reminiscent of the borrowed womb philosophy of the Japanese *samurai* class (Neuss-Kaneko 1990).

10 This term is still much in use, although its meaning has become redundant. In fact, one cannot do *nyūseki* when marrying anymore but rather sets up a new *koseki*, as opposed to the pre-war system when *nyūseki* meant that in most cases the woman entered the *koseki* of her husband's family or, less commonly, that the man entered the *koseki* of his wife's family (Satō and Kaibara 1990). The common use of the term *nyūseki* indicates the remaining prevalence of thinking along lines of the *ie seido*. Usually the woman used to enter the *koseki* of the family of the house she married into, of which a patriarch, the father or grandfather of the groom or the groom, is the head. Wedding ceremonies are still announced as if the main feature was the linking of two *ie*: they are announced as the wedding ceremony of *ie* so and so to *ie* so and so (*naninani ke to naninani ke*).

11 According to Japanese law, no difference is to be made in allocating public housing between Japanese nationals or foreign nationals living in Japan (Pe san. 1991). Apart from this it is rather perverse that a city like Osaka which prides itself on being 'international' does not allow those without Japanese nationality to live in its finest houses.

12 For instance Shussei Sabetsu no Hō Kaisei o Motomeru Onnatachi no Kai (Women's Group that Strives for Reform of the Laws of Birth Discrimination) and Kongaishi Sabetsu o Tatakau Kai (Group that Fights Discrimination against Extramarital Children; Josei no Jōhō o Hirogeru Kai ed. 1991).

13 Hendry (1987a: 16), referring to Seward, gives the example of a former emperor who was born illegitimately. This is not a good example at all because the laws as they apply to the rest of the Japanese people do not apply to the imperial family. The imperial family does not have a family name or a *koseki* (Satō and Kaibara 1990: 82). In legal terms, marriage in the case of the imperial family is common-law marriage and if general Japanese law applied, all emperors would be illegitimate.

14 Recent past refers to the Meiji, Taishō and Shōwa periods, i.e. the period from 1868 until 1989. Before the Meiji period most people did not have family names and if they did they were not supported by a bureaucracy that kept records of them. *Koseki* were invented no earlier than the Meiji period (Idota 1993: 15–17). Before then there was the *danka seido,* which demanded that all households belong to and register at the local Buddhist temple.

15 Tom Gill, who conducted research with *hiyatoi rōdōsha* in Kotobuki, made me aware of the fact that men who flock to areas like these in order to have sex with day labourers, are called *yogoresen* (dirt lovers).

# 4 Trying to Fit: Homosexuality and Feminism in Marriage

This chapter investigates how people are coping on a personal level with a system that does not fit their needs and on the other hand does not leave them untouched either. Given the existence of marriage and its position in society, how do those whose feelings or ideas disagree with marriage cope? While some marry and try to be as close to 'normal' (*nōmaru, futsū*) as they can, others do not marry and try to find alternative ways to live, usually calling that 'normal' as well. In their view, it is people who have *omiai* or otherwise try to bring their lifestyle into agreement with social constructions that do not fit their personal needs who are weird (*hentai*). Some of those who are married later decide that they made the wrong choice and opt for divorce. Others remain married while the marriage becomes void in the sense that human contact ceases to exist beyond the absolutely necessary. This chapter discusses how homosexuality and feminism combine with marriage.

## Male Homosexuality and Marriage

From the end of the Second World War and well into the 1960s and 1970s, it was very uncommon for men who reached marriageable age to remain unmarried. This was a period in which marriage had become widely regarded as the only way of life and was practically the only way of life.[1] Even nowadays many have difficulty in warding off pleas and urgings to get married by their families, superiors or friends. Most homosexual men in their 50s and above have been or, indeed, are still married. The cases of two gay activists illustrate the inescapable nature of marriage in Japan for this generation.

Tōgō Ken, gay politician and publisher of gay magazine *Za Gei,* is a descendant from ancient nobility and his father and his step-grandfather were both members of parliament in the pre-war period (Tōgō 1981: 18–45, 1984: 9–11). In line with his standing, Tōgō worked at a bank (Lebra 1993) in the 1950s and eventually, at 24 years of age, was forced to marry. An *omiai* was arranged for him and he agreed without even looking at his future bride: 'As I didn't want to marry at all, I couldn't care with whom.' Tōgō came out as gay in the late 1960s and participated in elections, campaigning in traditional Japanese female attire. This led to him and his children being ostracized by his family. His daughter claims never to have seen any of her cousins, aunts or uncles since her father came out. His marriage was still not legally dissolved when I met Tōgō in Tokyo in December 1991 because his wife refused to give her consent and, as discussed in the previous chapter, one cannot divorce someone who has done nothing wrong without this consent.

Another leader of gay activities, Minami Teishirō, was also forced to marry, when he was 35 years old, and also has children. He had more luck than Tōgō because his wife agreed to a divorce after their marriage had been void, in the sense that they had lived separately and hardly ever saw each other, for a long time. By then Minami had already set up his own gay magazine, *Adon,* but this was not widely known. Although Minami these days appears on television and in the print media frequently, he does not believe that his children know that he is gay because his relationship with his children was severed after his divorce.

People who are less strong-minded than these two men are more common and Minami is likely to be right when he says that the majority of men who visit Japan's major gay-bar area in Shinjuku in Tokyo, comprising about 200 bars, are married white-collar workers, who visit Shinjuku on their way from their jobs to their homes (Lunsing 1994a).[2] Most patrons stay for only a short while, one hour or two, and then hurry off to catch their trains home.[3] While there are some indications that the number of homosexual men who marry while being aware of their homosexuality is declining somewhat, other material suggests that the number of those wanting to marry is still high (Lunsing 1995).

Data from a survey published by Occur (Ugoku Gei. 1992) indicate that about 30 per cent of their sample of young gay men want to marry. As this sample consists of young gay men visiting gay bars in Shinjuku and members of gay organizations, this figure is definitely low compared to the overall situation. Many gay men do not visit gay bars and some even live totally isolated from other gay men. In their cases, resistance to marriage demands much more energy than for those who are part of some gay network. Moreover, the sample in question is very young, with a majority in their early 20s, which is an age at which marriage is not yet a very pressing problem.[4] Other surveys by the gay magazines *Sabu* and *Za Gei* equally suggest that many gay men still seriously think about marriage if they are not already actively involved in seeking a spouse.[5] Furthermore, of *Za Gei*'s sample, over 40 per cent had been married, with over 70 per cent of those being over 40 years old. Equally biased are the figures of Ōta who, with a research population of 100, found that 41 were or had been married, data which he gathered among participants of a gay network in the 1950s (Ōta 1987: 79). In relation to this it is also noteworthy that second-hand gay magazines are widely available from second-hand shops because many men discard them before their marriage. As an interviewee who tried to establish a documentation centre in connection with *Adon* said, often they send them back to the publisher.

As reasons for wanting to marry young gay men in *Sabu* mentioned the desire to have children most, followed by the wish to comply with the demands of *seken*, those who make up one's daily environment, and parents. Young men in gay groups I participated in mostly do not wish to marry, but there is a strong tendency to recognize that they are still young and are liable to change their minds later on when pressure may increase. In general they wish, however, to remain unmarried, the question rather being whether this will be feasible when confronted with mounting demands by *seken* in their later 20s. Indeed, at a meeting of Fain Kurabu (Fine Club), a group of a similar composition to that of Occur's survey and the groups referred to above but mostly in their late 20s and early 30s, a majority of 13 out of 24 were seriously thinking about marriage. In this particular group, there appears to be a negative correlation between seeking marriage and having had sexual experience with a woman, having had sexual experience with a man at an early age and thinking of oneself as charming (*miryokuteki*).[6] This suggests that the meeker and less experienced are more likely to opt for marriage.

Three groups I conducted research with in Osaka and a group in Tokyo discussed the question of marriage, and in gay magazines (especially *Barazoku*) and *minikomi* (*DON!*, *Behold*, *Kick Out*) it featured in special issues. While Occur, probably the most ardent politically active gay group in Tokyo, condemns homosexual men who marry, calling it *gisō kekkon* (camouflage marriage), other groups are less dogmatic. At meetings of OGC and JILGA I met several married gay men and in the other groups in Osaka, which largely consist of young gay men, marriage is a serious topic of discussion. While OGC's Hirano

Hiroaki opposes marriage for gay men, this may be understood as opposition to marriage in general. He opposes not only marriage of gay men but marriage as such, whereas most other gay groups tend to oppose marriage of gay men to women while at the same time regarding the acceptance of same-sex marriage as a goal to strive for.

Romantic and true love (expressed by *renai* while the partner concerned is called *koibito*) appears to be very much the ideal, for which reason the castigation of gay men who marry women is also understandable because it flies in the face of this ideal. In a vehement statement, Yukidaruma (Snowman, a nickname, 1993) attacks men who use being gay as an excuse for cheating on their wives because 'society (*seken*) does not permit heterosexual men to have mistresses' either. A heterosexual man who told about his feelings towards his wife at a meeting of the men's liberation group, however, desired, much like many homosexual men, that his wife would consent to him having love and sex relationships with other women, which was not made into a point of moral concern there. *Kick Out* published an issue in which marriage for gay men was supported theoretically with the argument that in a society that does not accept homosexuality, gay men can hardly be blamed for going with the flow (Masakami 1992). Thus, within gay circles much animosity exists around the theme of marriage.

The fact that, as discussed in chapter three (p. 73), the rate of marriage among men has declined considerably, to the extent that in 1995 over 22 per cent of men aged between 35 and 40 years had never married (Sōmuchō Tōkeikyoku ed. 1996: 48–9), suggests that a decrease in the percentage of gay men who marry is to be expected. Furthermore, among those who do marry, there appears to be an increase of those marrying a woman who knows of their homosexual preference (Lunsing 1995). Homosexuality is not something constantly present in the sense that people always know where their preference lies. Thus, men who find themselves wanting to share their sexuality with a man, may already be married. In my sample of married men who acknowledge their homosexual desire or activity I discern four types.

## Marriage of Convenience

Not very common is what one could call the total sham. In this case the marriage is between a man and a woman who both know that the man is homosexual but decide to marry, even though they do not want to share their lives. They may decide to live apart (*bekkyo kekkon*), or even decide on a date for divorce by contract before they get married (*keiyaku kekkon*: contract marriage). This subtype is based on the assumption that if you have been married once, there will be less pressure to marry again. You have given it a try and thus you are now in a position to argue that marriage does not agree with your personality.

## Friendship Marriage

More common than sham marriages are the second type: marriages in which the wife knows about the man's homosexual preference but still wishes to live with him and share her life with him to a varying extent. The men may want a mate to share their everyday life with, a housewife to take care of the household and/or a mother to give birth to and take care of their children. Many homosexual men see this as an ideal arrangement and also some women choose to marry a homosexual man on these terms because it gives them the status of a married woman without much of the burden, such as demands by the husband to have sex. Moreover, in negotiations preceding marriage they are in a stronger position to exert pressure on the man to meet any demand they might have than they would be with a heterosexual man.

When emotional ties and companionship play a major role in these arrangements, they may be referred to as *tomodachi kekkon* (friendship marriage) or, less commonly, as *kyōmei kekkon* (brother–sister marriage). A novel which has been made into a movie of the same title, *Kirakira Hikaru* (Twinkle), depicts such a situation (Ekuni 1992). The protagonists, Mutsuki, a gay physician, and Shōko, an alcoholic woman working as a translator, did not wish to marry but were pressured by their parents to have *omiai*. When Mutsuki right away speaks his mind, Shōko becomes interested. Together they work out that marrying each other might be a good way to avoid further harassment by their parents. Shōko makes sure that Mutsuki continues his relationship with his lover, whom she appears to be very fond of, even when her parents find out about Mutsuki's homosexuality and demand a separation of the lovers. Shōko works it all out to the effect that Mutsuki's lover comes to live in an apartment in the same building as theirs.

In the case of an interviewee it worked out less well. He married a friend who was about ten years older than himself, which led to criticism from his business relations because she could not have children any more. Nevertheless, he persisted and the marriage took place. She knew he was gay at the time of marriage, which for her was a reason to marry him. He explains:

> I was urged to have *omiai* and arrived at a period in which I didn't have the strength to refuse but I didn't want to marry in that way. I thought it would be good to marry, even though I am gay (*gei*), you might say in order to fit the structure, to take the form of marriage and live together (*kyōdō seikatsu*) as partners, and I married. A female friend

> asked me if I wanted to marry her even though I was gay because she didn't want to marry a heterosexual man (*futsū no otoko*) but would be fine in a marriage with a gay man. So we married. (. . .) It was a woman who didn't like sex very much. She knew my feelings quite well and I also understood her quite well, so we married thinking that it might work out fine.

It seemed nicely planned but it was evidently not talked through thoroughly enough: when he started an affair with a male lover, she realized that she was not getting what she had expected. She had wanted to spend more time together with her husband, who now increasingly left her alone in order to see his lover. After many fights she made him choose: either he had to break off his relationship with his lover, or she would divorce him. The outcome was divorce. He cared less than he expected. He had grown older and stronger (*tsuyoku narimashita*) in the sense that he had gained the strength not to yield to social pressure. As he had been married once, pressure to marry again could be countered more easily. He had experienced marriage and could judge it to be not his way of life, something he would use whenever his business relations brought up the subject of remarriage. On a number of occasions I met gay men in the company of their wives in gay bars, in Tokyo as well as in Osaka. Most of these cases appeared to be of this type. The wife had married the man while knowing he was gay. Although the man was known to be gay by other people present in the bars, they usually would not discuss this until after the couple left. While they were in the bar together, the man often posed as heterosexual.

## Deceptive Husbands

Much more common are cases in which the man marries his wife without letting her know about his sexuality, the third type. He may think that by getting married he can change his ways and become *nōmaru* (normal), that is heterosexual, or he may think it is a bad thing for him to do but pressure from people around him – his parents, his superiors and colleagues at work, or his friends – make him feel that there is no other way out. A man who married at the age of 35 under pressure of what he called *shūi* (environment), which in his case points in particular at the people he works with, said about his wife, to whom he was introduced by mutual friends:

> I don't know whether she knew [that I was gay when we married]. I did not say it, we didn't talk about it. (. . .) From the atmosphere [I think she might have known], but I don't know.

This marriage ended in divorce after two years, because it was clear that the marriage 'didn't work'. When they decided to separate, he talked to her about his homosexuality, but she did not tell him whether she had known all along and he did not ask. This man tried to adapt to a heterosexual lifestyle during his marriage and 'of course' did not have affairs while his marriage lasted. Another man who decided as a 27-year-old that it was time to marry and become 'normal', after he lost a lover, also did not tell about his past:

> Before we married I didn't talk [about my homosexual past]. She didn't know anything about it. (. . .) From the

> beginning I didn't like having sex with women but it was not that I couldn't. Well, she became pregnant and we couldn't have sex and I started going to gay bars again. I corresponded with a boy (*ko*) I met there (. . .) and eventually started an affair with him. Then the child was born and finally I hadn't had sex with my wife for over a year in total. (. . .) My wife started to find this strange (*okashii*), she began wondering why we didn't have sex after the child was born. She asked me to have sex because you're a couple and it's only natural. I excused myself saying that I was too tired . . .

His wife kept pressurizing him and eventually he ended up telling her that he was gay (*homo*), leaving it up to his wife to decide on the consequences. She did not accept his homosexuality and made him go to a psychologist but the psychologist merely said that there was nothing wrong with him and that homosexuals have the opportunity to live a very interesting life not available to most people. This was unacceptable to his wife who then demanded a divorce. The man has not seen his daughter since, which is his main point of regret. He would like to marry and have a child again but this time with a woman who accepts his homosexuality.

A small group hardly consider their wife's happiness and marry in order to be able to lead a double life. In these cases there is always the fear of being found out, which limits the possibilities of having homosexual relationships. A man who married and thought he had a very good relationship with his wife, was found out (*barashita*) within a year because lovers kept calling him at home. She demanded a divorce. He is still looking back on his happy year of marriage. What this indicates is that it is often not easy for a married man to have homosexual relationships. Even giving a phone number can be very hazardous. For this reason married men often do not even tell their names to sex partners. Often their homosexual affairs are limited to short excursions to parks, cinemas or prostitution quarters (Domenig 1991) which makes it all not very different from heterosexual marriages in which the man also may go and find his sexual pleasures outside the home. Masakami Junichi, writing in *minikomishi Kick Out* (1992), uses this fact as a defence for gay men who are married. Many married gay men, however, do not have sex with men at all. Not having a gay sex life was common among my informants and similar cases can be found in abundance in gay magazines.

In *Barazoku* a man described how he was more or less lured into marriage, to which he offered little resistance. A friendship with a female colleague at work led to the usual gossip and before he knew what was happening he was married to her. He tried to adapt to a heterosexual lifestyle, although it was all very 'dark and heavy-handed'. He had continued to hide his homosexual feelings ever since he discovered them at the age of 11 but as a 28-year-old he was seduced by a man who told him that there was nothing wrong with enjoying homosexual contacts while being married. These words sounded like 'the devil's whisper'. He started to hate himself and decided to do 'the right thing' and divorce. While feeling terribly guilty towards his wife, he decided this was the only way to live honestly (Mayoeru Sarariiman 1990).[7] Another man, also in *Barazoku*, writes about his 'secret pleasure' of visiting a gay sauna in Tokyo a couple of times a year, something he started doing only when he felt he had fulfilled his duty as a husband and father and had reached the age of 50 years. He never had sex in the sauna, except for one time, when he masturbated a young man. Otherwise his 'secret pleasure' was limited to watching (Yukio 1992).

A man who married because he wanted very much to have children and for the sake of *seken* continued to have lovers, even after his wife found out about his homosexuality. He wishes very much to stay married because he does not want to lose his daughter but since his wife found out their relationship has changed. He finds it particularly *tsurai* (painful, bitter) that he and his wife do not even share the same bedroom any more. When he told this at a meeting of OGC, Hirano Hiroaki was quick to remark that that is not uncommon in marriages in which both partners are heterosexual either.

## Latent Homosexuality

Another common type of marriage of homosexual men, the fourth, is that of those who do not realize, or acknowledge, that they are attracted to their own sex at the time of marriage. Only after marriage do they come to realize that that 'dark feeling of longing inside' for physical contact with men that they had in their teens, as one interviewee described it, was not something that belonged to a passing phase or something that had nothing to do with their sexuality as such but a longing that would keep recurring time and again. Men in this predicament often label themselves as bisexual, whereby the love they feel for their wife is often of a very different nature to that of their feelings for men. With their wives they may find stability, warmth and comradeship, which may be expressed by the term *aijō* (affectionate love). With male partners, if they have any, they find passion and lust, which makes the accompanying feeling closer to *renjō* (passionate love). In the words of an interviewee, who spoke about what he called his *baisekushuariti* (bisexuality) at meetings of OGC as well as the men's liberation group:

> What I often think is that I love her because she is my wife. On the other side I feel attracted towards men. But it doesn't go so far that I want to divorce her. If you ask whether I have a love relationship (*aijō kankei*) with her, at this point I hope to be excused. (. . .) I mean I don't love a particular man to the extent that I can live with him or have such a love relationship (*renai kankei*). And I already am married to her, we are talking about me being married. I didn't marry against my wish and I didn't marry because I wanted to . . .

This man married his wife when he was 29 years old, half a year after they were introduced to each other by a colleague. At the time of the wedding he did not know that there was such a thing as homosexuality, apart from in the *geinōkai,* the world of television and show business, but when he later happened to find a gay magazine he remembered having felt a strong attraction towards men and becoming excited when looking at pictures of male nudes in his adolescence. He (re)discovered his appetite for the male sex not long after his children were born, a not uncommon pattern. After this discovery he placed advertisements in gay magazines to find a lover but apart from some contacts of short duration and low intensity, these efforts were not successful.

He participates in meetings of OGC, often accompanied by one of his children, and his wife knows that he goes to a group but, according to him, she thinks nothing of it because he has always been going to all sorts of meetings and always has been involved in voluntary activities and movements. In the gay group's meetings, however, he is castigated for 'hiding behind the guise of bisexuality' and 'deceiving his wife', although he hardly deceives her in the sense of being untrue because he has had no sexual relationships with men. Moreover, he is comparatively a very progressive husband. He claimed to take upon himself many household tasks, in particular the laundry and washing up. In the men's liberation group, where he also told his story, reactions to his story were marked by a lack of understanding. His story was generally considered as weird (*hen*) and incomprehensible and not much effort was made to understand things better. This reflects the ideal of fidelity that is generally upheld in feminist circles and which men involved in the men's liberation group support without much questioning.

While in the case of men who deceive their wives knowingly divorces are common on being found out (*barashita*), in the case of those who deceived themselves rather than anyone else the marriage may continue after the man has been found out or told his wife. After all, the couple is likely to be in some sort of intimate or close relationship. The television series *Dōsōkai* (Alumni Association), aired by Nihon Television (Kuia Sutadiizu Henshū Iinkai ed. 1996a) in the autumn of 1993, gives an example of this. When the wife, Natsuki, is searching for her husband, Fūma, in the gay quarter of Shinjuku, she discovers that her suspicions are right, while looking at a television screen in the bar beneath a love hotel where she is invited for a drink by a *yakuza* boss. As it happens, the boss, who has an appetite for men, is just looking at the video-screen that shows live how Fūma has sex with his lover. This leads her to start thinking of Fūma and the loneliness he must feel and to stop being selfish and think only of her own problems, as she evaluates her attitude until then.

This is a somewhat extreme situation and not many Japanese women would react like that, especially after so crude a confrontation, but positive reactions do occur: I met a married couple in a gay bar in Osaka and it appeared that they were married and that the man had only later discovered the attraction he felt towards men. In fact it was the first time he had visited a gay bar and because he found it a rather frightening and intimidating prospect, he asked his wife to accompany him. Tomorrow, though, he promised to come again, alone. A man I met at a gay Christmas party in Tokyo said that he had quit being a Catholic priest because he felt dissatisfaction with the church and that he had married when he was 30 years old. When he married he did have homosexual feelings but he did not know what to do with them. Later he came into contact with other gay men and started meeting them. His wife, he said, knew he was at a gay Christmas party and understood (*wakatte kureta*) that he had a need to go to such gatherings.

A female interviewee married very romantically in Guam, after eloping with her boyfriend, whom her parents forbade her to see. After three years of marriage, her husband told her that he needed a man. He said that he loved her and needed her by his side but that at the same he time needed a boyfriend. He called himself bisexual (*baisekushuaru*) and explained the word bisexual as referring to someone who needs to have relationships with people from both sexes concurrently. Initially she believed him and found this all very interesting. She started reading everything about homosexuality she could find and together they placed an advertisement in a gay magazine in order to find him a lover. Everything seemed to go smoothly, until he started to give his attention increasingly to his lover while ignoring his wife. She was not at all happy about this and in a major effort to attract attention attempted suicide, making use of sleeping pills. In her suicide note she wrote:

> We are a married couple. I thought we were lovers. Now that we are not any more, I don't have the confidence to live on. I can't see dreams and goals in a future with you. It is totally dark. (. . .) I don't want to live on without the energy of love coming from you. (. . .) When I think of you tears come to my eyes, I must be a happy person, but I am tired of the unreturned love. Forgive me for not being a good wife.

She continues by writing to his lover that she, as the wife, knows that the feelings of her husband for him are true and concludes by wishing him happiness with her husband after her death. The suicide attempt was aborted when, according to her, her husband came home earlier than expected to find her unconscious. He took her to the hospital to have her stomach pumped. The suicide attempt gained her some attention but it did not last. However much he repeated that he really needed her, that he could not live without her, she felt increasingly neglected, a feeling which was exacerbated by his sneaking out of the house under all sorts of pretexts in order to phone his lover and by his not being open about his activities. Furthermore, she was concerned about AIDS. He did not practise safe sex because he felt that true love was worth dying for. She decided to try and live on her own. This was a grandiose fiasco; altogether she slept one night in the apartment they had rented for her at much expense.[8] She decided to return, or rather to continue, to live with him, trying to make the best of both their lives and that of his consecutive lovers. Although he said that if the relationship with his first lover came to an end, he would probably not look for another, as it turned out he found himself a new lover within a month of losing the first one.

A positive point she kept relating about her husband loving men was that it gave her a chance to meet many 'interesting people'. In order to talk about how she felt she had placed advertisements in gay magazines herself and thus made contact with a number of people with whom she gradually developed interesting friendships: mainly married gay men but also other people who were interested in talking about their own problems related to sexuality and marriage. She did not believe that her husband was bisexual but rather that he was homosexual, considering the difference in the attention he gave her and his lover.

The idea that homosexual men cannot have sex with women may be supportive of the idea men may construct of themselves as bisexual. Many gay men think themselves that they are unable to have sex with women but it rather appears that, if they do their best, they can, often by closing their eyes and thinking of men (Morioka 1979, Tamura 1988). Nevertheless, some men believe that they must be bisexual because they are not unable to have sex with their wives. This interpretation of sexuality is based not on preference, attraction or lust but rather on experience, which, indeed, would mean that a large number of Japanese men are bisexual.[9] In the gay magazine *Sabu*, however, a letter was published about the contrasting case of a man who married his wife who 'fortunately' became pregnant during their honeymoon:

> Since then we have sexual intercourse about twice a month and my wife does not desire more than that and in me about twice a month the desire to have sex comes up. Probably, if I would have

> continued seeing men (*otoko asobi*) after marriage, it wouldn't be like this. This way of putting things may be impolite towards my wife, but if my needs reach their limit, she fulfils the role of plaything (*omocha*) satisfactorily. People (. . .) tell me that I must be bisexual (*ryōtō*, lit. double-sworded) because I can do it with women as well as men, but I must protest. I am not bisexual. (Anonymous 1991)

Among my informants, most married men who had engaged in homosexual activities before marriage or had acknowledged attraction to the male sex did not believe that they were bisexual, even though they thought that they managed to sexually satisfy their wives. They rather believed that they were homosexual, even in the cases of men, like the one quoted above, who had no sexual contacts with men. The group of men who try to become heterosexual upon marriage or see themselves as bisexual is rather small compared to this. Moreover, this group tends to be very unstable. Men who try to become heterosexual usually recognize or rediscover their homosexual preference after children have been born, if not sooner. Many men who see themselves as bisexual tend to make a strong separation between the quality of their feelings for men and for women, which indicates, according to critiques by many gay groups and individuals, that bisexuality is not the right term with which to characterize them.

Men who see themselves as bisexual and whose feelings for men and women do not show this difference of course also exist. In general, I found that their position was readily accepted in most groups, like the case of a young man who, in a discussion on marriage on a cassette-tape recorded by Kamigata DJ Club, says that he would only want to marry a woman he really loves but that that is perfectly possible because he is not fully homosexual (*kanzen na homo*) but rather bisexual. This is accepted by the men appearing on the tape after they discussed the prevalence of men 'who pose as bisexuals' (Kamigata DJ Club 1992: side 2).[10]

It appears that the situation of male homosexuality in marriage in Japan has much in common with that described for North America by Gochros (1989) and Humphreys (1971) or for Australia, New Zealand, Finland and Sweden by Ross (1983) in those cases where men hoped to become heterosexual, did not acknowledge their homosexual desire at the time of marriage, or wished to hide their homosexuality. What is different in Japan is that there are also marriages in which the man recognizes his homosexual desire, which is accepted by the wife, or in which the man does not have many qualms about hiding his homosexual desire from his wife. In North America, northern Europe and Australia such constructions appear to be less feasible due to the importance attached to the contents of marital relationships, due to heterosexual couples being expected to present themselves as lovers. Further, the incidence of men with a clearly acknowledged homosexual desire who marry is most likely to be higher in Japan than in the other areas but so was, until recently, the overall incidence of marriage. The term *gisō kekkon* (camouflage marriage), as used by Occur, does not describe marriage by gay men in Japan in an adequate way. Most homosexual men want something more out of marriage than hiding their homosexuality, such as friendship, warmth, children and, most of all, a guarantee against loneliness (Lunsing 1995).

## Feminism and Female Homosexuality in Marriage

Although I originally intended to divide female homosexuality and feminism in relation to marriage into two separate sections, when writing drafts the overlaps turned out to be very large and a number of cases could belong equally to both sections. One of the reasons for this is that many lesbian women are also feminists, certainly in the wider meaning of women with independent ideas about how they wish to live that are not determined by *jōshiki* concerning marriage as discussed in chapter three. Some lesbian women, indeed, consider being *feminisuto* (feminist) of more importance to themselves than being lesbian and, as this section intends to clarify, in relation to marriage feminism may supersede or precede the importance of homosexual desire.

While conducting my fieldwork in Japan and when presenting papers based on my fieldwork, some heterosexual women who fitted my definition of feminist expressed great doubts about the feasibility of combining feminist and lesbian women in one framework. While these doubts have to do with general academic ideas that hold that one should limit the scope of research to one clearly defined group or theme, I believe that they also may partially stem from feminists' fear of becoming socially less acceptable by being associated with homosexuality. Let me, therefore, state clearly that most feminists are 'fully heterosexual (*kanzen na hetero*)', which is a way of putting things that is prevalent in Japan.

The majority of lesbian women over 30 years of age I interviewed had been married to a man in one way or another, i.e. *hōritsukon* or *jijitsukon* (legally or not), and had been living a heterosexual lifestyle previously. Some also had children. Even if they recognized their attraction towards women at the time of marriage, like gay men in their 50s and 60s, they had not perceived remaining unmarried as feasible, for economic reasons and above all for social reasons. One of the main features was that they did not know of other women with homosexual feelings and as a result they did not know what to do with their own feelings. Women who lived without men were not visible and the idea that they could live on their own was inconceivable. This is largely true for the *gakusei undō* (student movement) generation, that reached marriageable age in the late 1960s and early 1970s. Feminists of the generation that developed from discontent with role patterns in the *gakusei undō* in the 1960s, whose movement generally is called *ūman ribu*, had usually married and in many cases divorced once demands posed by married life became incompatible with their feminist activities.

The only figures available on the prevalence of marriage among lesbian women are produced by a survey that was conducted among lesbian networks and in lesbian bars in Shinjuku. These results are inevitably skewed because the women reached by the survey are obviously more confident in their homosexual preference than other women, otherwise the survey would not have reached them. The sample consists of 234 women of whom in total about 23 per cent had been married but the figure is kept low by a large percentage of women in their teens and 20s. Of those in their 40s, over 60 per cent had been or still were married (Hirosawa and Rezubian Ripōto Han 1991). I know of no figures on the prevalence of marriage among women who are involved in feminist activities but, given the high incidence of marriage in Japan, it is safe to say that a majority are or have been married. As a 41-year-old interviewee, who labelled herself as *feminisuto*, said: 'In my generation there was no question of getting married or not.' I discern four types of feminism and female homosexuality in relation to marriage.

## Opportunists

The first is that of women who have a clear goal with their marriage and adapt their choice of husband to it. The *feminisuto* mentioned above is a case that fits this type. She married in the middle of the 1970s to a man who was considered to be far below her standing. His family found this a reason to check up on her thoroughly because surely there must be something terribly wrong with her if she chose to marry someone so downmarket. Her choice, however, was determined by the fact that the man she chose was very amenable to her wishes and accepted her demands about her continuing to pursue a career. Although she also takes upon herself the brunt of the housekeeping – she is adamant that she loves to cook – her husband makes no problems when she goes away on a voyage related to her professional activities. As she is unable to have children, that aspect of the relationship has become a non-issue. This case has much in common with the two cases of academic women, described by Joy Hendry (1992b) who, as she stresses, were dependent on passive support by their husbands and fathers and active cooperation by female relatives in order to be able to pursue their careers.

A 36-year-old lesbian woman married mostly because she wanted to have children but also because a different way of life was not considered to be feasible at the time. She did not know very clearly whether her husband knew she was lesbian and she herself claims not to have been very certain about it when they married either, notwithstanding the fact that she had had lesbian affairs previously. After having been expelled from a girls' college, because she had confessed her love for a classmate, she was so hurt by the inimical reaction to her feelings that:

> From then onwards I tried not to talk about it. (. . .) Still, at the time there were

> a lot of women I liked. With all my might I tried to avoid getting close to them, I tried not to become intimate with girls (*onna no ko*). At the same time I had very close gay male friends. (. . .) Later I did it with heterosexual boys (*otoko no ko*), I had some small affairs but there was not someone I really liked very much. So I thought, let's quit for a while. (. . .) I couldn't become very heterosexual and there was not a man I liked that much and so I decided to make a child, I loved children.

Her major reason for getting together with a man was her wish to have children and that is what she did. At 27 years old, however, she met and fell in love with a lesbian woman and decided that, having already her desired child and having suffered enough, it was time to start following her feelings. She now told her husband that she wished to separate because she was lesbian and she wanted to go and live with a woman. Her husband, about whom she had very little to say, had been necessary to father her child but after that goal was achieved, he could go. By then it was the mid-1980s and in Tokyo lesbian circles, connected to feminist groups and a commercial lesbian bar circuit, had come into existence, making a lesbian lifestyle more feasible in her eyes. This woman has now become one of the most active lesbian networkers in Japan.

Another interviewee who mainly wanted a child became pregnant and, while scolding her for being so careless, her boyfriend decided that he must do his duty and moved in with her to help care for what was, after all, also his child. After some years of living in a somewhat rocky relationship, the woman became involved in the Women's Labour Union in Osaka because she had been dismissed from a company for refusing to put up with the sexual harassment she was expected to accept, such as continuous remarks and questions about her sex life. Through her contacts with the union she learned to see that her husband could hardly blame her for having become pregnant, as he did not use a condom at the time. She started to counter his deprecatory remarks towards her and, unable to provide her with a response that could satisfy himself, he became violent. They both agreed that this situation could not continue and separated. However, she already had what she had wanted in the first place: her child.

Having clear ideas about what is sought in marriage obviously influences the choice of partner and the structure a household is going to take. While the three cases above are very dissimilar in the sense that the first woman maintains that she loves to be with her husband, the second separated from him in search of her true feelings and the third dumped a husband she did not want in the first place, they are similar in the sense that all three knew what they wanted of marriage and achieved their goals.

In Japan as well as in Europe, I found a number of Japanese lesbian women who had chosen to marry a foreign man. For instance, one woman married a Frenchman only to find that he was no better than Japanese men and divorced him, while another married an Englishman with whom she had two children before she divorced him. Likewise, relatively many feminist women marry foreign men. The reasons behind this phenomenon are that foreign men are generally believed to be more liberal in their attitudes towards women and that foreign men can be more easily handled when in Japan because of the advantage Japanese women have compared to foreign men in dealings with Japanese. Marrying a foreign man also opens the way to living abroad and leaving Japan, possibly never to return.

Related to this is the phenomenon of women who wish to marry in order to become independent of their family. Marriage may be perceived as the only way to escape from the influence of parents. The gay magazine *Barazoku*'s 'Kekkon Kōnā' (Marriage corner: marriage advertisement section) lists such cases. The fact that advertisements seeking marriage by lesbian women tend to come from rural areas more than do those by gay men could indicate that some women see marriage as the only way to get some power over their own life. The total sham, as I called the first type of marriages of gay men, is indeed sought relatively more by lesbian women than by gay men, and lesbian women tend to seek material benefits rather than companionship in marriage (Lunsing 1995). As cases of feminist women show, heterosexual women may also want to marry rather to have the status, to get away from their parental home or to have children, than because they wish to share their life with a man. The *keishiki kekkon* of Shōko in *Kirakira Hikaru* (Ekuni 1992), whose marriage is described in the section on male homosexuality and marriage, also fits wonderfully well into this type. Indeed, contrary to the ideology of the *kekkon bessei* movements, who wish to keep their own names after marriage, I found that some women, even some that label themselves as *feminisuto*, actually want to marry, precisely in order to free themselves of their father's name (Yamada 1993) because they do not wish to be associated with their father any longer.

## No Choice

The second type of marriage is that of feminist and lesbian women who know that their ideas or feelings are not compatible with marriage as it is constructed in Japan but who feel that they have no choice but to marry and so they try to play the role of a good wife in the traditional sense. As Kakefuda Hiroko, who writes about lesbian life in Japan, told me, the most prevalent of the problems mentioned in letters she received in reaction to her publications (e.g. Kakefuda 1992a) was marriage. The mostly young writers wanted advice on how to combine being lesbian with marriage, or, in particular, with becoming a good wife. One interviewee sees marriage as inescapable, while at the same time she is certain that no man can cope with having a sexual relationship with a woman as aggressive as herself. In lesbian and gay circles she refers to herself as bisexual. Being the *chōjo* (eldest daughter) of a house without male offspring, she sees her role as spouse to the successor of the family business clearly ahead. Nevertheless, at the same time she is very clear that she does not think she can have a successful relationship with a man. For one thing, their lack of breasts makes men rather unattractive to her. Her vision of her future role in life demands, however, that she is at least bisexual and copes with having a relationship with a man.

This type is also represented by a woman who did not wish to marry and resisted as long as she could but in the end grew exhausted with being forced to go through one *omiai* after another and settled for a man who at first sight did not appear too repulsive. Fortunately, as she said, not long after their son was born the man died of a heart attack, so that she was alone once again. This concerns a woman who is now in her early 60s. There was no indication whatsoever that she might not be heterosexual: all she wanted was not to have to serve some man she did not care for. With serving her son, however, she had clearly much less difficulty. The idea, had her husband lived, of having a 70-year-old man in the house, seemed too horrific to consider. It would rob her of her freedom, even if it would mean that she would have much more income to spend. Now she managed with her savings and pension to travel abroad frequently, usually on her own.

A woman answering the survey among lesbian women mentioned above married through *omiai*, while she knew that she had a sexual preference for women:

> He is a kind (*yasashii*) man but there is not much love (*aijō*). For some reason I can't like him very much. If he is around every day my head starts to hurt. I don't remember how often I thought of divorce. As we live separately now we can go on without divorce. If he comes home, he is not around very long, so that I can avoid sleeping with him by saying that my head or my stomach hurts . . . (Hirosawa and Rezubian Ripōto Han 1991: 271–2)

This marriage appears to be the reverse of that of a homosexual man who marries without informing his wife. While at the time it seemed a good idea for this woman, by the time she wrote this, she had come to regret her marriage. However, since her husband is not much at home, she can cope with remaining married. While she knew beforehand that she did not like men, her education and her surroundings had made her believe that 'to marry a man and have children' is what makes one happy. Children, however, she does not mention having and as for marriage, it did not make her happy.

## Latent Feminism or Homosexuality

The third and, according to my findings, most common type of marriage is that of women who do not know of their homosexual preference or of their ideological differences with marriage. For them, marriage is the only way of life and the idea of other lifestyles never crossed their minds. Successfully socialized into believing Japanese *jōshiki* that marriage is the natural way of life for all women and that being a housewife is their road to happiness, they marry only to find out later that marriage is not all that blissful. This disenchantment may come quickly, as in the case of women who divorce within a couple of years, or it may take a long time, as with women who divorce after having been married for about twenty years or more. While some women almost instantly feel that there is something wrong with the role they are given in marriage, others need inducement from outside. In a majority of these cases divorce is the final result.

Among lesbian interviewees a common pattern was to come into contact with another lesbian woman, often at feminist meetings but also in other contexts in daily life,[11] and fall in love, after which it was usually only a matter of time until the divorce stage was reached. Among heterosexual women it usually involved some sort of activity outside the home, which might be professional or political, related to feminism or not. This would become incompatible with the demands of married life after which a divorce was eventually seen as the best solution. In very few cases did the husband possess sufficient adaptive capabilities to make continuation of the marriage feasible.

Bubu, a heterosexual woman, related that she had been a very good and successful housewife. Even though her husband did not bring in much of an income, she was always praised by her in-laws for making do so well. For her husband, however, this situation became unbearable. His lack of success as a provider led to an inferiority complex and eventually he started an affair with a less perfect woman. The couple divorced and to her own surprise Bubu was much happier with her newly gained independence. At the time of my fieldwork she worked as manager and actor of the performance group Dumb Type and felt that she was finally doing something she really liked. In Dumb Type's performance *S/N* she said that she was working as a prostitute, which had become her main source of income. She said that the first time she felt like a prostitute was when she let her ex-husband have sex with her even though she did not feel like it. In retrospect, she sees her married life as boring and uninteresting and the only reason she could cope with it so well was her enormous ability to adapt to situations and play the required roles.

Matsuo Megumi, a heterosexual woman who now manages an art gallery, likewise tried to be a good housewife and was also quite successful in that. First she worked only part-time at an art gallery and that was easy to combine with marriage. When the owner of the gallery decided to quit, however, she felt that it was important to have a gallery for young talent and decided to start her own gallery. As she was now the main responsible person, she did not succeed in being home in time to prepare her husband's dinner every evening. He rapidly grew discontented with this situation and because his attitude gradually became unbearable she decided to go and live on her own. She waited to get a divorce for eight years until her husband finally gave in and dropped his demand for the *isharyō* (compensation money) to which he was legally entitled because she in the meantime had other lovers. Partners who have been 'wronged' can refuse to consent to a divorce or demand compensation. In this case the compensation demanded was so high that in practice it amounted to a refusal to give consent. Having to pay the money he demanded was for financial reasons out of the question for the woman, so the divorce had to be postponed until he dropped most of his demands.

One interviewee had not married her husband legally but intended to do so one day. She was thus part of a traditional *naien* relationship (common-law marriage), which is underscored by the fact that she even used her husband's name. Moved by the fate of an old newspaper seller, she started a movement against the decision of the Osaka city government to wipe out newspaper sales stands in Umechika, the extensive underground shopping centre and pedestrian area in Umeda in Osaka, connecting three railway and three subway stations. Her involvement in this movement inevitably meant that she had less time to devote to housekeeping and as her husband wanted a nice home to return to after his working day, he grew increasingly discontented. They ended up in divorce, *rikon*, as she calls it, but she is still generally known by her husband's name, as that is the name she used from the start of her social activities and it would produce complications if she were to change it.

Another woman, who described her sexuality as *tada no sukebe* (just lewd, just a lecher), was mainly oriented towards men but also had sexual experiences with women. She had been married to a man without giving much thought to what the contents of the marriage would be and, even after having been confronted with the realities of married life, she did not particularly want to divorce her husband, with whom she also had a child, but she wanted to lead her own life, which appeared not to agree with her husband's ideas about marriage:

> [If you are married] it is as if you and your partner have to become one thing. While I resisted this very strongly, he did no such thing. So, when I went to work on my own or just thought independently about things, he became very dissatisfied. And I don't know if you call that love (*aijō*) but I could not

> handle it. (. . .) I went out to work and lived fully (*sei ippai*) but he seemed to be unable to endure (*gaman suru*) that.

This eventually led to fights and they started to talk about divorce. He found another lover, whom he married after the divorce. She thinks that he found someone who suits him very well, a woman who took over the mother role he expected her to assume, a woman who tells him how wonderful he is and does not go out to work or have her own interesting activities. The only problem that remains is that he does not want to see his son. She explained that he became ill at ease whenever he was confronted with her and seeing their son was too much of a confrontation because of his connection to his mother.

Another woman married with the idea of becoming a good housewife and a wise mother but after giving birth to two sons and a period of trying to comply with the demands of the role she had taken upon herself, she could not deal with it any longer. She renegotiated her marriage to the effect that the relationship with her husband became purely functional as parents to their children. Household expenses henceforth were paid equally by both, making this a case of *kateinai rikon*, that had been thought over carefully and worked quite well. She had had a wide variety of odd jobs but more recently had found better paid and more stable employment as a hostess. In the first years after the renegotiation she had several affairs with men but recently she had fallen in love with a woman and within a short span of time she came out in the national media on the occasion of the first Lesbian and Gay Parade in Japan in Tokyo on 28 August 1994, in which she participated in the company of her children. Eventually she divorced her husband and went to live with her female lover. Education of the children is shared by all involved.

A *feminisuto* married before she was interested in feminism. When she did become interested and started to go to meetings, to study and to work, she had several upheavals in her married life because her husband needed to adapt to the fact that she was going out to work and thus would not always be in when he returned from his work. Eventually he swallowed his discontent and nowadays he even takes on tasks like cooking and vacuuming. The relationship of this couple is not very close. According to the interviewee her husband is more like a guest of the family who comes to stay at the house she shares with her children. Nevertheless, that is no reason to change the arrangement. They are not bothering each other and can live happily side by side, while ignoring each other's presence most of the time. In fact, she feels much closer to a female friend, with whom she 'can talk about anything, even the most personal, even about sexuality'. This relationship, of which her husband and sons are well informed, is so close that she equates it to a love relationship. She thinks that if she had not been married already, she might have preferred a lesbian lifestyle.

A woman, writing in Kakefuda Hiroko's lesbian *minikomishi Labrys*, married before she discovered her feelings for women. She maintains that she is bisexual and thus does not have many problems in relating sexually to her husband, but there are also regrets. Nevertheless, she had to marry in order to be able to leave her parental home. The major problem, however, is that her husband needs to be made to feel superior:

> Because we are both selfish (*wagamama*), there are too many collisions and mostly I end up becoming neurotic and being hit until I lose consciousness. It makes me feel that it is just a matter of time.

She wants to quit this marriage but thinks that she lacks the strength to take such a step because she married and became neurotic precisely because she lacked the strength to take her life in her own hands (Y.A. 1993).

The cases described here are likely to represent a large number of Japanese women who are married today and continue to be representative for some time to come. However, the case of the woman who attempted suicide, described in the section on male homosexuality in marriage (pp. 135–6) would not belong to this group because her ideas are not at variance with *jōshiki* concerning the role of women in marriage. The type described here is likely to be the most common because it is a direct product of *jōshiki* concerning the education of women in Japan (Higuchi 1986). Existing dominant *jōshiki* is, however, under fire because increasingly mothers see it as important for their daughters to learn skills that will enable them to be independent of men (Hendry 1986a: 92).

## Disappointment

As a fourth type there are women who initially tried to fit the first type, in the sense that they tried to have the husband accept a married life that would fit their desires, but who found after marriage that there were more barriers to overcome than they expected. Some married women, who may not want to refer to themselves as feminists, nevertheless have egalitarian ideas about the position of women versus men and they often find that marriage brings them a lot of unwanted changes. Even if they are quite confident in the egalitarianism of their husbands and they are sure that they will impose no limits to the freedom for which they negotiated prior to marriage, relatives, the neighbourhood and friends, or *seken*, often turn out to impose constraints. They feel that they are expected to behave as a *yome* (bride) towards the outside world. They have to appear to cook and clean for their husband and to participate in neighbourly gossip with the housewives in the *danchi* or other housing environment (cf. Imamura 1987, Hiromi 1992). Furthermore, family and friends often develop an overwhelming interest in the children that are as a matter of fact expected to follow upon marriage[12] and would not hear of the couple's decision to plan to have them later or not at all.

In other cases the husband turned out not to be as egalitarian as he presented himself before marriage. Thus some informants are in distress about the ongoing demands of husbands to have children, while before marriage it had been agreed that they would not have children, and about demands of husbands that the wife spends more time at home, especially when he expects to be returning from his job (cf. Imamura 1987) and wants dinner on the table. Most of these cases I encountered ended in divorce, after the wife decided to live her own life, even if it meant that her husband became grumpy or, in some cases, violent. His misbehaviour consequently made divorce a desirable option. Whether it concerns common-law marriage or legal marriage makes not much difference, except that in the former case it is usually easier to reach an agreement about dividing possessions and care for the children.

A 33-year-old designer who now sees herself as lesbian, although she did not at the time of marriage, grew dissatisfied with her husband who had agreed that they would share household chores equally:

> My work became interesting and I had to do the housework and my work and I began wondering why on earth I was doing all this. (. . .) We had agreed initially to share everything but the man gradually became a sluggard

> (*namakemono*) and I had to do it alone. (. . .) Gradually our feelings came to be alienated from each other.

After three years she had enough of this and decided to divorce him, to which he consented. It was not until four years later again, that she became lesbian, which suggests that her divorce had little to do with her sexuality. Although she had always felt something was not quite right (*nanka chigau*), she did not know that there was such a thing as female homosexuality, so she merely tried to adjust to reality as she knew it. Her divorce was rather the result of a desire to pursue her career, something the husband did not support sufficiently. While she initially had wanted children, her husband's attitude put her off the idea.

Another 33-year-old interviewee, who is now one of the central figures of the singles' network in Osaka, lived with a man with whom equality was expected:

> [When I lived with him] he didn't say it directly but he wanted me to obey him and he showed this in his attitude without saying it clearly but he showed it. When I nodded in agreement with whatever he said he was happy but I didn't really agree and I felt that this was useless and decided to stop doing that. (. . .) Whatever I did, as long as I nodded in agreement there wasn't a problem but as soon as I confronted him . . .

While the man did not actually demand that she did anything in particular, this woman, who was rather set on being honest and open, found the implicit demand that she show a demure attitude unacceptable. Although the man had appeared to be very progressive and there was no discussion of making their cohabitation legal, his attitude demanded that she put herself below him, if only by the ostentatious activity of nodding, which became insupportable. Most women might never have noticed that this man demanded her to act in a subservient manner because they are socialized in a way that makes them act more subserviently than this man needed. Nevertheless, if a woman does not comply with what men expect of them, which may not be voiced, problems are likely to occur because many men cannot deal with women standing up to them, which has been a recurrent feature throughout the cases described above. Furthermore, a heterosexual male divorcee I interviewed gave his violent behaviour as the reason for his divorce and, likewise, another man was seeking counselling because he could not express his feelings, which led him suddenly to beat his child or scold his wife, which surprised even himself when it occurred.

Most but not all lesbian women had felt alienation in the sexual relationship with their husband, or in some cases a clear dislike of having sex with him. However, since they believed that to be not uncommon because many women do not like to have sex with their husbands – an observation that is supported by findings in the *More Report* (Moa Ripōto Han ed. 1983: 510–13) – they did not think anything of it. At most they thought that they should try harder and be more like other housewives who were, compared to themselves, perceived as more enduring (*gaman suru*). For mainly heterosexually oriented women the problem was not very different. Many clearly resented the way their husband thought sex was to be conducted. Resistance to this led in some cases to the husband becoming violent or in one case even to rape, which according to Japanese law does not count as rape because it takes place within marriage (Fukushima 1991b:

104–5, Tsunoda 1992: 37–40). Tsunoda and the *More Report* clarify the implications of this by giving various examples of women who do not like to have sex but 'the more I refuse the more he gets excited, so I understood that it was better not to resist' (Tsunoda 1992: 39), 'it is the duty as a married couple' or 'if I don't give in, he'll become unpleasant' (both Moa Ripōto Han ed. 1983: 513).[13]

It is remarkable that no criticism is voiced towards married lesbian women by those who strongly disapprove of married homosexual or bisexual men. Gay activists and feminist activists criticize the men but tend to be supportive of the women, if an opinion is voiced at all. The exception to this is Ogura Chikako (1988) who criticizes all married women, picking out especially those who regard themselves as *feminisuto*, which, according to Ogura, cannot be combined with marriage. Furthermore, husbands appear to be little concerned with their wives having a lesbian lover. In several cases in which the man was made aware that a woman was lesbian, the heterosexual man did not regard that as a reason for not asking her to marry him. Kakefuda Hiroko discusses this phenomenon and sees it as an indication that female sexuality is not taken seriously and that female homosexuality is not seen as threatening to the male prerogative because in the end she remains at the disposition of the man (Kakefuda 1992a: 141–2).

Most married women in my sample who established contact with lesbian circles, feminist circles, or who developed other interests that made a change in their lifestyle necessary, eventually wanted to divorce. Apart from two cases – a lesbian woman who left her children with her husband because he was very fond of them and a feminist woman whose children chose to stay with her husband – they could keep their children. Given the situation in Japan, where until as late as the 1960s the majority of children were officially allocated to the father,[14] this is most likely to have happened with the consent of the father. If the father opposed the arrangement and exposed his wife as lesbian in court, I do not believe that she would be likely to win custody, even though most children are nowadays allocated to the mother. Financial problems turned out not to play such an important role because, having the gratification of an emotionally more rewarding lifestyle, it seemed that financial needs could be adjusted enormously, once the choice was made.

While there are differences between feminist and lesbian women in relation to marriage, in both cases the expectations of the role of the housewife often form the major reason to opt out of marriage. While lesbian women may stress their sexual preference and heterosexual feminists their role in the household, a considerable overlap is present. Although feminists may have a heterosexual preference, often they do not find emotional and sexual satisfaction with a husband who is not educated to please and esteem women, or they find that the husband has no regard for their intellectual capacities and is unable to adapt to a housewife who stopped being only that and started to do something that does not fit in with her role in the household as he sees it.

## Comparing Men and Women

Lesbian women who positively see themselves as lesbian and have contact with lesbian networks are less likely to opt for marriage than gay men in a comparable situation. Although pressure on women to marry is definitely stronger than on men, especially the indirect pressure provided by the economic discrimination against women, lesbian women feel that they have much more to lose. The type of marriage some women opt for fits that of the platonic *keishiki kekkon,* which is discussed in the section on male homosexuality and marriage. They want their husband to know and to accept that sex is out of the question. Unlike gay men who often desire companionship and a warm home (*atatakai katei*), lesbian women tend to want the outer form and economic benefits but as little of a relationship as possible (Lunsing 1995).

Itō Bungaku, the heterosexual editor of the gay magazine *Barazoku*, suggested that it might be a good idea for gay men to marry lesbian women. This, however, seems not to work very well, as Itō admitted when I asked him. Women who think of themselves as lesbian usually do not want to marry, except in order to achieve financial security or an official status that might alleviate pressure from the family. They tend not to follow *ippan jōshiki* (general *jōshiki*) about marriage but see possible personal advantages in complying with a system they generally do not believe is right for them. Gay men wanting to marry, on the other hand, tend to follow *jōshiki* quite closely. In marriage they seek things like children or warmth and security in old age (ibid.). Mismatches in marriages between gay men and lesbian women are thus likely. They are less likely in the case of gay men who marry heterosexual women who, if they choose to marry a gay man, are more likely to provide the warm home many gay men desire (ibid.).

Among both lesbian and feminist women, dissatisfaction with the unequal division of household tasks and the wish to pursue activities outside the home in many cases increasingly strained the marital relationship which eventually led to divorce. The difference between male and female homosexuality in marriage is great. While women are much more likely to do whatever they think is expected of them and are more likely to discover some sort of emotional gratification in marriage, for men the wrapping aspect appears to be more important, the possibility marriage gives them to appear towards the outside world as 'normal'. This may seem contradictory to the reasons for gay men and lesbian women to seek marriage but it is not. In the rarer cases in which openness in a relation is achieved, men turn out to expect a warm home and women are less eager to provide that. However, in the more common cases that the feelings are hidden, the opposite occurs: gay men tend to avoid being home and lesbian or heterosexual women tend to try to be 'good housewives'.

Without exception the single women with children (*boshi katei*) I spoke with did not think of remarriage. They were very happy having made the decision to divorce and even though financially they were usually barely getting by, this was a minor problem compared to that of having a husband who expected to be waited on. Indeed, in the cases in which the husband became violent, it is not hard to imagine that women felt that they can do better without a husband. These women thus chose to be single while taking upon themselves the role of the mother. Single mothers often have or wish to have lovers but do not generally want to marry or even live with a man. One such interviewee, though, married in 1995, notwithstanding her earlier voiced opposition towards marriage. The reason appeared to be a reconciliation with her parents, which she did not wish to risk by cohabiting without being 'properly' married. The fact that women tend not to want to remarry contrasts sharply with single fathers who usually want to remarry as soon as they find someone willing to take on the role of mother for their children (Kasuga 1989). The presence of children is a reason to remain married and to keep hiding one's sexual preference commonly voiced by men, who fear the loss of contact with them. Female informants never mentioned children as being of much influence in decisions in this area.

## Conclusion

The major difference between homosexual men on the one hand and homosexual women and feminists on the other in relation to marriage is that homosexual men tended to look back on their married life with regret and may aspire to remarry. Among the women I interviewed there were none who aspired to remarry and all were quite content with having put married life behind them. Of those still in marriage, all men I spoke with wanted to continue, even though many things might be difficult and unpleasant, while among women there were many who contemplated divorce. Homosexual men discussed in this chapter generally did not have ideas about emancipation and equality between husband and wife, ideas that were quite prevalent among the women. As will be discussed in following chapters, however, among homosexual men who do not marry emancipatory and egalitarian tendencies are more prevalent.

## Notes

1 As discussed in the introduction (p. 6), an extraordinary feature of Japan between the 1940s and the 1980s was that over 98 per cent of both sexes married (Keizai Kikakuchō ed. 1992: 29).

2 Minami related this on several occasions and another core member of his organization, JILGA, said the same thing again on television in a programme of Fuji television, which centred on the activities of Occur but included other groups as well. This programme appeared on television in Osaka in October 1992.

3 Western gay men who visit Shinjuku Nichōme might find the contention that the majority of patrons are married to be an overstatement because the bars that are frequented most by foreigners tend to be atypical in the sense that fewer Japanese visiting them tend to be married than those in other bars. Furthermore, they tend to be younger and more open about themselves, often under the influence of foreign lovers.

4 Ugoku Gei. (1992) interprets the fact that one-third of their sample stated that they want to marry as proof of a considerable decrease in the number of gay men who aspire to marry. However, here they disregard the bias in their sample, even though elsewhere they discuss it. Besides, as there are no comparative figures on the wish to marry among gay men in earlier times, such a conclusion cannot be drawn from the survey. It seems rather to be an example of wishful thinking.

5 In *Za Gei*, a rather radical magazine that is more explicit in its pornography than any of the others and that discusses questions regarding the *tennōsei* (emperor system) and forms of discrimination that are thought to be related to it, the annual survey of readers shows no decline in the numbers wanting to marry since 1989 (Za Gei Henshūbu ed. 1992). In the gay magazine *Sabu*, which is, compared to other magazines, relatively more oriented towards sadomasochism and macho men, just under 30 per cent of single respondents to the survey wanted to marry (Nakajima 1991).

6 This group held a small survey among themselves at a party in an *izakaya*, a Japanese-style eating and drinking place, in Kobe. Replies were written on a piece of paper. People did not discuss their answers with each other and were anxious to prevent others from seeing what they wrote. The results of the two tables the people were sitting at were compared to

each other. While at the table I sat at a majority did not want to marry, most people at the other did, which correlated with answers to the other questions in the way described.

7 Mayoeru Sarariiman means 'puzzled company man' and here is used as a nickname.

8 In the Kansai area, where this couple lives, one has to pay about six months' rent key money, of which merely half is received back after leaving the place, which makes renting a place for only one month horrendously expensive because one ends up paying at least four months' rent.

9 Compared to the figures Kinsey *et al.* (1948) gave on sexual activities of American men this is not at all remarkable. As Kinsey showed, 37 per cent of American men had engaged in homosexual activity up to the point of orgasm sometime in their lives. The Kinsey data have been criticized because in the sample university students and criminals were over-represented (Gebhart and Johnson 1979) but the results have been roughly confirmed by follow-up research. Ross (1983) refers to Gagnon and Simon (1973) whose research data show that 30 per cent of men had homosexual contact to orgasm. Singer and Deschamps (1994), in their *Gay and lesbian stats*, discuss both these results as well as those of Smith and Garner (1976), among whose sample of male athletes 40 per cent had homosexual contact to orgasm, a *Playboy* survey (1983), in which 35 per cent of male respondents had the same, and Fay *et al.* (1989), according to whom the figure was 20.3 per cent. They also present other, less spectacular, figures but they are less convincing because the samples are smaller and a lot of critics have pointed out that the methods were rather disputable.

10 This series of tapes is called *Midnight Minx*, but pronounced 'Midnight Mix'. Kamigata DJ Club makes these tapes and

sends them to hundreds of listeners, many of whom live in rural areas.

11 Other places for chance meetings between lesbian women mentioned by informants were a regular nightclub, the local neighbourhood and an English language class. Hashimoto's much-praised story about a woman meeting and eloping with a lesbian woman was set in the transport cafe where the main protagonist worked, while the woman who came to seduce her was a truck driver (Hashimoto 1987: 126–85).

12 Hendry (1986a: 14) mentions that she was confronted with this herself when doing research before she had children, while being married.

13 This puts the contention of, for instance, Lebra (1984: 305) that rape is much rarer in Japan than in the United States, which she apparently based on the number of rape cases recorded by the police, in a dubious light. Apart from the question of whether Japanese women are as likely to go to the police as American women in a case of rape, it is of course easy to keep figures low by not calling rape large categories of sexual activity that are no different from rape, but it has little to do with what really goes on. The statistical data clearly cannot be compared.

14 In fact this meant in many cases that they were brought up by their grandmothers. This indicates that the influence of the *ie* with its patrilineal structure persisted for a long time. See for instance Ueno (1990a) for a detailed discussion.

# 5 Private: Alternative Lifestyles

This chapter discusses why people may remain single and how experiments with alternative relationships and living patterns develop from the point of view of those directly concerned, including discussions about relationships that may occur in networks or circles. Two lifecourse routes can be discerned for all categories this book is concerned with. One is the route of marriage and divorce, whereby some have not yet arrived or indeed may never arrive at the divorce stage. The other is the route of remaining unmarried throughout, whereby relationships and living together with lovers are optional. People remain unmarried for various reasons, ranging from the impossibility of marrying because of the shortage of men after the Second World War to political rejection of the marriage system, including *jijitsukon*. Homosexuality and feminist ideas are obvious features among those who reject marriage but others come to reject marriage only after realizing that they probably will not marry. Such a realization or the ideological rejection of marriage opens ways of experimenting with alternative forms of relationships and living.

## Singles: *Dokushin, Shinguru*

The oldest known network of singles in Japan is Dokushin Fujin Renmei (Single Women's League), an organization of single women founded in 1967. Some of its central figures claim that members could not marry because so many of the generation of men they expected to marry died in the battlefields of the Second World War (Dokushin Fujin Renmei. 1977, 1987, Tani 1982). Interviewees and informants of this group, however, are of all types of singles. There are those who could not marry because their fiancés had died in the battlefields and they would not settle for less than someone they 'really' loved, those who wanted to marry very much but never found a husband, even though they tried everything they could think of, possibly including joining this group, and there are those who never wanted to marry. This is confirmed by a survey among single women of the concerned age cohort conducted by Ōkubo Sawako of Dokushin Fujin Renmei (Ōkubo 1977). According to Ōkubo, a matchmaking office the league maintained for a while did not result in any marriage. There is nevertheless a case of a member who married. She had not joined the league in order to find a husband but when a man asked her to marry him she decided to agree because the security the league offered made her confident that she would have a place to return to should the marriage go wrong. In this sense, Dokushin Fujin Renmei took over a role that might otherwise have been fulfilled by the parental home (Ōkubo 1987).

While the percentage of single women in this age cohort is slightly higher than that in the cohorts before and directly after them, leaders of this group systematically produce over estimations of the number of 'war widows', as they sometimes call themselves.[1] Such a strategy was apparently thought to be necessary in order to receive sympathy from the media and the Japanese people. In the 1960s a woman could not very well say that she was happy to be single. Such a line of thinking did not become acceptable until the late 1980s and is still not widely recognized. Nevertheless, a considerable number of Dokushin

Fujin Renmei's members now say that they are happy with having remained single, although they were aware of and troubled by society's prejudice and discrimination against them (Ichibangase 1971: 69–70, Naruse 1977, Tani 1982: 131–62). This is underscored by the fact that they simply felt that they could not say that they positively chose to remain single. The titles of two booklets produced by the league indicate that a change in this attitude has taken place. While the title of the booklet published in 1977 referred back to the war and those who never came back (*Wadatsumi no Koe o Towa ni*: Voices of the ocean for eternity; Dokushin Fujin Renmei. 1977), the title of the publication of 1987 refers to the joys of being single (*Hanayaka ni Shinguru Raifu*: Joyful single life; Dokushin Fujin Renmei. 1987).

This change in attitude came with an increase of media attention for people, initially women but later also men, who remain unmarried following an increase in the rise of singles in their 30s and 40s. As discussed in chapter three (pp. 93-4), not only has the average age of those who marry risen to 28.4 years for men and 25.9 years for women in 1990, a trend that started in 1970, when the trend towards marrying at a younger age, visible from 1950, was reversed (Keizai Kikakuchō ed. 1992: 23–5, 408), but also has the number of men and women who have remained unmarried in their 30s and 40s reached a level that was unthinkable only ten years ago (ibid.: 26–9, 409).

These trends are more conspicuous in large urban areas, and may be reported in a sensational manner, for example when the headlines on the front page of the quality newspaper *Asahi Shinbun* were trumpeting that of men in their 40s in Tokyo one in five was unmarried and in Osaka it was one in ten (*Asahi Shinbun* 1992). In general those who see this development as a problem blame women who refuse to marry, possibly because they were influenced by feminism, while single men tend to be portrayed, rather sadly, as men who cannot marry (Genshi Shuzaihan ed. 1991). This is widely believed to be a result of women having become strong and men weak, which itself is an idea that has become almost *jōshiki* in the late 1980s (Watanabe 1989, 1991, Nakamura 1991).

While figures for those who do not marry include those who live in *jijitsukon*, who thus might still be seen as married, there is also a growing trend for unmarried people to leave the parental home and live by themselves. The total number of single households passed the 9 million mark between 1985 and 1990 in a continuous rise from about 6 million in 1970. This rise is considerably more than the increase in the number of single elderly persons, which is about 700,000 over the same period and which is a major focus of attention because of its problematic character, caused by a shortage of services to assist them (Sōmuchō Tōkeikyoku ed. 1992: 18–19).

The couple discussed in chapter three that lived apart in *jijitsukon* were eager to explain that they, just like most of their friends, were not married and thus fitted my research topic but a single woman who was part of this circle of friends, when interviewed privately, disagreed vehemently with this. According to her, there was not much difference between being married with or without setting up a *koseki*. It amounted to the same thing and their situation could definitely not be compared to hers because she was really single and living alone.

Support for this idea can be found in Ebisaka who defines singles as people who live by themselves, possibly with children. He adds to his definition that those who are married but temporarily separated because of their jobs (*tanshin funin*; Tanaka 1992, Shiina 1994) are not included because they fit the system of marriage, nor are those who live together in *jijitsukon*. Singles can have one or more lovers but are not included if they live with them (Ebisaka 1986: 37–8). This is further supported by Yoshihiro Kiyoko's books on single women (1987) and single men (1988), which also exclude cohabiters, and Matsubara Junko's book (1988) in which cohabitation is not considered at all. Aoki Yayoi, however, includes in her *Shinguru Karuchā* (Single culture; 1987) cohabiting couples. Apart from Matsubara, whose argument is that it would have been better if the women discussed in her book had married, these books tend to describe singles who are happy and confident with being single and to overlook the fact that there are also unhappy singles who would rather be married. Here I define singles in a wider sense than Ebisaka, by including unmarried people who live with their parents. Among my informants three different routes of remaining single can be discerned.

## Single by Circumstances

The most common and obvious reason for people to remain single is that they happened not to find somebody they wanted to or could share their life with. For one thing, the *koseki seido* may make marriage impossible. Many Japanese still think today that *koseki* include criminal records, psychiatric patients and bankruptcies in the family and that as a consequence having a brother, sister, father or mother tainted by such features damages one's chances of marrying into a 'good' family. For this reason people may abstain from becoming too close to someone they feel attracted to because they do not wish to be exposed as being related to people who possess one of these features. Although *koseki* do not list such features any more, they can be found out through them; for instance, criminal records are linked to *koseki* and less scrupulous civil servants may mark *koseki* to indicate that a criminal record is related to it because it is convenient when files on people are needed (Satō and Kaibara 1990: 122–3, 151).

The wish to investigate a partner your child wants to marry is officially not a ground for being allowed to look at someone's *koseki* but unscrupulous lawyers and detectives frequently find ways of access to *koseki* and compile files on them (Idota 1993: 177–8). Particularly if someone is discovered to be of *burakumin* (Japanese outcaste) descent, parents of the partner may effectively oppose marriage (Satō and Kaibara 1990: 91, Tsuji 1992). *Buraku* descent can be deduced from looking at *koseki*, especially in the Kansai area, where *buraku* areas are generally known. Thus the *koseki seido* may prevent marriages that are desired by a woman and a man on personal grounds from taking place because the parents will not accept the match. Although parents legally have no say in this once their children are 20 years old, it is still customary for children to ask for parental consent and they may defer to parents' wishes, even if they do not agree with them (DeVos 1986a).

A second major cause for remaining single because marriage is impossible can be found in the ideal of romantic love. A very clear case is that of an interviewee who grew up in the strong belief that she, as a matter of course, would marry one day and become a housewife and have children. She fell in love with a man she could not marry because he did not want to marry her. As a result of this love, however, she decided that she could not settle for someone she did not really love. Although she wanted to marry and have children, she did not want to have *omiai*. Thus she remained single as a result of what she saw as remaining true to her feelings. Other interviewees fell in love with a man who was already married, which made marriage impossible. This way of remaining single is shared by many homosexual people. Hase *san*, introduced in chapter three (p.

112), was very clear that he could not possibly marry because he did not wish to deceive a woman and make her unhappy. He had always thought that, being homosexual, it would be wrong to marry. At the same time he happened never to find a male partner he really loved or, when he did, the other party did not love him. As a result he had lived alone since he left his mother's home. For similar reasons many gay and lesbian people have remained single.

Many gay and lesbian people, however, were positive that, while they could not marry, they would want to live and share their lives with a same-sex partner. Even some people in the singles' movement clearly stated that they would rather be married, although usually they would not want to set up a *koseki* and thus have a *jijitsukon*. Women in particular are of the opinion that the *koseki seido* must be opposed; men are less adamant about this. Men often seemed to give lip service to this idea because they know that this is the prevalent political stance among the independent women they see as desirable partners. The relationship based on equality and mutual love that is usually the ideal among this group, makes the possibility of *omiai* unthinkable. As a result they are restricted to meeting potential partners in their work or personal life, where chances are often limited. According to Higuchi (1984), this is an increasing problem because many *OL* (Office Ladies: mostly young women who do odd jobs in offices; Kelsky 1994, Carter and Dilatush 1977) nowadays work in offices where, apart from a male supervisor, only women work, whereas they used to work among male colleagues. Marriage as a result of meeting through the singles' network did not occur to my knowledge.

## Single without Intention

A second category of singles are those who really want to marry and have made much effort, often including *omiai*, in order to find a spouse but did not succeed. In some cases they are still hoping and trying, in others they have given up on the idea and decided to make the best of their single life, in the latter case usually with a very positive view about living alone from then onwards. In this category could also be included people who became single after a spouse died as well as those who were divorced at the instigation of their partners, such as homosexual men who, when their homosexuality was discovered, felt obliged to accept their wife's demand for divorce. For this category being single is never a positive choice but after a while it might come to be accepted as a fact of life and possibly embraced in a positive way. Further, people may decide on a reconsideration of the idea of marriage once they come to accept the idea that they may not marry. A 28-year-old woman said:

> Well, sometimes I think that it might be good to live together with someone, if it was for a limited period. If it was for ever, I think that would be tiresome, hard to bear (*shindoi, tsurai*).

This interviewee claimed that she had always been against legal marriage but that she would consider cohabiting. At other points in the interview, however, she claimed to be very happy living alone and not to want to share an apartment with a man. After we discussed her friends and other relationships and considering her behaviour towards me, I felt that she was rather lonely and in search of friends and a lover. A story about a previous love relationship with a man, who had been mentally disturbed and had received much support from her before moving elsewhere and severing all contacts, strengthened my feeling that if she found a lover, she would most likely agree to live with him, or possible even marry him, if that would be his wish.

Similarly, a heterosexual man in his late 30s did not tire of talking about how interesting his life as a single man was. He had many hobbies and engaged in various activities, such as *shimin undō* (citizen's movements), artistic pursuits like painting and writing and the singles' network. While engaging in these activities he had become acquainted with many interesting people a regular married *sarariiman* was not likely to meet. When I asked him about the loves in his life, however, the hitherto very friendly and positive atmosphere changed, while he admitted that never in his life had he had a lover. He tried to remain positive about his life but his attitude towards me had changed not to recover. When talking of the future, it also transpired that he really would very much like to get married, but only to a woman he met through his activities, most of whom do not want to marry. Such interviewees indicate that Yoshihiro's books on singles (1987 and 1988) are more directed to drawing a positive image of the lives of single people in Japan than to giving a true representation. As a method to give counterweight to prevalent negative images this of course has its value, and the fact that such a need is apparently felt indicates all the more how powerful these negative images are.

## Single by Intention

Finally, there are of course the die-hards, those who will not marry or live together, not even if they encounter the proverbial prince or princess on a white horse. Some may not even want to have close relationships, like a member of the singles' network, who has sexual relationships with women but thinks it is wrong to trouble them with personal problems and claims that he is capable of abstaining from breaking wind when in the company of a sex partner. This he sees as a virtuous way of avoiding embarrassment to the woman he is with. Embarrassing and troubling people one has sexual relationships with in his view would be a corruption of the purity of a relationship marked by individuality and independence. It is more common for singles of this category to want to have more emotional and personal involvement with lovers but none of them want to live together or be bound economically in any way.

The wish to keep their independence is the most important reason for choosing to remain single, especially in the case of women but also among some men. Even *jijitsukon* is not perceived as an alternative to *hōritsukon* because the surrounding people, neighbourhood and friends, will regard one as part of a couple. A single woman lived for a large part of her life together with her lover but always kept her own apartment, so that she always had a place to be alone. Further, they made sure that they were not seen as having a permanent relationship in their neighbourhood. This woman was introduced to me by a colleague who did not know of this arrangement and presented her as a die-hard single.

A heterosexual male interviewee, who definitely did not want to marry, said that the example of his brother's marriage had brought him to this decision. His mother, whom he 'hated very much (*tottemo kirai*)', treated his brother's wife very badly and he did not want to cause any woman to be treated like that. This is reminiscent of DeVos's contention that people may refuse arranged marriage and engage in a love marriage to hurt a parent (1986a), which today is probably largely outdated because the influence of parents has decreased and they are more likely to agree with love marriages. Hence, in order to hurt parents one may have to take a step further and refuse to marry altogether. Although my interviewee wondered about problems like illness and old age, he enjoyed evenings out and having fun with girlfriends very much and did not want to forego such pleasures in favour of marriage. Nevertheless, he also told of a woman he loved very much and he was not certain whether he would refuse to marry her if that would result in the discontinuation of their relationship. Particularly among women the idea of having a partner in the house is not thought to be desirable, often based on experience, like the 33-year-old interviewee quoted in the previous chapter, who decided that she could definitely not bear to live with a man. A woman who was 20 years old in 1945 and managed to remain unmarried for her entire life, said:

> When I was 20, everybody talked of marriage, which meant that you'd have to do the household work and cook for the rest of your life. I don't like cooking (. . .) , it was this sort of feeling. But it's a long time ago, at the time I didn't know a thing about feminism and such but I wouldn't go for [marriage]. I never even considered getting married, I always thought it to be disadvantageous for women. If I'd been a man, I might have married.

When asked about children, her answer was similar; she would have liked to have children if she had been a man with a wife to take care of them. Being a woman, however, children would have been too much of a hindrance to her autonomy. Since she retired from her job she had been sharing an apartment with another woman, which she likes much better than the times she lived with men, as she did for shorter periods previously.

This category includes those who divorced because they wanted to and cases like the woman discussed in the previous chapter (pp. 145-6), who was quite happy when her husband, whom she never wanted to marry, died suddenly at an early age. In this category one also finds many homosexual people. While one male interviewee thought he could not live together with most people because it would be too stressful, he did not totally exclude the idea. However, he still felt that he must be free to engage in other relationships. Another interviewee stated that he could not live with his lover because their lifestyles were too different. While he always made a mess of his room, his boyfriend was very neat. Living together would produce too much strain on the relationship. This manner of arguing that emphasizes the stress of living together and the advantages of living apart can be found among all die-hard singles, heterosexual as well as homosexual, female as well as male. It is more common among women, lesbian as well as heterosexual (Chō 1992). While men generally hoped to be understood by a woman, women often did not count on being understood by a man and thus thought they would be better off single, rather than living together with a man whom they saw as being in need of change without him being aware of what and how, or even that he was in such need.

## Alternative Lifestyles

This section discusses features concerning the sharing of living space in groups, same-sex couples and other relationships that differ from marriage in the legal sense as well as in sense of heterosexual *jijitsukon*. In addition, lifestyles and relationships of single people are discussed. There will be seven parts: group living, male same-sex relationships, promiscuous gay men, female same-sex relationships, promiscuous women, alternative female–male relationships, and Tsutamori Tatsuru: relations denying gender boundaries. It concentrates on the internal features of relationships rather than their relation to the outside world.

## Group Living

Ochiai Keiko's novel *Gūzen no Kazoku* (Family by coincidence; 1990) is an account of the life of a number of people who are living together in a spacious house. The only *ketsuen kankei* (blood relationship) that exists is the one between a mother and her son. Otherwise all characters are related by nothing but friendship and love. The house is shared by a gay couple, one of whom inherited the house, a single woman, two single men and a divorced woman with child. Such living patterns are statistically negligible, with 77,000 non-family households (*hishinzoku setai*) in 1990, up from a low of 62,000 in 1980 (Sōmuchō Tōkeikyoku ed. 1992: 19). It remains unclear how reliable these statistics are because people may be registered differently from where they actually live. These figures would include most same-sex partners living together and some, not many, of the people in heterosexual *jijitsukon*. The fact that having children of under 6 years old receives a horizontal line in the table, which indicates that such a thing is not deemed possible, means that most *jijitsukon* couples must be counted under family households (*shinzoku setai*). Single-mother households with one or more children comprised in 1990 well over 2 million and single-father households 425,000, both rising continuously and significantly since 1970 (ibid.).

One of the groups I found to be living in roughly the situation depicted by Ochiai, consisted at the time of my visit of a married couple with a child sharing a household with a single man, which they called a kibbutz. There had been more people previously and, indeed, the house was spacious enough to easily provide room for three times as many. Internal strife, however, had made people leave and the latest news that reached me about this household was that the couple with the child had also left. Similarly, an experiment of communal living of two heterosexual couples, a single woman and two children did not last because the men could not adapt to this way of life. They wanted their wives to be at their personal service, not at that of the group. The experiment continued all the same, without the men who left (Fujimoto 1982).

Another group consisted of three lesbian women who lived in separate rooms in a house. This situation developed gradually. The first woman of the group moved in when a friend left. As she was looking for a place to live, the landlord agreed to rent it to her. When other rooms became vacant, the landlord agreed that she could choose friends to share the house with and thus it became a house where a group of lesbian women lives. In another case a group of gay men shared a spacious house in Osaka, which was inherited by one of the men. The owner preferred to have foreigners living in his house because Japanese often gave trouble as a result of their lack of directness in expressing any complaints they might have and instead sulked in silence until they burst into a rage.

The owner apparently lacked *omoiyari*, empathy, which has been presented as a characteristic Japanese trait (Lebra 1976: 38–49). If he had more of it, he would have understood from the silent sulking that something was wrong and taken steps to prevent emotional outbursts from materializing. *Omoiyari* is something that has to be developed by relating to people. By relating one learns to understand the different moods and ways of non-verbal communication. This understanding then is to be used in order to make the other feel at ease.

It has been suggested that Japanese who have to deal with people they do not know and in relation to whom their status role is not clearly defined, must develop patterns of behaviour to which they are not used in everyday life, where usually their roles are clearly set, be it at home, at school, or at their jobs. In these set roles they are (*de aru*), rather than do (*suru*), as Maruyama Masao (1987: 154–80) pointed out. In relation to people one does not know, however, rapport has to be developed in some way or other without any clear rules determining how to behave. One cannot just be (*de aru*) but rather has to act or do (*suru*), to be creative. Following this line of reasoning, it is obvious that many of the relationships discussed here are under stress because of the absence of clear rules for behaviour.

As Ōkubo Sawako of Dokushin Fujin Renmei said, it is very difficult for Japanese to cope with living with people they are not directly related to, especially once they have become used to living on their own and developed their own particular way of doing things without having to negotiate anything with others. For this reason, efforts to establish homes where single women could live together have rarely been successful. Putting up with habits of other people without the need to is not something many people are prepared to do. This is a problem among people who are forced to live in institutions for the elderly, where conditions usually are such that rooms have to be shared, which makes it inescapable to find ways of dealing with others (Bethel 1992). Further, the social pressure to continue and put up with others, which may play an important role in sustaining marriages, does not exist in the case of non-kin groups living together, which makes it easier for people to quit as soon as there is something they do not like, and such things inevitably occur.

## Male Same-Sex Relationships

Here also lies one of the reasons for the short duration of many relationships between gay men. Among my informants three months was generally considered to be a long time. A young man said that he had been together with his lover for three months, upon which I remarked that this was a dangerous period and, indeed, the next time I met him the relationship had ended. Reasons why relationships were broken up were often unclear to the people involved. In a number of cases the other suddenly refused to talk, to the point of throwing the phone on the hook when being called. In one case, two lovers chanced to meet each other in a gay sauna, which is a place where men go to have casual sexual contacts. After this episode my interviewee decided to end formally a relationship in which alienation had already grown considerably before this event. In fact, with hindsight he thought that he only entered the relationship because he wanted very much to have a lover, rather than because this particular boy (*ko*), as he referred to him, really was his type. This method of rationalizing the ending of past relationships is one many interviewees used.

In almost all gay circles I participated in, discussion of what type of person one could love occurred regularly. The first question was whether he should be younger or older, after which qualities such as physical build, i.e. fat, athletic, slim, slender or muscular, usually followed. Of importance were further what he wears, for instance jeans or a suit, what kind of occupation he has and whether he is masculine, androgynous or feminine. Gay bars may even be divided along the lines of what customers like. There are, among others, bars for young men and those who like them (*wakasen bā*), for older men and those who like them (*fukesen bā*) and for fat men and those who like them (*debusen bā*; Lunsing 1994a). Thus, a first selection of prospective partners is based solely on outward appearances, after which character may be considered. It appeared that most gay men had quite definite ideas of what their type is and usually practice agreed with this quite closely. Many, however, do not succeed in finding their ideal lover.

A survey by the gay magazine *Sabu* shows that of 186 respondents 56 had experienced living together with a man. This figure is greatly boosted by the fact that of those in their 40s about three-quarters had the experience, compared with only a quarter of all other age cohorts (Nakajima, K. 1992). The percentage of those having experienced cohabitation in Occur's survey of 300 young gay men was 20, and of these most relationships only existed for a couple of years, which does not say much because it concerns mostly young men (Ugoku Gei. 1992: 364).

In the few cases of gay men living together I encountered while conducting participant observation, I witnessed that there was usually a division of tasks that resembles the traditional male–female division in marriage. In this light one might wonder what the grounds are for Hirano Hiroaki's criticism of *Rasen no Sobyō* (A spiral sketch), a documentary film that depicted exactly such a relationship. I rather saw this as a very realistic depiction of relations as they exist. The relationship in the film was in fact modelled on the relationship the two main actors had at the time. While Hirano could not deny this, he, having embraced feminist thought, had ideological reasons for attacking a depiction of yet another relationship that resembles a heterosexist relationship.

Thus the film missed the chance of showing that other ways of role division are possible. Hirano's critique was all the more valid because he appeared in the film himself and had made the director promise that its depiction of homosexuality would agree with his ideas (Hirano 1991). One elderly gay couple I met by chance, on the other hand, seemed to be close to Hirano's ideals. While they were both rather feminine in their behaviour and speech, there was nothing to indicate any division of role pattern along heterosexist lines. Their age also suggests that egalitarian gay relationships are not necessarily a novelty but may have existed all along, albeit largely invisible to most people.

Occur's leaders advocate the idea of equality in relationships. A gay couple, who were members of Occur, that was selected to appear in a television documentary, exemplified equality between the partners, dividing tasks in a way that is common among egalitarian heterosexual couples. Itō Satoru also describes his relationship with his partner as egalitarian and characterized by an absence of role patterns along the lines of those in heterosexual relationships. When Itō's ageing mother moved in they had to divide the four rooms of their apartment: one for each of the three persons and a living room (*ima*) for the couple was the outcome (Itō, S. 1993: 153). Having a room of one's own was often mentioned as a condition for considering cohabiting with a lover among gay men, including those who had never experienced it.

In January 1994 the quality newspaper *Asahi Shinbun* published an article as part of a series on the United Nation's Year of the Family in which a gay couple were depicted as 'sitting in silence together, just like a heterosexual couple', which shows a feature that is thought to be positive in couples: they are so closely related that they do not need to talk; they know what the other thinks and feels. This is of course not always true, either in the case of heterosexual couples or in the case of gay couples. This belief has, however, greater consequences for gay couples, for whom chances that drifting apart may lead to a separation are much greater than for heterosexual couples. As a young gay interviewee, who had lived with a lover for two years, said, it was not in the first place the role division, in which he took upon himself most of the household tasks, that made him want to separate:

> He was involved in various left-wing movements. In these activities, there seem to have been several struggles during meetings and because of that he got in a bad mood. (. . .) Because the meetings didn't develop as he liked, he got angry and consequently he got angry at home as well. (. . .) I tried to talk to him about it and to make him understand that I didn't like his attitude but he didn't understand. On top of that he was terribly jealous and he got very angry when I'd go to meet friends (. . .) and so our feelings became gradually estranged.

The fact that his partner increasingly did not listen to what he had to say, that he took his presence for granted, was the major point of dissent, combined with his partner's jealousy of his friendships. Only after I asked specifically, did this interviewee say that he also disliked the fact that in practice he did all the housekeeping. Just as in the case of some of the women in the previous chapter, the fact that there was no possibility to discuss dissatisfaction with the way things were was the major ground for stopping living together. In contrast to most cases, however, this interviewee now has a relation of friendship with his previous lover. The idea that talking is not necessary clearly gives an edge to the more masculine of two partners and the only way of countering this is to make him or her see that something is wrong. If he or she is lacking in *omoiyari* this may be extremely difficult. If he or she refuses to recognize this, the choice between separation and accepting the situation appears to lie with the more feminine side. *Omoiyari* seems to be a quality instilled in and expected of women more than men, as examples in chapter four, where women had difficulty with men expecting things of them without discussing the reasons why, also indicate.

Somewhat different from this case is that described by Taira, who half lived with a lover when he was a student. Half, because he kept his own apartment where he, however, did not stay often. His lover was a *sarariiman* and, as it made sense that whoever had the time made dinner, Taira always made dinner. He ended up having to wait every day for a phone call from his lover to tell him when he would be coming home, so that he could prepare dinner in time. The daily insecurity produced by having to wait for these calls, made Taira think of questions like that of whether his lover was seeing other men. Gradually he lost contact with groups and friends he used to spend much time with and he started feeling very lonely. After Taira graduated, however, he moved to an apartment near his lover's, so that he could always go home and so that there was no need for him constantly to know when his lover was home and when not. This changed the relationship, which Taira now hopes to develop further, while learning to know himself better as well as his lover (Taira 1993).

In Taira's case, the existence of a widespread problem may be found, that of dependence in relationships. Taira obviously was oriented towards his lover to an extent that made him neglect his other needs. Doi Takeo (1975) referred to 'the pathology' of *amae* in homosexual relationships in which usually, but not always, the younger of the partners assumes the position of dependence in relation to the other, usually older, partner. Occur appears to have adopted this idea and condemns such relationships and Kawamura *san*, who is related to the Kansai-based gay organization OGC, also discussed his relation as problematic because his lover is acting as emotionally dependent on him, something he finds hard to comply with and would prefer to change (Miller 1992: 177–8). Other informants have fewer problems with lovers being dependent on them or themselves being dependent and take it as a fact of life. Especially some informants who are in their 40s do not mind having a younger lover act emotionally dependent, as long as this lover is reliable. This relation of dependence among gay lovers is often mistaken as a typical Japanese characteristic. In the international groups in Japan in which I participated, I found that relations between Japanese and Americans were more clearly characterized by dependency than relationships between Japanese, and that the dependent one could be either the Japanese or the American.

Of course dependency violates the ideal of equality in relationships and as such it does not agree with, for instance, Occur's ideas of how a gay man should be, which is based on what they believe to be usual in America. Therefore Kanda, a member of Occur, even condemns relationships between people of different age, adding that in advertisements in Japanese gay magazines the terms *aniki* (older brother) and *otōto* (younger brother) are widely used (Miller 1992: 178). There are three reasons why I believe this to be a misrepresentation of particular characteristics of gay relationships in Japan. First, family terms are widely used in referring to people one is close to and there is no term for a brother of the same age. Second, in advertisements in European gay magazines, like *Gay Times* in England, there are equally many advertisements from people who explicitly seek a lover who is younger or older. Third, among the couples I found and heard about in Japan there was no indication that age difference plays a larger role than in other countries I know, including the Netherlands. Dependence can be a temporary feature, as in the case of Taira, and the roles of the dependent and its counterpart may be switched at some point in time.

More problematic are the following relationships which were unsuccessful because of attitudes of one of the partners. A man had several relationships that did not last for long for various reasons. In one, his partner was so concerned that anyone might discover the relationship that he only wanted to be together in his lover's private room. He did not want to be seen with him. This put so much stress on the relationship that my informant decided to end it. In another case, his lover was living with another man, who fulfilled more or less the role of housewife. My informant disliked this arrangement because the relationship always had to progress in secret, so that his lover's lover would not find out. This relationship also ended after a short time. Other relationships ended because they became incompatible with the marriage of one of the partners, or because one of the partners was transferred in his job. These endings of relationships are all strongly influenced by social circumstances, combined with a partner who fails to stand up for his love.

Two couples of men I found to be living together were not lovers but friends. While in both cases they were both homosexual, their relationship was based on friendship rather than love and they had love and sex relationships with others independently. This solution to overcome the difficulties of living with a lover was one that appealed to many informants, especially those who were in their 30s. The rationale behind this is that it is desirable to live with someone but when sex and passion are the base of a relationship, it is difficult to sustain being together on a daily basis. Therefore living with a friend can be a good solution. It is a solution that is not very different from a man and a woman sharing a house in a platonic relationship, which is one of the types of marriage discussed in the previous chapter. In addition to this, I found men who started to cohabit as lovers but now describe their relationship as one of close friends (*shinyō kankei ni natchatta*), while love relationships (*koibito*) may be enjoyed on the side.

A survey on differences in lifestyle and ideas between heterosexual and homosexual people and between women and men, conducted by students of a Yajima seminar class of Chūō University, questioned Occur members as the homosexual sample, which was compared to students of Chūō University. Here, the ideal of equality is clearly espoused by the homosexual sample, with 89.2 per cent of gay men answering that they expect household chores to be divided equally and 80.6 per cent of lesbian women, compared to 47.9 per cent of heterosexual men and 51.6 per cent of heterosexual women (Chō 1992). Most couples I observed were in their 50s or older and it may be the case that among younger generations the ideal of equality is more widespread. At the same time, however, I found that gay and lesbian people who are not related to Occur have less set ideas about how a relationship should be and are more open to experimenting with a variety of role patterns, lifestyles and relationships, unbound by preconceived ideas about equality and the like.

## Promiscuous Gay Men

The men discussed in this section are different from those in the section above not because they are necessarily more promiscuous but because they do not desire a one-to-one relationship. They prefer the idea of promiscuity. Among gay men the ideal of *ippu ippu sei* is strong. In its usual written form with the characters meaning one-man–one-woman-system, *ippu ippu sei* refers to heterosexual monogamy. It can, however, also be written with characters meaning one-woman–one-woman-system or one-man–one-man-system, while the pronunciation remains the same. In these written forms the meaning is homosexual monogamy. Although monogamy is not the correct term here because it does not concern marriage, *ippu ippu sei* is widely understood by gay men and lesbian women to refer to exclusive relationships. As noted in chapter three (p. 96), even the word *kekkon* may be used and understood to refer to same-sex relationships. The ideal of *ippu ippu sei* is supported by publications on the prevention of AIDS by the authorities who have stopped presenting gay men as a risk category but have continued to point at other categories as being likely to carry HIV, such as foreigners, prostitutes and people who have sex with many or, more precisely, an indefinite number (*futokutei tasū*) of people rather than in a steady (*tokutei no*) relationship. The authorities appear not to be able to understand what is wrong with this, even when told (Hirano 1992).

AIDS information in the gay magazine *Adon* also stressed that one should be careful when having sex with someone other than a steady partner, thereby closely following Japanese bureaucracy. What a steady partner is, however, is not determined, giving rise to the problem of people having a different 'steady' partner every three months and using it as an excuse to engage in unsafe sexual behaviour. Moreover, no attention whatsoever is paid to the problem that a steady partner might also be having sex with others or to what those who do not want to limit their sex life to one partner must do. Even in 1996, safe sex according to the information provided in gay magazine *Adon* is limited to using a condom or no insertion of the penis in anus or mouth, without discrimination: 'Sex with many people without a condom is dangerous!! Let's stop that!!!' Thus, *Adon* fails to inform people about the low risk of oral sex or mutual masturbation and, by pointing a finger at those who have sex with many partners, supports the idea that one needs to have unsafe sex with more than one partner before being at risk. The radical gay magazine *Za Gei* does not fail to provide correct information every now and then (e.g. Aide Suisse. 1992) but its readership is much more limited. The other magazines tend to offer information about AIDS sporadically.

Sapporo's gay group, Sapporo Miitingu (Meeting), published a discussion about the stress on 'steady' lovers in relation to AIDS prevention and came to question the idea that sex within the *ippu ippu sei* is safe as a dangerous idea and to propose that there is no reason not to engage in multiple sexual contacts as long as one has safe sex (Mino 1992). Indeed, many informants, like one of the married men discussed in the previous chapter, thought that if they really love someone, risking AIDS does not matter, which is obviously a very dangerous stance when people 'really love' another person every couple of months. That HIV spreads comparatively slowly within gay circles in Japan is most likely due to two factors: many gay men do not or very rarely have sex with other men, i.e. have sex mostly or exclusively with themselves, and sexual practices among gay men tend to be limited to mutual masturbation and oral sex rather than anal sex (Takamizawa 1979, Itō, S. 1993: 132–5, Saitō and Fushimi 1993: 155–61).

Another problem related to gay men wanting to have more than one lover or multiple sexual contacts is the disapproval it may meet with in many gay circles. In a bar in Tokyo the *masutā* (bartender) was discussing a man who had not visited the bar for some time. The reason for this was that his lover was temporarily abroad and that the man did not feel like going to gay bars alone because that would entail the risk of being courted or becoming fascinated by another man. This stance was highly valued, while the *masutā* checked how I reacted, knowing that I had more than one relationship simultaneously. Some people criticize Japanese gay men for being squeamish about sex, like Pasukaru Nishi (e.g. 1992) who poses as a child of Japanese and French parentage and in his pornographic writing of fantasized experiences in France often criticizes Japanese for being boring and not given to lust.

Ozaki (1993) and Ogura (1993) describe the situation in gay saunas, where men have casual sex possibly with more than one man. Ozaki suggests that it might be a good place to work on spreading knowledge about safe sex and thereby to make gay saunas safer places than most. Ogura describes a night in the sauna and stresses the need for manners, i.e. the need for safe sex. An informant said that he does not feel capable of having a sexual relationship with one man for an extended period because his lust for men is very much related to the thrill of the unknown, a phenomenon that has been described by many European novelists (e.g. Busi 1989, 1990, 1993, Genet 1977, 1978, Hollinghurst 1989, Warren 1986a, b, 1987) as well as gay thinkers (e.g. Hocquenghem 1978). Here it concerns sexual contacts instead of relationships, although relationships might result from these contacts.

Onitsuka Tetsurō advocates *rankōgata*, which originally was a derogatory term for promiscuity but is nowadays also used in a positive manner by more radical gay men and others, following the reasoning of Douglas Crimp (Tazaki 1993b: 58–60). The ideal is to always be available for new encounters that may develop into relationships (Onitsuka 1993). Onitsuka's position seems to be gaining currency in Japan, where an increasing number of gay informants expressed a wish and, indeed, on later encounters appeared to experiment with more partners and a wider variety of sexual activities. Fushimi Noriaki was among the interviewees who expressed this wish but he, at the time of the interview, had promised his boyfriend that he would not engage in any other relationship or have sex with anyone else and therefore he could not follow his desires. This promise resulted partly from anxiety relating to AIDS. Onitsuka, on the other hand, developed his ideas about *rankōgata* as a result of activities related to the AIDS prevention law proposal, which appeared to be mainly directed at harassing prostitutes.

Ōhama Hōei, the man responsible for the law proposal, aligns himself in his explanation of it explicitly with the National Front of France and the Christian Social Union of Bavaria, while unremittingly discussing the problem of the prostitute who continues working while being HIV-positive and ignoring the men who are HIV-positive and continue to go to prostitutes and demand unsafe sex (Ōhama 1988: e.g. 106–28). This reasoning cried out for reactions and served to bring together many people who were concerned with sexuality and gender-related themes, including women's liberationists, lesbian women and gay men (Lunsing 1994b, 1999b). Condemning people who became HIV-positive through sexual contacts as immoral is a practice some scholars and others persistently engage in (e.g. Iwai 1993, Matsuoka 1993).

Onitsuka's propagation of *rankōgata* may be a powerful method of making people understand that it is not so much with whom you have sex but what form of sex you have and how you protect yourself that makes the difference between being highly at risk of becoming HIV-positive or not. His propagation of *rankōgata* does not mean, however, that he is actually having sex with many different people. It means that he is in principle open to having sex with whomever he might meet. The late Furuhashi Teiji, on the other hand, said in Dumb Type's performance *S/N* that he had sex, of course safe, with at least a hundred men, since he tested HIV-positive. He also stressed that he became HIV-positive because his thinking about love was outdated. He became infected by having unprotected sex with lovers he loved very much. His case underscores the idea that limiting sexual activity to partners one loves very much, which is the basis of those advocating sex only with steady partners, does little to prevent AIDS. Furuhashi stressed that love nowadays requires that one thinks about protecting oneself and those one loves.

## Female Same-Sex Relationships

Compared to gay interviewees, many of my lesbian interviewees lived together with a woman and in a number of cases they even, usually unexpectedly, turned up together for the interview. It appeared that lesbian women are generally more successful in maintaining long-term relationships than gay men. A number of reasons for this can be pointed out, internal as well as external. There appears to be less general awareness of the existence of lesbian sex, so that lesbian women are relatively untouched by social condemnation of their relationships. More important is that among lesbian women there is less focus on one ideology or other of how a relationship should be, and more awareness that a relationship is something that needs time and effort to develop. There is more time and attention given to the feelings of partners which are accepted as they are rather than only accepted when they are agreed with, which suggests that women are socialized to employ more *omoiyari* (empathy).

Even in the survey conducted among members of Occur this is visible. Among lesbian women only 3 out of 31 do not want to share household chores evenly but prefer to have their partner do most. Further, the percentage of lesbian women who want to live together is considerably smaller than that of Occur's gay men (Chō 1992). This might suggest that they are more aware of the implications of any decision on these matters and therefore have more realistic ideas about the choices they make. Of a survey among 234 lesbian women a mere 14.9 per cent live with lovers and 35.1 per cent live alone. The rest live with their parents or are married. At the same time, however, about 50 per cent have a steady partner (Hirosawa and Rezubian Ripōto Han 1991), which is a percentage that is not nearly matched by any survey on gay men.

Two lesbian interviewees in whose home I stayed were obviously quite egalitarian in relation to the division of all tasks. They both cooked and both sat with the guests when they felt like a break from cooking. This couple also performed sadomasochistic lesbian shows in which one was usually the masochist but not always: the roles could change halfway through the performance. When I interviewed them together, it was the one who mostly played the underdog on stage who was initially most responsive and talkative, but gradually the other started talking more and eventually almost took over totally. A couple of lesbian interviewees who work as carpenters also turned up together at a station in a Tokyo suburb. During the interview the same thing occurred. The one who started answering most left more space for the other to speak later on. In both cases mentioned here, the interviewees did not only live together but also worked together. While the first couple would have nothing to do with feminism, the second saw themselves as feminist more than as lesbian women.

Sharing household chores equally does not mean that both do everything equally. An interviewee said that her lover usually returns from her job earlier than herself and that it thus is purely logical that her lover makes dinner, something they both dislike doing. My interviewee, however, as a rule clears the table and washes up afterwards. In this case there is a major difference in income, for which reason the richer one pays about two-thirds of the rent. If she did not do this, her lover would not be able to live with her. Thus, social and financial facts may influence relationships and the scope of equality that is feasible.

Among the lesbian women I spoke with it was not common to adhere to the *ippu ippu sei* ideologically. Although informants in relationships were in practice often quite true to each other, in general it was agreed that if one or the other were to fall in love with another woman this was to be respected:

> The mutual idea is: please, if you like, go ahead. If you meet someone else you like, please feel free to go with her. But at the moment I don't have the time to start loving someone. I don't know why but I just don't have such a desire at all. (31-year-old interviewee)

This may be related to the fact that for many lesbian couples companionship is more important than a sexual relationship. As some interviewees said, they had been living together for such a long time now, that they did not see the other as a lover and were uncertain what to call their partners and how to define their relationships.

One couple was interviewed separately, while they knew I was interviewing both. In this case I was surprised to find that their ideas agreed to a great extent. Neither saw their present relationship as the one they would pursue for the rest of their lives and they were quite open to meeting new lovers but enjoyed what they had while it lasted. When I met one of them two years later, it transpired that the other had engaged in a relationship with another woman and that they had had a triangular relationship for some time. This, however, became the focus of much gossip in lesbian circles in Osaka, which complicated matters because it affected relationships with their friends. In the end, her girlfriend moved out to live with her new lover.

One lesbian couple, however, was in company characterized by a close bond of silence. They would not talk about their relationship, which seemed to be greatly dominated by the partner who did all the talking. This was the focus of some gossip but it did not influence their lives much because they were exclusively oriented towards each other and as a result they were almost fully emotionally independent of what other people might think or say. Others seemed to be perceived as dangers to their relationship and there was much jealousy if one even spoke with another woman for longer than a few minutes. Similarly, another interviewee thought that her lover had difficulty with her activities. She managed a place for lesbian women to come and have tea and to play music and show art. According to her, her lover was very anxious about her meeting many other women she might be charmed by. When I interviewed her lover, however, she did not agree that she felt any such threat whatsoever.

In the case of lesbian couples with children, it appeared that the major problem consisted in the relationship of the woman who was not the natural mother with the child and the way the child might perceive the relationship of her mother to her lover. Mostly the mother's lover would not play the role of mother but rather switched between the roles of an older sister to the child and a lover to the mother. In one case the mother's lover and the child had a very difficult relationship with many fights. When the mother was away on business travels for a fortnight, however, they managed to cooperate with each other very harmoniously. Upon her return, though, the child had an enormous fight with her mother, which my interviewee, the mother's lover, interpreted as the child releasing the stress that had built up during her mother's absence. This was the same explanation as the mother herself had provided in an earlier interview. My interviewee did not herself like children in particular but because she loved the mother she had to find a way of becoming friends with the child.

Lesbian relationships may come to an end for similar reasons as male gay relationships and heterosexual relationships outside marriage, for instance because one of the partners marries or moves. Other relationships usually end when one of the partners finds another lover, when the passion has gone, or as a result of the jealousy of a partner who has many other friends and interests. Nonetheless, in the latter cases women may stay together for the sake of the companionship they have achieved and the lifestyle they may have become used to.

Not all women who live together are sexually attracted to each other. Some heterosexual women also prefer the company of women to that of men. In *feminisuto* circles, i.e. among more academic feminists, they are often referred to as *sōsharu rezubian,* social lesbians. The most well-known example of this is that of Komashaku Kimi, retired professor of Hōsei University and Konishi Aya, anarchist. Their age difference has led to some criticism, Konishi could be Komashaku's mother. This example, that has been described elsewhere (e.g. Ueno 1988a: 81–3), has given many other women ideas. I found many heterosexual women who thought it desirable to spend their old age together with a close female friend, among them many who were married. Opposed to this, writer Matsuo Hisako, who had many contacts with women of the all-women Takarazuka Revue, said that some Takarazuka women have intimate friendships while working with the revue but once they retire from it often marry and become heterosexual housewives.

## Promiscuous Women

Among lesbian women I found some examples of much openness as to what lifestyles could be feasible. Contrary to gay men who think that they can become heterosexual upon marriage, they see no problem with having heterosexual relationships while remaining lesbian. Even though they may not like men as a category, they are sure that there are men they can love. A 26-year-old woman, who defines herself as lesbian, definitely does not want to marry legally but believes it to be possible that she might live together with a man (*dōsei suru*), something she had experienced before:

> When I was at high school I had a girlfriend and we became close but after we graduated we became separated and it ended. At that time I met a boy I liked a lot. With him everything was also totally platonic. Until then I didn't know much about boys. There weren't many men nearby and I never had male friends. But thanks to him, I came to understand that I don't dislike all men.

> Among us [lesbian women] there are those who hate men and among such [gay] men there are also those who hate women. But I don't have that because of this [experience]. I had it a bit before though.

With this man she had no sexual relationship and he knew that she was attracted to women and accepted that. Together they would discuss the beautiful women they saw around them when they were in town. Although she is adamant that she is lesbian, this in her viewpoint does not exclude the possibility of loving a man, although the chances that she will are small because her eyes only search for women and the fact that she has experienced a close relationship with a man makes her all the more certain that she prefers women.

A 28-year-old woman also had a male lover before she had female ones and while she at the time of the interview clearly identified herself as lesbian, on later occasions she was less decided. Later again, after she appeared as a lesbian woman on stage in a performance and found a steady lover, she was very definite about being lesbian. When I met her at the European Lesbian and Gay Pride Parade in Amsterdam in June 1994 she was joking about her being a *rezubian no obasan* (lesbian aunt). As her attention is drawn towards women wherever she goes, she had now decided that she was lesbian. Another lesbian interviewee even said that she had a short affair with a man while she was having a steady relationship of eight years with a girlfriend. When he started to talk of marriage, however, she quickly brought an end to it.

Another woman who now was in a long-term relationship with a woman, had previously had several relationships with men. While her lover had always seen herself as lesbian and had had previous relationships with women, she had never considered the possibility of loving women until her present lover courted her. She did not define herself as lesbian and thought it very possible that she might have a male lover sometime later, although her experience had taught that it was much easier to remain true to herself in a relationship with a woman. The woman she has a relationship with pays attention to her as a person, unlike the men who tended to see her rather as a woman, which operated to push her into a feminine role, more precisely, that of the housewife. She strongly objected to labelling people in general and thought that it would be best to take everyone as a person one must get to know before making any judgements about her or his qualities. Both she and her partner agreed that it might be interesting if one or the other would find a female lover they then both could share, trusting that the other would choose someone likeable.

The *tada no sukebe*, introduced in the previous chapter (pp. 149–50), had more than one relationship at the same time. One of them was with a woman she saw as very strange because she was trying with all her might to be like a man or, indeed, to be a man. She liked to enjoy her sex life in whichever way it developed and thought that she must always be open for new encounters and experiments. This was a view shared by a female Buddhist priest, who lately had come to present herself as bisexual because at a *gasshuku* (overnight group trip) of a women's network she learned that she could also love women. People in this context are not divided into men or women but into people one is attracted to and people one is not attracted to and both can be found among men as well as women. In general women adhere to this idea more than men. As a survey among university students by a Yajima seminar class shows, the percentage of women who are eager to try sex with the same sex is about double that of men (Oshima 1994). Some lesbian women, however, said that they have become tired of women who are interested in having sex with a woman but do not decide that they are lesbian. Calling themselves *rezubian separetisuto* (lesbian separatist), they want to organize weekends exclusively for women who label themselves as lesbian.

In a similar way, a woman who saw herself mainly as heterosexual did not like to have relationships with men. She liked to have sex with them and use their bodies in that way but did not want to listen to anything they might have to say because experience taught her that this was usually very boring. She found it preferable if they had left before she woke up in the morning, so that she did not need to have breakfast with them or make them leave. She also had a sexual relationship with a woman which lasted for a while but in the end was not satisfactory. While she did enjoy having sex with her, she kept feeling lust after men. Feelings like hers have lately been described by two female Japanese writers, who are quite popular among young lesbian and feminist women (Saitō 1991, 1993, Matsuura 1987) and whose work is comparable to that of Pat Califia (1988). Written from the standpoint of women, they contain a high dose of explicit sexual description and sadomasochism, whereby women and men each play both roles. The interviewee mentioned above said that she was fond of Matsuura's work and that she also liked soft sadomasochism, and, indeed, I discovered handcuffs when I was staying in her apartment. Nonetheless, shortly before embarking on a voyage around the world she fell in love with a man, which made her postpone her travel plans for several months because she wanted to enjoy his company just a little bit longer.

A feminist woman, who does not like to use the label of *feminisuto* for herself but otherwise fits rather well into the general perception of *feminisuto* as academics involved in women's studies, found a singular solution to organize her love and sex life. She has more than one male lover at the same time and sees the lover she wants to see when she feels like it. While one is good for intellectual discussion, another is better for sex and a third good to have fun with out drinking. As she has many aspects of herself to all of which in her opinion no man can answer adequately, she needs more than one man. She explained the organization of her feelings by referring to a painting by Dali, that of the woman with drawers in her body. For each of her lovers she has a separate drawer and whenever she is with one she opens the appropriate drawer and lets out the attitude that fits with this lover. This orderly way of organizing her love life also prevents her from becoming obsessed with one man and when all her lovers are locked up in their drawers, she still has other drawers to open up other parts of her life, such as her profession, on which she does not want her love life to have any influence, a position that is typical of many *feminisuto*.

## Alternative Female–Male Relationships

The woman described above would also fit into this section but because the position of the men in her story was almost not discussed and, because she claims to make her own choices independent of what her lovers may think, I decided to place her in the section of promiscuous women. In the discussion where she explained her lifestyle, another woman, who saw herself as a *feminisuto* and is generally recognized as such, spoke of her difficulties in maintaining a love relationship with a man. She had been married before and also had children but, since she could not keep herself from focusing her whole life on him and expecting him to comply with her desire to find everything she sought in lovers in one man, this relationship became insupportable. It neither agreed with her feminist ideas nor with her life as an academic. Moreover, her husband was incapable of being the perfect man she desired. They broke up and later relationships followed the same pattern.

This continued until, she reported, she found a solution in a relationship with a foreign man who lives overseas. The simple fact of a limitation to the possibilities of seeing him prevents her from seeking everything in him she sought in lovers who lived in Japan. She can still be romantic but reality makes total indulgence impossible. To this she added that she believed foreign men to be easier to deal with than a Japanese '*ossan*' (short for *ojisan*: literally uncle but also middle-aged man or man from about ten years older than oneself), a word that is increasingly used to typecast Japanese men of middle age and older, who are thus presented as rude, boring, self-centred creatures outside the league of people one wants to deal with.

A male interviewee who lived in a Tokyo suburb had an open relationship with a woman who was also the mother of their daughter. They did not live together but had a steady long-term involvement. He had been greatly influenced by the ideal presentation of the open relationship between Sartre and de Beauvoir and he claimed that he and the mother of his daughter had other relationships and that this progressed on an equal and unproblematic basis. Living apart was not only in agreement with ideological ideas but also practical because their lifestyles differed greatly. While his lover had a day-time job, he worked as a writer, often long into the night. During her younger years the care of the daughter fell mainly to the mother but once she started to attend school she would often go to her father's house, where she could be welcomed easily because it coincided with the time of day he usually did not work much. In the evening she would then go to her mother's where she spent the night and was woken up and provided with a lunch box before going to school again. After the mother died the father moved to live partially with his daughter while keeping his working place separated. Lunch boxes are now prepared by a friendly neigbour.[2]

The ideal of free love that was the base of this man's lifestyle was not entirely new to the Japan of the 1960s. Itō Noe, anarcho-feminist of the 1910s also believed in it, as did her main lover, anarchist Ōsugi Sakae. They, however, were not wholly successful in accomplishing this lifestyle. Ōsugi's legal wife probably felt some objection – she wrote that she was not a *nyū ūman* (new woman), unlike Itō (Hori 1913, Sievers 1983: 177) – but she could not stop them. When their relationship started, Kamichika Ichiko, a feminist friend of Itō and an ex-lover of Ōsugi became very jealous. These feelings drove her to stage an incident in which she slit Ōsugi's throat, almost killing him. After this, Kamichika was arrested for attempted murder and the relationship between Itō and Ōsugi appears to have continued (Arahata 1978, Itō 1978a, b, Ōsugi 1978a, b) until they were arrested and strangled in a police cell on the occasion of the Kantō earthquake which destroyed Tokyo in 1923 (Sievers 1983: -186).

Male interviewees who believed in free sex found it hard to find women who agree with their ideas. One eventually settled in a *jijitsukon* relationship and the other in practice spends most of his time without a lover. While he sees himself as emancipated, he thinks it is difficult to find women who want a relationship on the basis of total freedom for each. He calls his problems, in an article he wrote, the Nausicaa complex (*Nausika konpurekkusu*), a name he derived from a popular Japanese comics heroine who is a strong and independent woman. According to his theory, progressive men who want a relationship with a woman who is their equal cannot find such women because many of the strong, independent and politically active women, who are not all that common, do not want a relationship at all (Shida 1992).

In Kyoto I participated in a circle where sexual freedom was a much-discussed subject. This was, however, not always directly related to discussing one's own sex life. At a New Year's party, a woman told me that she wanted very much to know about the contents and importance of the relationships her boyfriend had with other women. When we asked him to tell us about them, he did not answer but became silent. When we asked again he moved over to the other side of the room. Likewise, another woman whose boyfriend had another female lover found it impossible to cope with the fact that he acted towards her as if he was not seeing anyone else, while everybody knew that he was. As he refused to discuss it with her, she finally ended their relationship on the occasion of her moving house to another city.

## Tsutamori Tatsuru: Relations Denying Gender Boundaries

Tsutamori Tatsuru used to be a freelance writer specializing in motorcycles and the world of motorcycling in Japan. Pictures of him through time show a total image change, from a motorcyclist with an unkempt beard, to a beautiful woman (*Popeye* 1993). He said that he went through much turmoil, trying to deny his male sex, before he finally ended up accepting himself the way he became, i.e. a highly androgynous individual whose sex organ happens to have the shape of a penis. These developments were accompanied by changes of profession. He worked as a female seamstress, a help in the kitchen of a dance hall, a nude model, a bar hostess and took upon himself the role of housewife. His changes and the accompanying development of his ideas are described in three books and some articles he published during these changes (Tsutamori 1990b, 1992, 1993).

When I interviewed him, he was living with a woman and taking most of the housekeeping upon himself. He was acting the role of a housewife who did some writing on the side. He told me his history, about which he was just writing a book that appeared later (Tsutamori 1993). When he started to use make up and wear women's clothes, the relationship he was engaged in with a woman had gradually deteriorated and they separated, which set him off on a period of several years of moving from place to place and job to job, while he was trying to discover how he could deal with gender ascriptions that no longer made sense to him. He contacted Watanabe Tsuneo, who wrote a book which discusses the increasing difficulty of being male and various problems concerning men who feel that the male role has become insupportable (Watanabe 1989).

Tsutamori had come to hate his own physique, especially his penis, because the discussion of penises among *feminisuto* had increasingly given him the idea that he had better have it cut off (Hashimoto and Tsutamori 1990). As he saw his penis as repulsive, Tsutamori was not able to have sex with a woman until his new lover referred to his penis as a clitoris and said she liked it, which made Tsutamori see that one's physique does not really matter all that much. Instead, one's feelings and emotions are the core of a relationship and if those feelings are not sexist and discriminatory against women, a penis does not need to stand in the way of achieving mutual sexual satisfaction (Tsutamori 1993). Likewise, a lesbian couple, of whom my interviewee was halfway through a sex-change operation and still had a penis, also found a way to enjoy sex together. And when Hashimoto Osamu suggests that he might refer to himself as lesbian (1992a), he does not mean that he has a female physique but that his feelings may be similar to those of lesbian women.

During the interview Tsutamori said that he had experienced sex with men but that, in general, he preferred women because their bodies are softer, just like the 'bisexual' woman discussed in the previous chapter (p. 145). He thought that he should always be open towards new relationships and not be afraid to hurt other people. By trying to avoid hurting other people one would most likely end up creating an undesirable situation for all people concerned. If one avoids engaging in a relationship in order to avoid hurting someone else one is already involved with, this will inevitably increase the demands placed on that relationship because its costs have risen. A final result is likely to be that the relationship becomes insupportable. Tsutamori teaches that one should always be honest towards oneself and others and recognize one's feelings and act upon them, without fear of hurting oneself or others. The expression of fear of hurting or pain he dismisses as a way of excusing oneself for not following one's intuition, and that he calls 'stupid (*bakabakashii*)'. Likewise, Hashimoto discusses the contradiction between the recent value attached to 'true love' and the persisting condemnation of love affairs when one already has a relationship, which, in the case of being married, is called *furin* (immoral, unethical). If love is a good thing, how can it be bad at the same time, he wonders (1992b: 86–90).

Among transvestite men I found that many seek sexual relationships with women or, alternatively, with other transvestite men. They have a dislike of non-transvestite men and masculinity. Others, on the other hand, may feel attracted to masculine and macho men, to which they oppose their own femininity. One case of a man, using the female name Shimada Toshiko, who used hormones to grow breasts and who dresses and makes up to look perfectly feminine, has become particularly well-known because he was interviewed by Fushimi Noriaki for his book *Kuia Paradaisu* (Queer paradise; Fushimi 1996: 37–52). In this interview he says that he likes his penis very much and tells about his relationship with a man who may look more masculine than himself but has a much more feminine character. In the same book one finds a number of people, including gay men and lesbian women, transvestites, transsexuals, and a hermaphrodite with relationships in which gender boundaries have effectively become void because those concerned have crossed them and there appears to exist no relation whatsoever between their acquired gender attributes and what gender attributes they seek in their partners.

## Conclusion

Among my informants, lesbian women tended to live in couples much more than gay men, although they often do not adhere to the *ippu ippu sei*. This indicates that men, no matter whether they are gay or heterosexual, are generally less critical of the marital system than women and adhere more to the ideal of exclusivity in love relationships. Heterosexual feminists are more in favour of the *ippu ippu sei* than lesbian women, which suggests that lesbian women have a more liberal attitude towards developing alternative lifestyles. Ways of thinking about *ippu ippu sei* do not appear to have much influence on what lifestyles people actually have. Lesbian women who have decided to pursue a lesbian lifestyle have longer-lasting relationships than gay men.

Heterosexual singles tend either not to have love relationships or to have shorter, less compelling ones, although there are exceptions. Particularly among the younger generations of women one can find relatively many with a free attitude towards sexuality, love and living patterns, and a readiness or even eagerness to experiment. This is more true for women who label themselves as lesbian than those who do not label themselves but they exist in both cases. Among men, such examples can be found but they are much rarer. Men are, overall, less successful at achieving their ideals and have less inclination to discover personal alternatives and to experiment. Their ideas about relationships tend to be more in agreement with general *jōshiki*. Nevertheless, a wide variety of lifestyles is viable and exists in Japan.

## Notes

1 Ōkubo Sawako, who is one of the founders of Dokushin Fujin Renmei, when I interviewed her, mentioned a figure of 2.5 million, which is the approximate number of soldiers who were killed in the battlefields. Fujiwara (1972: 285–6) and Yoshihiro (1987: 140) mention about 3 million war victims in total and Ienaga (1982: 233) mentions 658,595 civil victims. While Tani (1982: 27) mentions 600,000 women as the figure concerned, statistics show that in this age group there were about 247,000 unmarried women in 1990, which is 3.7 per cent. While this is higher than in the age cohorts before and directly after theirs, among women who are twenty years younger the percentage of unmarried women is already higher (Keizai Kikakuchō ed 1992: 409). The surplus of 200,000 men before the war had changed into a shortage of 1.5

million after, while the population grew by 14 million (Sōmuchō Tōkeikyoku ed 1992: 8–9).

2 Lunch boxes became a topic at a seminar class with Ueno Chizuko in which Kasuga Kisuyo's book on single fathers was discussed (Kasuga 1989). An episode in this book concerns the sad story about children whose fathers could not make perfect-looking lunch boxes. This I found rather ridiculous and so did a Chinese participant of the seminar. The Japanese women participating in the seminar, however, were moved to tears by the episode, including Ueno. Ueno's conclusion was that Kasuga apparently had touched a tender spot in the emotional realm of many Japanese women. That lunch boxes are important and not having a lunch box that looks as nice as that of other pupils may make one feel left out, is the point. The Chinese participant, who was male, and I thought that it was ridiculous that it was taken for granted that the fathers could not make a decent-looking lunch box.

# 6 Dealing with Society: Practical Problems, Passing and Coming Out

This chapter discusses strategies employed for coping with a social environment that often has little consideration for people whose lifestyles, feelings or ideologies are at variance with its norms. First, practical problems and strategies people may employ to cope with them are discussed. Housing and work are foremost examples of necessities and the distribution of these may be based on *jōshiki* concerning how one should live. Those whose lifestyle does not agree with *jōshiki* may take into account problems resulting from discrimination when making choices of where and how to live and what type of work to choose.

Strategies of dealing with surrounding people, such as family, friends, colleagues and classmates, vary from trying to keep people ignorant about one's lifestyle to explicitly informing people. While, for instance, remaining single is not doing something, rather than positively doing something, many single people feel that this not doing something demands a lot of their energy. Most people employ several strategies simultaneously, depending on specific situations and relationships. First, 'passing' in combination with 'compartmentalization', a strategy in which particular parts of one's life are kept completely separated from other parts (Goode 1960), is concentrated on. This strategy may agree very well with general patterns of conduct in Japan in which roles particular to contexts may be valued more than intrinsic and independent identities (Valentine 1990, Hendry 1992c, Bachnik 1994). Thereafter, the problematics and implications of coming out and being revealed (Davies 1992) are focused on.

## Solving Practical Problems

### Housing

A problem is posed by difficulties in finding a place to live. Public housing is, according to the Public Housing Law (*Kōei Jūtaku Hō*), only available for people who are related legally, i.e. by marriage, by adoption or by birth, and for women over 50 years of age and men over 60 years of age, or handicapped people. The age difference between women and men is the result of political activities by Dokushin Fujin Renmei, a leading figure of which, Ōkubo Sawako, fought for recognition of the plight of women who remained single as the result of the Second World War and had difficulty finding affordable housing. At the housing department in Kyoto's city hall a civil servant explained that I definitely would not be allowed to live in public housing because I was single and neither handicapped nor over 60 years old. A reason he 'forgot' to mention is that I was non-Japanese. As the case of the Korean Pe *san* (see chapter three, p. 118, note 11) shows, access to public housing is more limited to foreigners than to Japanese. I found single people under 50 without a handicap living in public housing in Kyoto, Osaka and Tokyo. A 28-year-old Japanese woman was living by herself in a public housing apartment in Kyoto. In Tokyo I found a similar case of a 34-year-old man.

Both apartments were rather old and small, with one room and a kitchen, which makes them hardly acceptable in terms of present-day housing standards for families. Moreover, 'old' in the context of Japanese housing is usually perceived as synonymous with dirty (*kitanai*), which makes these places undesirable in the eyes of people who care about status more than money. Therefore older and smaller apartments are likely to become increasingly available to single people and by implication also to same-sex couples because there is nothing to keep a partner from moving in. A man who lived alone in a *danchi* in Osaka stayed there after his wife demanded a divorce and moved out and a woman in a similar apartment had lied that she was going to live there with her sister, who lived with a boyfriend elsewhere but agreed to live there legally so that her sister could obtain a *danchi* apartment. Once a couple move into a *danchi* they do not need to stay together. If one leaves the other can as a rule stay on.

As a case in chapter three (p. 111) suggested, private housing can only be rented at the whim of landlords or ladies who often do not want two men living together in their apartments and may become quite annoying if the second one moves in with the one who rented the apartment alone originally. Even giving birth to a baby may be a reason for eviction because landlords or ladies may think that children will damage the house and cause trouble (*meiwaku o kakeru*) to other tenants because of the noise they make. In the case of single women having a baby, the landlord or lady may also decide that her moral standards are such that he or she cannot let the woman stay (Onodera 1982). Many contracts explicitly state that children may not be born and pets may not be kept.

While in the case of young students landlords or ladies have less objection to two men living together, once they are past student age, which in general is believed to end at about 22 years old, landlords or ladies are likely to refuse male couples. For female couples this problem is not so great because it is widely accepted that women often do not have an income that allows them to live on their own. Sharing with a friend is seen as a logical way for women to save money. Neighbours might, in the case of two men sharing a house, start to gossip, whereas in the case of two women this is less likely. Lesbian women benefit in this respect from the fact that the existence of female homosexuality is much less known than that of male homosexuality. One lesbian couple living together even thought that the neighbours believed that the one who looked less feminine, because she was taller and her hair shorter, was a man.

Nonetheless, there is a well-known case of two women who live together (see chapter five, p. 195) that is being criticized. In this case the ages of the women differ by twenty years and therefore, as a friend of them said, their cohabitation is considered by some to be 'unnatural (*fushizen*)' or 'distasteful (*iyarashii*)'. The apartment is owned by the two women, who may set a new trend because many women would like to share housing with other women in old age (Ueno 1988a: 81–3). In cases where finances are available, same-sex couples, as well as singles, may buy an apartment and thereby eliminate a problem that otherwise would become progressively more difficult to overcome because landlords increasingly dislike renting their apartments and houses to elderly people. Indeed, among those who expect to remain single there appears to be a relatively large number of people who buy apartments, which they regard as a security for old age. As long as they can take care of themselves they have a place to live. If that becomes impossible, they can sell the apartment and use the money to pay for care. However, as a single female civil servant, who owns a two-room apartment, clarified, this is not always an easy decision:

> To tell the truth, I bought this *manshon* (apartment) with a mortgage of 35 years. When I have paid all that back I'll be 75.

> Because in Japan it's very expensive they can't sell unless they spread the mortgage over such long periods. (. . .) Halfway through I'll probably retire. And then I can probably pay off everything with the retirement bonus. Compared to other women, I definitely think that I'm privileged in the area of money.

## Work

The civil service is one of the career options in which women can be sure to receive a decent income which is not lower than that received by men. This interviewee even thought that she was better off than a man with wife and children doing the same job, for whom life was more difficult financially, and that she was better off than female friends who work for companies, where initial wages may be higher but pay rises for women lag behind and pressure to retire early may soon mount (Saso 1990: 37, 80). She feels that the mortgage binds her to her job. While during the interview she felt free to criticize sexism at her workplace and discrimination against singles, homosexual people and single mothers by the bureaucratic system because I promised her anonymity, she felt bound by the mortgage to remain silent about this in other contexts because criticizing the system might cause her to lose her job. Since civil servants are legally bound to refrain from political activities related to their work and may not criticize the system,[1] she felt that buying an apartment forced her to continue to apply regulations she thinks are wrong. For this reason Satō Bunmei resigned from his job at the population registration department of the ward office of Shinjuku in Tokyo when he found that it was impossible to criticize, let alone change, the system from within.

Those who choose positively to live outside marriage rather than just not finding a partner to marry, can live as they please, apart from economic constraints like having to have a job in order to earn a living. Income, however, does not have to be all that high, as was pointed out by many informants, if only one forsakes the idea of having to live up to standards many Japanese take for granted. If, for example, one waits to buy new brand named clothes until prices go down in the sales one can save enormous amounts of money and still have the same clothes. Further, not having children is a great economic asset because it saves many millions of yen one might otherwise feel compelled to spend on their education and such. Indeed, the financial burden is prominent among the reasons the Japanese give when asked why they believe the birth rate has declined lately, closely followed by a supposed shortage of child-minding facilities (Keizai Kikakuchō ed. 1993: 26).

It is also important to find the right job. If one does not wish to marry, it is better to avoid working for a conservative company. Some progressive companies for instance nowadays have gay men who came out as gay in their jobs, which does not appear to influence their position in any way. These companies interfere very little in the personal lives of their employees, who as a result enjoy much freedom. A man working for the international telephone company ITJ said that there were no problems related to being openly gay there and the same was said about Japan's largest cosmetics company, Shiseido, which could, though, be a feature of a local branch. Both men were, however, in their mid-20s which makes it unclear whether their marital status might hamper them in climbing the career ladder in future years.

In general being a *kōmuin*, a civil servant, gives more security in this respect because a *kōmuin* cannot be fired because of personal circumstances that do not relate to her or his working capacities, which in the case of companies does occur. Indeed, the civil service has been known for a long time to provide a good job opportunity for single women. Already in the first half of this century the civil service was known as an occupation where lesbian women were relatively concentrated (Robertson 1992). Teaching at universities is also a good option but such jobs may become more difficult to obtain in years to come, due to a decline in student numbers combined with the large number of graduates of the generation born in the 1960s.

Those working in creative professions, where the atmosphere may be very liberal on the one hand or very conservative on the other – consider for instance the artisan world of Kyoto (Haraven 1992) – were divided between being very free and easy-going and very troubled. Informants working in designing and kimono painting in Kyoto could be divided into those who made it an independent occupation and therefore were bound to *tsukiai* (personal relationships) with suppliers and buyers, which made them feel that they needed to comply with *jōshiki* to a great extent, and those who worked for others and had much more freedom in their choice of lifestyle. In the modern arts the atmosphere is generally very liberal but it is very difficult to make a living. Most painters and performance artists I met derived their main income from doing *arubaito* (underpaid, unstable jobs such as waitress and shop assistant).[2]

An option open to those who wish to live outside mainstream society is offered by the *fūzoku sangyō* (the pleasure industry) where one can work in positions from bartender and host or hostess to stripper or prostitute. All the people I asked who worked in gay bars claimed that their parents did not know about the nature of their jobs. They might have told their parents that they work in a bar, but not what sort of bar. Women and men working as hosts and hostesses, strippers and prostitutes alike, usually try to hide their occupation from family and often friends outside the industry (Kanematsu 1987, Kakinuma 1991, Louis 1992, Lunsing forthcoming). Some people may perceive working in the pleasure industry as their only way to make a living. Particularly in the case of transvestites and transsexuals it is difficult to find a mainstream occupation (Kuroyanagi 1992). There are bars where women work as men (*Cross Dressing* 1992) and where men work as women (Kuroyanagi 1992). Some gay and transvestite men made a show-business career out of it, such as the gay twins Osugi and Piiko (Sugiura and Sugiura 1992) and transvestite singer Miwa Akihiro (Yamaguchi 1985: 31–3, Miwa 1992). Karūseru (Carousel) Maki is a transsexual singer who changed her sex from male to female. Apart from the women with temporary intimate relationships, mentioned in chapter five (p. 196), there are also some women who continue a lesbian lifestyle after leaving the all-women musical theatre Takarazuka. Although in publications on Takarazuka any reference to sex and sexuality of the stars is avoided (Robertson 1992), people with inside knowledge confirmed this 'secret' that is more or less public knowledge in lesbian circles.

While most interviewees had not given much thought to discrimination problems when choosing a career, one gay man decided to take it into consideration. He was to have been employed by a major bank in his home town but at the last moment decided not to accept the job, for two reasons. He did not want to live too close to his family and the branch he was to have been employed at was in his home town. More important than that was that he thought it most likely that if he did not marry his career opportunities within the bank would be limited. Single men's careers end up in side-tracks in banks because they are not trusted to be mature enough to deal with large sums of money. Instead he chose to work as a civil servant for the metropolitan government of Tokyo, where being single is not much of an issue.

## Coping with *Seken*: Going Along with it or Ridiculing it

A major problem for the people discussed in the previous chapters is that many people think nothing of interfering in other people's private life, especially when it comes to marriage and finding spouses. Even if one shows clearly that one is not eager to marry, all sorts of people may come up with prospective spouses. A common method of coping with the demands of *seken* and family employed by those who do not wish to marry is to have proposed *omiai* but to turn down the candidates every time. While this may be time-consuming, it serves to satisfy parents, superiors or friends because one appears to be doing something about finding a marriage partner. A 31-year-old interviewee who works as a *sarariiman* had such a problem:

> In the end you can't refuse, if such talk comes from a superior. It's part of being *sarariiman*. (. . .) But I ended up behaving very impolitely towards the woman concerned. (. . .) I didn't want her to think that I might be interested and ended up creating a very unpleasant atmosphere. I knew what I was doing and I think it was very impolite to let myself go like that.

This man reproaches himself for behaving unpleasantly, not for not refusing to have *omiai* because that would have been impossible in his eyes. The cost of refusing to have *omiai* may be high: I found two cases of men who were dismissed because they refused to have the *omiai* their superiors proposed. Many people, however, find having *omiai* without any intention to marry an immoral activity. One interviewee only once had *omiai*, though he did not want to marry because he was gay and did not want to make a woman unhappy, which he saw as the inevitable outcome of such a match. He turned her down but as it turned out she was attracted to him, which made him feel guilty for having raised false hopes. After this episode he decided never to consent to having *omiai* again and made clear to his parents that he chose not to marry. A 30-year-old female interviewee had had many *omiai* and saw them as a chance to meet people in various walks of life, although she was not sure whether she wanted to marry at all. She did not rule out the possibility of meeting a man she would want to marry but she estimated the chances to be very low. Her mother, who arranged the *omiai*, usually chose quite interesting men for her to meet but she invariably deemed them not suitable for marriage. Two years after the interview she sent me a letter in which she expressed growing distress over the question of whether she should marry.

A heterosexual man, who wanted to marry if he could only meet the right person was still single at the age of 36. His parents showed him pictures of women so that he might have *omiai* but this he always refused because he thought that such 'feudal (*hōkenteki*) practices' were not of this time and he felt that marriage should be based on love and equality. When his parents kept proposing women and showing him pictures he clearly showed his anger about their persistence, after which, according to him, they thought it wiser not to bring up the subject again out of fear they might lose him altogether. A female interviewee in her 60s said that whenever her mother, who was widowed during the war, so much as brought up the subject of marriage, she would react by saying: 'Get married yourself (*jibun de kekkon shite*)', and thereby she managed to avoid marriage. Other people are more subtle but also keep refusing to have *omiai*, which is after all something they cannot be forced to have.

One of the major difficulties expressed by those who are not married is the fact that many people think nothing of asking for an explanation: 'Why aren't you married?' or: 'Why don't you want to marry?' The question of whether you are married is often a kind of greeting, rather than an expression of real concern. In this sense it often is a vital part of making initial contacts develop smoothly, which Hendry describes under the heading of the wrapping of language: it is not the actual content of what is said that matters but rather the intention to be congenial expressed by words that do not have much importance otherwise (Hendry 1993a: 64–5). People over 30 years old are usually expected to be married but are still asked. If one is married, the next question is whether there are any children. If one is not married, the next question, or rather insinuation, is that surely there must be a loved one with whom one expects to marry shortly and thus the ice is broken in many an uneasy introductory conversation.

If one gives all the 'wrong' answers, however, that is if one is single and has no prospect of marriage in the near future or if one is married for over a year but without children, this is likely to keep the ice intact or make it freeze even harder. People whose answers are 'wrong' may be shut out of the group in the same way that people are shut out of groups because they do not use the level of politeness or the vocabulary that binds groups (Hendry 1991). This is an example of discrimination in everyday life against unmarried and childless married people. The concept of discrimination in everyday life is derived from the concept of 'everyday racism' (Essed 1984), which fits the situation of singles and childless couples in Japan very well. It is a form of discrimination most people who transgress are not aware of. People who are subjected to it often come to accept it as a fact of life, until one day they may burst into a rage at one or other last straw, which in itself might not even be worth discussing. This happened to a gay interviewee who in a rage severed all contacts with his father when he started talking of marriage. Likewise, a lesbian interviewee thought that she would probably burst into a rage one day and say that she was lesbian if her parents would not leave her in peace. A member of Occur dubbed this form of discrimination 'gay harassment'.

A common strategy employed by almost all singles to cope with this form of discrimination is to avoid family gatherings. A man who dislikes being asked about his marriage prospects by his family avoids going home on occasions such as *shōgatsu* (New Year), when most Japanese families gather and celebrate, a common pattern among many interviewees. Others go on *shōgatsu* but that is the only occasion each year. Especially in the case of single women, the family may even prefer them not to come home at all. Tani (1982) provides some examples of this and an interviewee said that her family preferred her not to come home because she was *mura hachibu* (ostracized) and her family would rather avoid having other villagers reminded of her existence. She related this story with pride and was quite happy that she did not need to visit her parents. While for those who moved away family may be relatively easy to evade by not visiting them, other people in the daily social environment have also to be dealt with somehow. For many informants *uchi* (inside), be it the parental home or the workplace, is not a place where they can relax and show their real feelings, as it has so often been described (e.g. Lebra 1976, Hendry 1986a, b, Bachnik 1994, Kondo 1994).

A typical method of dealing with situations in which one is expected to comply with *jōshiki* concerning marriage was often described by informants by the word *gomakasu*, which means avoiding answering a question, ideally in such a sophisticated manner, that the questioner does not notice that one is evading the subject. It may also refer to an effort to avoid giving a direct reaction to criticism and divert the attention to a less dangerous area, ideally without clearly appearing to avoid giving an answer. This behaviour can be understood as a polite way of avoiding difficult situations and as such fits very well with the concepts of *tatemae* (public face) and *honne* (real feelings; e.g. Smith 1983, Moeran 1989). While ideally the other should not see through the evasion, people often do, but what is said should make clear that the subject had better be put to rest or *gomakasu* may even make it impossible to pursue the subject any further. *Gomakasu* is used to ensure that people's feelings are not upset by hearing things that do not correlate positively with their worldview. In this sense, it can also be understood as a warning not to continue the line of conversation.

Some Japanese are very sophisticated in *gomakasu* and those who are not are not likely to end up in a high position because *gomakasu* often is the only way to avoid awkward situations. Some informants would give the relative sophistication of people from the Kansai in this field as a reason why there are so many successful politicians from that area. Ueno (1988a) writes that in Kyoto people ask, after having been given a *honne* answer: 'What do you mean?' According to Ueno they cannot be satisfied with one answer, whether it is *tatemae* or *honne*, but need both to make up their minds as to what to think of it. Kyoto people, in contrast to Tokyo people, perceive as the real answer something that is not actually said but lies between *tatemae* and *honne*. Ueno's difference between Kyoto and Tokyo was not apparent among my informants but in the Kansai area as well as in Tokyo many informants originated from elsewhere. The two cases in which people changed their stories, were both people who lived in Tokyo.

The Japanese style of communication has been called affective and intuitive as opposed to the instrumental style in Western languages. The Japanese style of communication is said to be determined by *awase*, a style in which the speaker attempts to adjust himself to the feelings of his listeners (Gudykunst and Ting-Toomey 1988: 112–13, referring to Okabe). *Awaseru* (to go along), the verb of which *awase* is a stem, is another term informants used in describing their way of relating to problematic but significant others. Research comparing American and Japanese students has shown that Japanese students tend to be more reserved and formal towards others and to have 'a larger private self that is hidden or unknown' (Barnlund 1975: 50–2), which combines perfectly with the tendency to *awaseru*. It also combines perfectly with the idea that the use of polite language is not so much determined by verticality in relationships as it is by degrees of intimacy (Neustupny 1978: 200).

As many people think that people often tell lies (*usotsuku*), they may end up believing whatever their fantasy places in their heads rather than what someone says. The idea behind this is that anything anyone says may be a lie and for some people this even seems to go so far as to believe that everything anyone says must be lies because otherwise they would not have ventured to say them. This view implies that truths are preferably hidden at all times. In another light, it might also suggest that Japanese in general are relatively aware, although it may be unconsciously, of the shortcomings of language in representing reality.

A common, albeit somewhat clumsy, way of *gomakasu* is to repeat the question somewhat differently: '*Sā, dō deshō nā?* (Yeah, how would it be?)', which should make the questioner understand that the question is perceived as embarrassing. More adept examples given by interviewees as answers to the question why they were not married include: 'I'm still playing around (*asonde ru*), [I'll wait] a little longer until I am more adult' and: 'I haven't found the right one yet', both of which defer the problem to the future, and: 'The crown prince isn't married either, and I'm even younger', which redirects the attention to the crown prince who remained unmarried at the age of 33. He subsequently made this diversion impossible by marrying in 1993 but still offers implicit support to childless marriages, since he still has not fathered a child. A man who compared his family with the English royal family because almost every marriage ended in divorce, saw this situation as a gift from heaven. If his mother so much as hinted at marriage, he would point at the marriage record of his family and make clear that there seemed to be little point in marrying if, as evidence showed, the usual outcome in his family was divorce. He thereby avoided talking about himself and the reason why he did not want to marry: he was gay. In all these cases the people were quite decided that they would never marry if they could help it.

Others who are less adept at *gomakasu* end up being silent, something that happened once when I asked a gay man how he personally intended to deal with the problem called marriage, after we had been discussing the general situation for a while. He remained silent for over 10 minutes, until the situation had changed to the effect that someone else drew attention and a new subject came to be discussed. A similar method of avoiding unpleasant questions consists of walking away. Silence in Japan is a common method of expressing the unacceptability of a question (Morsbach 1973) but this is not always the case. In a group discussion with young gay men about coming out and marriage, one of the participants on being asked about his ideas reacted by saying that his head was spinning around from all the things the others had said and that he could not make sense of his feelings. Such a genuine disturbance of someone's mind should not be mistaken for *gomakasu*. If he had wanted to *gomakasu* something, it would most likely have been to hide his disturbance, the expression of which was very awkward.

Sometimes not giving a satisfactory answer may take a lot of stamina. In a crowded underground train a young man who stood right in front of me was recognized by a middle-aged woman, whom he addressed as *obasan* (aunt), a common term for younger people to use when addressing middle-aged women. She called him *niisan*, literally older brother, but commonly used to address young men. She asked him where he was going. When he said that he was going to meet a friend from Kyushu who was coming to stay with him in Osaka, her mind was made up to the effect that this friend was a lover. While he kept denying this and saying that they were *tada no tomodachi* (just friends), she kept insisting that they must be lovers all through the underground ride, which lasted for about 15 minutes, while he kept twisting and bending, trying to convince her that they were 'just friends'. Unfortunately, I could not make out whether this friend was female or male.

A gay interviewee said that he would *tekitō ni awaseru*, go along as fits the situation. When talk of women came up among his friends he also made remarks such as that he fancied one or the other and when the subject of marriage came up he said things such as that it was not his time yet or that he had not met the right one yet. He also made jokes in order to *gomakasu* any conversation that had anything to do with homosexuality among his friends in order to change the subject of discussion to another because:

> I don't want to talk about such things. I'm afraid to see everybody's reactions. On the other hand I'm also interested but I'm afraid [to know how they feel]. Although I sometimes think that I should have more confidence in them.

He avoids talking about homosexuality in general with the friends he shares his life with because it makes him feel uneasy. Due to the so-called *gei būmu* (gay boom), a boom of articles and television programmes about male homosexuality that started in 1991 with an article in the women's magazine *Crea*, talk about homosexuality has become less uncommon in Japan (Lunsing 1997), but many closeted gay men do not necessarily see this as a positive development. This interviewee also said that he felt 'pain in his heart (*kokorogurushii*)' about lying (*usotsuku*) to his parents when he went to participate in the activities of a gay circle. He would say that he was going to visit an old friend from his student days or that he was going shopping. He added that he always made excuses in silence for wronging his parents, indicating that rather than shame he felt guilt. It appears that Japanese are not always as free of feelings of guilt as has been thought (Benedict 1977).

The differences between *awaseru*, *gomakasu* and *usotsuku* are subtle. When asked, nobody could give a clear explanation but there appear to be differences in seriousness and situation. *Usotsuku* is used in contexts concerning very direct ways of deception, such as having *omiai* without any intention to marry or telling parents that one is going somewhere one is not really going. *Gomakasu* is used for ways of evasion that refer to something in the future, i.e. something that might eventually become true, even if it is most unlikely, and ways of diverting attention and *awaseru* is a matter of adapting what one says to the general line of discussion, even if one is saying things that are contrary to one's real ideas or feelings, one's *honne*.

Some gay groups developed a special vocabulary to talk in public contexts. Participants of the Kansai-based leisure circle DON! replace *gei*, which they may use in closed contexts, in public surroundings with *asshu*, the Franco-Japanese pronunciation of the letter 'H' in French, which in this case refers to *homo*. They also developed words to discuss men they see when in public contexts, such as *haipuri*, abbreviated Anglo-Japanese for high-school pretty, referring to a beautiful high-school boy, and *jei*, Franco-Japanese for the French letter 'G', standing for the English word 'good' and referring to men they find attractive. Lesbian women, when interviewed in public settings, often preferred to use the word *daiku*, Anglo-Japanese for dyke, to refer to themselves as lesbian because they thought that most Japanese do not know that meaning. In Japanese *daiku* means carpenter. Furthermore, many interviewees referred to homosexuality as *sono koto* (that) or similar vague descriptions. Part of this is due to people having difficulty using explicit terms for gay and lesbian (Kakefuda 1992a) but another reason is to prevent people who overhear the conversation from understanding what it is about. Even when I was invited by gay activist Tōgō Ken for dinner in a Kani Dōraku (Crab Pleasure: a crab restaurant chain) in Shinjuku, his aide tried to arrange for a separate room because otherwise our discussion might embarrass or upset people at the next table.

When meeting closeted gay men in a context in which they are not known as such, it is usually expected that one does not show that one knows the other. I was confronted with this when

I saw someone I knew from a gay circle at Osaka station, where we bumped into each other while trying to catch the last train. Given the late hour and knowing that he frequented the nearby gay bars, I assumed that he, like me, came from one of them and I went up to greet him. He reacted by anxiously looking beside me. When I looked around I saw that he was with someone else, a man who looked as if he might be a colleague. I walked on but stayed within eyesight. Later he glanced intensely at me while shaking his head briefly, indicating that the other was not 'one of us'. I smiled briefly and bowed my head in an effort to communicate that I understood.

Shortly before this episode he had related his anxiety about his use of language. As he often visited gay bars and liked to use *onē kotoba* (feminine, camp language and manner of speech) there, he sometimes ended up using *onē kotoba* at his job. This made him very anxious that his colleagues might suspect him of being gay. Another man, who I could only perceive as being obviously gay because his whole *shigusa* (manner of movement) and manner of speech were extremely feminine, including holding his hand in front of his mouth when talking, was not in the least concerned about colleagues thinking that he might be gay. He was closeted at his company and expected to remain that way. This may have been easier than it seems because many Japanese do not think of lesbian women and gay men as people whom they might meet in everyday surroundings and certainly not at a major company. On the other hand, a similarly feminine man was pointed out as gay by his colleague. It is plausible that the increased media attention for gay men and lesbian women may make people more anxious about being recognized as such.

While the much-cited psychologist Doi Takeo claims that Japanese are very adept at understanding the hidden meanings behind people's words (1985, 1986), in cases related to sexuality and the desire not to marry I found that listeners often are not aware. While this may be the goal of the speaker, it also gives problems in case the speaker wants to convey something about him or herself that does not agree with *jōshiki*. *Awaseru* may be forced upon people rather than them wanting to comply, simply because people fail to understand anything else. Hence, it may be very troublesome to make people see and believe that one is not joking. And even then people may not appreciate the significance of such revelations, as, for example, a female single interviewee who thought that her mother understood and accepted that she did not wish to marry discovered. When she took up the subject after years of having been a central figure in the singles' network in Osaka, she discovered that her mother still thought that she would probably one day find the right man for her to marry.

The case of a gay man who works at a major company provides another illustration. At company parties, called *enkai*, it is not uncommon for a man to dress like a woman to the hilarity of his colleagues. My interviewee did this once out of curiosity and won much acclaim for his sophistication. Consequently the master of ceremonies, who organizes such performances, continued to ask him to perform in female drag at *enkai*. While he came to dislike this, he feels he cannot refuse. Everybody thinks he is very good at it and some even humour him by remarking that he must be gay, to which he then replies in the affirmative. This, however, is understood as a joke and only adds to the hilarity. He does not intend to make them understand that he actually is gay but he finds it very *tsurai* (bitter, hard to bear) that he is forced to play this game. He was very worried about how things will develop in the near future because he was approaching his 30s. He feels uncertain whether he will be able to avoid marriage without exposing his homosexuality.

While most people feel that much stress is put upon them by the continual questioning about their marital status, I found some cases of people who ridicule the whole situation by giving whatever answer comes to mind. Some say things such as that they are married and their husband is off working in Iran or some other place far away, or that he died. Other possibilities are to ridicule the question by giving an answer like: 'Surely you don't mean to say you find me stable enough to have a marital relationship?' A woman said she was always thinking of answers to give the *ossantachi* (elderly men) who would ask: 'Why is a beautiful young lady like you not married?' She came up with the following answer: 'I was married but he died last week in a plane crash.' This may be a good method to end a conversation altogether because people are likely to be so embarrassed that they will not venture to continue. These tactics cannot, however, be employed very well when one is dealing with someone with whom one wants to continue or establish a relationship or even a conversation.

## Coming Out: To Whom, How and to What Effect

Revealing one's homosexuality is referred to in English as 'coming out', a term that is also used in other languages, for instance German. In Japan, the Anglo-Japanese expressions *kamingu auto suru* and *kamu auto suru* (to come out) have recently gained some currency and even singles, feminists and men's liberationists may use them to refer to the time they told their parents, their friends or colleagues, or the media, about the ideas that made them not want to marry or the political views that made them disagree with the roles of gender according to *jōshiki*.

The similarity between the different research categories proved to be strong here.

Coming out in lesbian and gay contexts has been divided into three parts. The first is the coming out to the self, the recognition and acceptance of one's homosexual feelings. The second is the coming out in lesbian and gay circles and the third is coming out to significant others (Edwards 1994: 26). Some people separate the first step from the others and regard them as essentially different (Davies 1992) because the coming out towards the self is a psychological, rather than a social, event. From an anthropological point of view, coming out has been likened to a rite of passage: the gay man or lesbian woman leaves general society to be gay or lesbian in lesbian and gay circles or networks and to come out of there reborn as a lesbian woman or a gay man who assertively presents this new identity (Herdt 1992). In this case, though, it often concerns a passage without a definite end because in many people's lives there are continually new significant others. A further step, which is prominent in Japan today, is coming out in the mass media, which implies coming out towards an unidentified number of readers or viewers. While not all these steps need to be taken in the order presented here, it is the most common order. Coming out towards friends is more common than and usually precedes coming out towards parents, and those appearing in the mass media often tell their parents beforehand.

Ueno Chizuko once suggested to me that lesbian and gay people in Japan 'do not need to come out' because Japan is a homosocial society, i.e. a society in which most activities take place within groups consisting of one sex only, as opposed to America where the need is felt because it is a heterosocial society, i.e. a society in which most activities take place in groups consisting of both sexes. While her argument may hold some truth in the case of women, who may have extensive networks in which they can discuss private matters, in the case of men there is nothing comparable, as men's liberationists have pointed out. As I also found, even in radical women's groups discussion about sexuality is extremely limited and while lesbian women may feel relatively at ease when they are among women, sexuality is typically not discussed. Moreover, it is not true at all that American lesbians and gays generally come out beyond lesbian and gay circles, which they call communities (Signorile 1994), which makes this opposition of America and Japan nonsensical.

Lesbian women and gay men in Japan who engage in debates concerning lesbian and gay politics invariably point at the importance of coming out in order to be able to do anything at all (Ugoku Gei. 1992, Kakefuda 1992a: 196–8). After all, if there are no people known as lesbian and gay, there is nothing to discuss apart from theoretical and philosophical ideas. Even the heterosexual publisher of the gay magazine *Barazoku* Itō Bungaku, who criticizes Occur for what he sees as Americanized behaviour and following American rhetoric of lesbian and gay politics and says that the Japanese situation demands different strategies, also stresses the desirability of coming out for lesbian women and gay men (Itō 1986).

Some lesbian women and gay men recognize that coming out is a rather unnatural form of behaviour but given the present situation, in which all people are as a matter of course expected to be heterosexual, or *nōmaru* (normal), unless they show themselves to be different, there is no choice:

> Why do we need to go this far out of our way and come out? There are many people who think: 'If you live as a serious (*majime na*) person, without making public such a personal feature,

> nobody would say anything,' or: 'I don't feel the need to come out myself.' Indeed, coming out is letting an indefinite number of people know about the personal and private matter that you are homosexual (*dōseiaisha*). But opposed to this 'very personal thing' there is discrimination and prejudice from society. And above all, homosexuals have to live while hiding the fact that they are homosexuals. If they don't do that, they get various disadvantages and are hurt. Discrimination exists in reality. (Morita 1992a)

While it may be all right to be gay or lesbian in a lesbian and gay context, many people feel that it is rather unsatisfying to limit the scope of one's friends to gay men and lesbian women and therefore the need to come out and make friends with heterosexual people is felt (Furukawa, K. 1993). Furthermore, as I found, the lack of people who come out is a major problem for young people who think that they are the only lesbian woman or gay man in their environment. For this reason, I believe that lives may be saved when more people come out. In the case of lesbian women, the near total absence of information about the phenomenon of female homosexuality often made people feel different from everybody else and very lonely. One interviewee, who grew up on Okinawa, attempted suicide for a combination of reasons:

> I used drugs, medicine. At the time I was troubled (*nayanda*) most, when I

> was at high school. Well, there were many things at the time. For instance, I'm a love child. That problem was also part of it, and because there were many things, I thought, well, I've had enough (*mō ii wa*).

Shortly after this attempt she joined a theatre company and went to Tokyo where she found the lesbian edition of *Bessatsu Takarajima* (1991) in which addresses of lesbian groups were printed. Hesitantly, she made contact with a group in Tokyo and since then she has become self-assured and has started to engage in activities such as writing for *Regumi Tsūshin*, a lesbian *minikomishi* and organizing lesbian dance parties in a club in Shinjuku. She describes herself as 'lucky' for having discovered lesbian circles. In her case, like so many others, meeting other lesbian women was a condition for accepting her own homosexuality. In a survey among 124 lesbian women, 38 had attempted suicide and 42 had seriously thought about it (Hirosawa and Rezubian Ripōto Han 1991: 234).

Suicide stories can also be found among gay men. In a documentary by Fuji Television on Occur, JILGA and homosexuality in Japan, one of the interviewees also says, while tears well up in his eyes, that at high school he was so depressed that he wanted to commit suicide. Shortly after this he established contact with Occur, who showed him that gay men are not necessarily weird and lewd people or transvestites. In 1986 a teenager committed suicide by jumping from the roof of a seven-storey building in Miyazaki after he was caught when stealing the gay magazine *Barazoku* in a local supermarket. It is assumed that he committed suicide out of shame for being caught with a gay magazine because 17-year-old shoplifters do not usually jump from high-rise buildings when caught. Another plausible assumption is that he stole the magazine because he was afraid to take it to the counter and pay for it, which would necessitate a confrontation with the salesperson (Itō 1986: 198–209).

Fear of buying gay magazines is a common problem. Most gay men think that salespersons will notice that they buy a gay magazine and conclude that they are gay. Therefore many travel far, often to a shop in another town, to buy a gay magazine. The same holds true for novels concerning homosexuality and for lesbian women buying, for instance, the lesbian issue of *Bessatsu Takarajima* (1991). In this sense, buying a gay magazine or other gay and lesbian literature or lectures may also be seen as a way of coming out. One interviewee solved this problem by pretending it was a game. In a popular game among youngsters in Japan participants are given awkward assignments to fulfil. He pretended he had been given the assignment to buy a gay magazine. Others buy several heterosexual erotic magazines and put a gay magazine in between in the hope that the salesperson will not notice or think that it is bought by mistake. Among all informants it was common to go in and out of a bookstore many times before making up one's mind to buy. After buying a hasty exit followed. While there are bookshops that specialize in gay magazines and gay clientele, they are difficult to find without a gay magazine, in which they advertise. The role of the lesbian and gay press in accepting homosexual feelings is very important for many people, but not always. A considerable number of gay men found gay magazines *iyarashii* (distasteful, disgusting) because of the nude pictures, which they saw as pornographic, and the pornographic stories in them (Lunsing 1995).

Women who do not like to be feminine or accept the gender roles assigned to them have similar difficulties with feelings of loneliness and the lack of information about feminist organizations. While I had no problem in locating Kyoto's women's bookstore, most people, even those living in Kyoto, were not aware of its existence. The same is true for Japan's two other women's bookstores, called Crayon House, in Osaka and Tokyo. Books by *feminisuto*, that are sold in bookstores throughout the country, are often found to be difficult and inaccessible (*katai*) and not to have much relevance to individual situations. Most informants, even if they bought feminist books, said that they seldom read any of them.

## Friends, Classmates and Colleagues

Occur's data from a survey of 300 gay men show that they are most likely to come out first towards close friends (39.9 per cent), followed by gay friends (12.7 per cent) with parents and brothers and sisters in the third place (6.3 per cent); 20.7 per cent told nobody and 13.3 per cent gave no answer (Ugoku Gei. 1992: 365). These results are supported by my own findings and by those of the Yajima seminar survey which also includes lesbian women and bisexual people (Taniguchi 1992). Further, there is a clear bias towards telling women rather than men. Similar results follow from research among lesbian women (Hirosawa and Rezubian Ripōto Han 1991) and my research showed that similar patterns can also be discerned among heterosexual singles and feminists who talk about their ideas and personal matters.

The decision to come out towards heterosexual friends, classmates and colleagues in general was determined by the question as to whether the person concerned could be trusted (*shinrai dekiru*) to treat the information in an acceptable manner and not gossip about it to others. Some tested people they considered revealing their sexual preference to by talking about homosexuality in general, others thought they knew, for reasons they could not identify, that they knew which of their friends would be supportive. Gay men usually tell at least some of their friends, women more than men, when they are at university or around the time they are 20 years old. Lesbian women tend to come out later and have a stronger preference for coming out to female friends. Singles and feminists usually do not seem to make much effort to establish themselves as such explicitly but talk about personal matters to people selected along lines similar to lesbian women and gay men.

As sexuality is rarely discussed seriously in Japan,[3] in order to talk about one's own sexuality in terms that differentiate it from what is perceived as normal, a major problem lies in the need to overcome the layers prohibiting discussion of personal matters. A relatively close relationship has to be established before sexuality can be discussed, otherwise it might even be considered impolite (*shitsurei*), or troublesome (*meiwaku*). Some interviewees mentioned these terms to indicate why they did not consider coming out or confronting people with their ideas about gender roles and sexism. When I proposed to a wholly closeted interviewee that he could talk about his homosexuality with a mutual friend with whom I had discussed her and my sexuality before, he thought that they did not have the sort of relationship in which he could trouble (*meiwaku o kakeru*) her with his problems (*nayami*). Another reason for not telling particular people is that they are thought to be incapable of understanding (*rikai dekinai*). Why they thought this, nobody really could explain. Feelings, rather than rational deduction, are important means of selection.

Those who talked to friends, colleagues or classmates about personal matters were in general not confronted by homophobic or sexist reactions. Typically the reaction amounted to next to nothing, for instance a mumbled: '*A sō na no* (oh?).' In other cases the reaction was very positive. People were interested to talk further about it and the relationship generally improved. A gay interviewee told a classmate he fancied that he was gay the first time he revealed his sexual preference to anyone. As it turned out, this classmate was also gay and the happy outcome of this was a love relationship. All surveys also show that the most likely reaction to revelation is positive,[4] which, given the selection of people to come out to, discussed above, is not surprising.

Sometimes people may feel compelled to tell about their sexual preference in order to prevent complications. This is especially the case when someone of the opposite sex develops an amorous interest. A woman, with whom I had gone to the cinema, was thought by another to be developing an affair with me. I first told the woman I went to the movie with that I was gay and she became one of my best friends in Japan. The next day I informed the woman who thought we were having an affair and she never spoke to me again. A 33-year-old gay interviewee told the following story about his experience with a female colleague who had her eye on him:

> One day I went for dinner with a girl (*onna no ko*) from my job. The food came and we were talking away in the restaurant. And this girl says all of a sudden that she had separated from her boyfriend (*kareshi*). I said it was terrible. But she said, not at all, there were reasons why she had to separate, three reasons. The first was that he was very nice when they started to see each other but the longer they were together, the more he became very violent. (. . .) The

> second reason, she always thought that this was not the way things should be but he saw another woman.
> (. . .) The third reason was that she had fallen in love. When I said that's good, lucky for you to have found someone and so on, she turned towards me. She looked straight at me and said, it's you. This was an enormous shock, and I was at a loss what to do. But since we had been talking so intimately, I thought I should come clean and said, to tell the truth, I can't have sex with women, I'm gay (*gei*), just like that. She shrank and looked down, she lost her spirits. I felt bad about myself, shocking her like that, but suddenly she looked up and smiled, saying that it was all right.

She meant by this that they could still be friends and, indeed, that is what happened. They enjoy going for dinner or drinking together and, according to my interviewee, have a relationship in which they can talk about anything. The only thing he regrets is that, while he is liked among women, among men he is less popular.

As Hase *san*, discussed in chapter three (p. 112) and chapter five (pp. 169–70), said, you cannot really call someone who does not know that you are gay a friend. Many lesbian, gay, feminists and single people who talked about personal matters found that it greatly improved and deepened their friendships. In fewer cases people lost a friend or what they had called a friend until then. Recognizing that they were faced with the choice of either having increasingly meaningless and superficial, or 'thin (*asai*)', relationships with people with whom they could not talk confidentially about matters that were close to their hearts, or revealing their feelings or thoughts at the risk of losing the relationship altogether, most thought it worth the risk, whatever the result. A 32-year-old lesbian woman from LIO (Lesbians in Occur), the lesbian group of Occur, thought that things had changed over the past ten years. Among young people, whose parents are of the generation of the student movements in the 1960s, it is increasingly acceptable to discuss subjects like masturbation or what form of sex one likes. Therefore, she thought that it had become easier to talk about homosexuality. She does not regard it as very special that she came out to her friends:

> I've always been out, ever since high school. At high school I didn't exactly say that I was lesbian. I only said things like I fancy that woman. I have always been told by people that they thought I fancied women. (. . .) In that respect I never met with negative reactions (*iya na me*: lit. nasty eyes). If I'd say I liked [women], I got reactions like, oh, there was a student like you last year in a higher class, or don't worry about it. I haven't [lost any friends by coming out]. Only, there were some who made comments like stop it, I'm not like that. If I confessed my love for her, there were friends who reacted like that. I was really fortunate. (. . .) If you make clear

> that you tell because you trust them, I
> don't think they will react strangely.

Telling people that you like someone rather than that you are gay or lesbian, is a common method of coming out, especially among young people. Kosaburō, a 31-year-old gay singer/song writer and caretaker at a day-centre for mentally handicapped people, told friends at his vocational school that he liked a particular 'boy' (*ko*). Among colleagues of his nursing job he also came out. If he was asked whether he had a girlfriend (*kanojo*), he said that he preferred men. Nowadays, in his shows, he always discusses his homosexuality and his songs are often about his loves. His shows are also visited by many of his heterosexual colleagues. At his job there are, nonetheless, also people who find the idea of love between men unthinkable. They seem to regard Kosaburō as someone with a handicap but he is not troubled much by them. They are a minority and he has decided long ago that being gay is nothing special (*nan to mo nai*).

Feminist women usually remain silent about their ideas unless they are among feminist friends. Eventually their circle of friends tends to consist increasingly of feminist women. In work situations it was usually seen as hazardous to vent opinions about sex discrimination. Indeed, several interviewees were dismissed or made to resign after complaining about sexual harassment or wage discrimination.[5] The topic of tea-serving – which has been much discussed in feminist circles as a prime example of discrimination against women in Japan and may lead to major conflicts in companies (Pharr 1990: 59–74) – was avoided by many because they expected that many of their female colleagues would attack them if they complained about women having to do it, saying that they like to serve tea. A 33-year-old interviewee who worked as a designer and said that she does not understand much of feminism, tried to discuss discrimination against women at her workplace:

> It's a small company. I asked all the time why do we have to do it like this, but there were never understanding answers. Always I got strange answers, answers I don't understand. (. . .) Their way of looking at things is after all totally different, seeing things from men's side or seeing things from my side. Therefore I felt totally misunderstood, and that's still the same. (. . .) They make you feel bad for saying it, only because I want to say that they should look at it from the idea of humans, and that we are all the same human beings, only that everyone has strong points and that [they shouldn't judge you] just because you happen to be a woman. I want them to see women as the individuals (*kojin*) they are, and like there are men who like doing the laundry or cleaning, among women there are those who don't like that. That's not because you are a woman, that varies from person to person.

Her frustration at not being able to talk about these things made her look for another job. This was notwithstanding the fact that her superiors had been very positive when she divorced because they thought that meant that she would continue to work. I rarely encountered women who were successful in questioning the way things are in their workplace. A woman who refused to wear a company uniform, because men doing the same line of work do not have to wear one and she saw it as an invasion of her privacy, was allowed not to wear it but at the cost of constantly being harassed for being uncooperative. Another woman who in a publication questioned the pressure applied to people who do not wish to marry and who do not wish to have children (Watanabe, Y. 1991), said that experience had taught her that it was useless to try and discuss such subjects with colleagues. They would only think she was being strange and stop listening to her altogether. There are many books on these subjects that are little read by people who do not already agree with the ideas expounded in them and there is little discussion among people with differing views.

If one does not mind being different and is not insecure when others think one is *hen* or *hentai* (weird or queer), life may be easier. A single man working at a small company was given a job in a room apart from the rest of the staff and was quite happy with this because he never enjoyed the everyday contact with his colleagues. A lesbian woman who worked at one of the major companies showed people she thought she could trust pictures of her female lover and avoided contact with those she did not like as much as possible. This was not always successful. On a company trip to Kyushu, a male colleague tried to kiss her and harassed her for turning him down. On her return, she filed a complaint with a superior and had him transferred to a position in which she did not have to see him any more. She never joined social events after hours, which usually are thought to be obligatory by people in positions like hers.

The difference between discussing homosexuality and feminism is striking. While lesbian women and gay men may be more closeted and isolated overall, when they come out they choose and find people with whom they can talk and in some cases the workplace may be quite accepting. Feminists may discuss the way things are organized at their jobs in relation to sex. In doing so, they often find doors being closed to them. This suggests that revealing a matter that can be regarded as purely personal, one's sexual preference, is less problematic than matters that have an explicit political component and are related to the division of tasks, acceptance of which would demand change in everyone's behaviour.

## Parents

While many gay men and lesbian women have come out among a selection of friends, parents, especially the father, are often seen as people who are not likely to understand because they are too old or their minds lack the suppleness to accept alterations to their *jōshiki* and thus had better be kept ignorant. In other cases it is expected that the shock would be too great for them to overcome, many even saying that they would die of it. It is not so much the reaction towards oneself that is feared but rather the problems it might cause to the parents. A major reason people gave for not talking about their homosexuality, and also feminist ideals or the wish to remain unmarried, was that they did not want to trouble (*meiwaku o kakeru*) the parents with their ideas or worries (*nayami*). Further, the love of a parent, usually the mother, for the child, was often given as a reason not to openly defy the parent's wishes. While motherly love in the Netherlands is ideally expressed by her utmost efforts to understand her child, whatever he or she may do, among Japanese informants motherly love was often rather felt like a burden and used to clarify why it is impossible to do anything one's mother might dislike.

Fear of parents finding out and upsetting one's lifestyle may be well grounded. The lesbian writer Izumo Marō recounts an episode in which she travelled secretly to Kyoto with a lover to stay with her and be away from her parents. The next day police knocked on her door and summoned her lover to go with them. Her lover's parents had arranged for her to be brought back home. Izumo's protest that there was no legal base for this action and that her lover was an adult person who could go as she pleased, did not help. Her lover did not resist and after having been threatened with arrest for obstructing the work of a police officer, Izumo let her go. On a second elopement, her lover's parents were on the phone scolding Izumo even before she was aware of her lover's absence from the parental house. This time, her lover wished to see Izumo once more before she married. She showed little resistance towards her parents' orders that she marry but insisted, nevertheless, that she wished to continue seeing Izumo every now and then, secretly (Izumo 1993: 133–6).

Mothers are by far the favourite of the two parents to discuss personal matters with. For gay men this is underlined by data in the survey by the gay magazine *Za Gei*, where the siblings knew in 25.8 per cent of the cases, the mother in 21.6 per cent and the father in 14.4 per cent, about their brother's or son's homosexuality (Za Gei Henshūbu ed. 1992). A survey of 312 gay men by *Sabu* confirms this, although there the overall rate of being known as gay by family members is lower (Takakura 1992). In a majority of the cases the respondents thought that none of their family knew (ibid., Za Gei Henshūbu 1992). A Yajima seminar survey did not distinguish between different family members but found that 49 think someone in their family knows as opposed to 105 who think nobody knows. Of those who think they know, 25 told them, 22 think they ended up understanding it (*wakatte shimatta*) and 2 had been asked and answered in the affirmative (Taniguchi 1992: 78). Of the lesbian survey, 27.0 per cent think their family knows, 10.7 per cent think they might know to some extent (*usuusu shitte iru*) and 60.4 per cent think they do not know (Hirosawa and Rezubian Ripōto Han 1991: 229).

In cases where people told one or both of their parents, reactions ranged from outright indignation and telling their child that he or she had no home any more, via urges to get married soon, to positive acceptance. The last is most common among my informants and according to surveys.[6] In one case the mother went so far as to buy gay magazines for her son, who himself was afraid to confront shopkeepers. Again, it should not be a surprise that positive reactions are more common because children of parents who are more likely to react positively are more likely to tell them. In some cases parents, on hearing that their son saw himself as gay, decided that it would be best for him to marry soon and that then everything would become all right. For this reason, in a group discussion with young gay men of JILGA in Tokyo my idea that coming out towards one's parents might be a way to stop them from urging one to marry, was refuted from the beginning. Other reactions were to tell the child to be discreet and keep this information from the neighbours and the admonition not to do anything weird (*hen*), which also refers to being indiscreet.

In this context it was evident that those who had only one parent because their mother never married, because the parents were divorced or because one of the parents had died, generally had much better relationships with that parent, including the ability to discuss their sexual preference or their ideas regarding marriage or women's or men's roles. If this is taken as an indicator of good parenthood, it suggests that it may be advantageous for children to grow up in a one-parent household, at least if personal understanding between parent and child is desired. In some cases it transpired that the single parent depended more on the child emotionally, which would have the positive effect of the parent being forced to try and understand the child. On the other hand, a 32-year-old lesbian woman felt that she could not easily leave her father to live on his own because of this dependence and because she thought that he could not take good care of himself, especially when it came to preparing food. About his knowledge of her personal life she said:

> I didn't really come out to my father. But he knows. Saying without saying is an enigma (*nazo*) of the Japanese. (. . .) Last year I went to the Gay Parade in San Francisco, with Occur. And because I had said that I was going there I was sent information about lesbian places, saunas and so on. My father found the letter. He thought it was addressed to him and opened it. When I came home it was opened and I thought, well, let's come out, but when my father returned and I said, welcome back (*okaeri*), he said, I didn't read the letter. (. . .) I didn't believe my ears. But he doesn't harass me about marriage and in the end he always says things such as that I must make sure that I can support myself. In that sense I'm fortunate.

Among lesbian women and gay men who think that their homosexuality has been found out (*barashita*) by their parents, finding letters or lesbian or gay magazines were often mentioned as the reasons. Kosaburō's mother once went to clean his room, which is something many mothers of single sons do, when he was out. When he returned, he found that his collection of gay magazines was gone. Since he had a whole shelf of them, he thought that his mother could not have avoided concluding that he was genuinely interested in them. If there had only been one, she might have thought that he bought it by mistake but one does not buy a shelf-full by mistake. All his mother had to say about it, however, was that she had thrown away the distasteful (*iyarashii*) magazines, which does not indicate acceptance. Similarly, an informant who was active in making a gay *minikomishi* returned home one night to find his mother reading it. She showed it and asked whether he intended to continue making it, which he confirmed. That was the end of the discussion.

A man who told his mother that he was gay thought that she did not accept it. She did not react at all. He thought that she did not want to be confronted with it again and that as long as he would be discreet, she would not trouble him. She conveys *omiai* invitations to him, which are offered by aunts and other relatives. He believes that his mother would be offended if he would be so indiscreet as to let other relatives know about his sexual preference. As long as it remains their little secret and nobody else knows, there is no need to talk about it. Later, though, he appeared as the discussion leader in a public forum on homosexuality, giving his full name and relating his own life history, which appeared in print afterwards (Uchikoshi 1995). He may have thought that it was unlikely for his family to come across this publication and he may have decided that even if they did, he is not really doing anything reproachable.

I also found some more positive parental reactions. The mother of one lesbian woman asked her whether she was *S*, which is a word that was in vogue in the 1920s and 1930s to refer to special friendships between women, as discussed in the introduction (p. 20). *S* is short for *shisutāfuddo* (sisterhood: Higuchi 1993a).[7] Other mothers praised their daughters' girlfriends when they visited together. The mother of a gay man also showed understanding when he confronted her with the fact that he had come from Osaka back home to Yokohama because he wanted to attend the hearings of the court case Occur had started against the metropolitan government of Tokyo because the Fuchū Seinen no Ie, a sort of youth hostel on the outskirts of Tokyo, refused to let them stay. As in the case of the parents who found a magazine or book, this coming out follows a lead, in this case a court case, after which the reasons for going there and his own homosexuality came to be discussed. On later occasions he brought a boyfriend home and they stayed together in his mother's house. A lead may also be found by parents in the way their child behaves. A hospitalized father was visited by his son:

> My father died last year, but [I came out] about seven years ago, at the time I was seeing a boy (*ko*) from Osaka. I lived in Tokyo and travelled up and down to and from Osaka. After about a year we separated and I felt really terrible. My feelings were such that I almost wanted to die. At the time I happened to return to Fukuoka, to my own town (*inaka*). My father was hospitalized. When I went to see him he saw my troubled face and asked directly whether something was wrong. If so, tell me, anything, please tell me, he said. I decided to tell. I told

> him, to be honest, I love someone and that someone is a man. My father understood what I was saying. He knew me from my childhood and had always wondered why I always played with girls but never had a girlfriend. Now his riddle was solved. My father's reaction was very simple, I really love what he said: (. . .) If you can change being gay, it would be better to become straight. If you can stop being gay, it is better to stop. When I asked why, it was because I would probably not become happy. (. . .) That was all. And in the end he said, among men, such things also exist. He meant that because he was also a man, he could understand my feelings.

This interviewee is now quite well-known in gay circles throughout Japan and participated in organizing many activities, including the Lesbian and Gay Parade in Tokyo of 1995. The father's remark that he should stop being gay if he can stems from fear that homosexuality could damage his chances of happiness. Such a reaction could also be explained as homophobia but this is not what my interviewee felt. In Japan, there is not much knowledge of what homophobia is and how it works and, indeed, of discrimination in general, which places this remark in a rather different light than when it is pronounced by someone in a Western European or North American context, although there, too, it is a common first reaction by parents. The second part of the reaction is one I have never heard in Europe. The acknowledgement of the father that, being a man himself, he also knows homosexual feelings is one that contradicts the idea that he is homophobic because a feature of homophobia is that people deny the possibility of homosexual desire in themselves, which is then fought by criticizing and refusing to understand those who acknowledge their homosexual desire (e.g. Harper 1992).

Among women I categorized as feminist, their failure to comply with parents' wishes can be regarded in the same way as coming out. In several cases this led to a severance of contacts with parents. A woman who decided to go and live together with the boyfriend with whom she was expecting a child, was heavily opposed by her parents and at the time I interviewed her, five years later, all contact was still suspended, although they live in the same town. In the meantime she had thrown out her boyfriend and she was contemplating resuming contact with her parents, also in order to give her daughter grandparents. Her parents had never expressed interest in the child but since she had now reached school age, she thought they might at last accept their grand-daughter. The *tada no sukebe*, who figured in chapters four (pp. 149–50) and five (p. 198), also lost all contact with her parents when she decided to divorce. She is quite happy with that because her father especially is, according to her, a very conservative man with whom she prefers having nothing to do. A woman of an older generation was equally heavily criticized by her parents for not getting properly married and pursuing studies in her 30s. She also has not seen them again.

All cases I found of parents who refuse to see their children again have two things in common. One is that it always concerns two parents living together and the other is that it always concerns women. Men who decided not to live up to their parents' ideals tend to meet with opposition also but their choices appear to be accepted more easily. Parents appear to accept that a son has a right to make his own choices, which may be related to the expectation that sons are going to be economically independent or to the actual independence of the son, which may make any efforts by parents futile. Nevertheless, there was no clear difference between how parents of economically independent women reacted and those of women who were not (yet) independent. In some cases parents wanted their son to get married properly, instead of living in a *jijitsukon*, but typically they would think that they just could not follow the younger generation's way of life. Furthermore, it appears that there are fewer men who openly confront their parents with their choices and those who do tend to have progressive parents, who show understanding and interest in the ideas of their children. Overall, parents' ideas appeared to be highly irrelevant to the lifestyles informants enjoy.

## The Media

Coming out in the media may be easier than coming out directly towards people one knows personally. People who read about it in magazines or see it on television may think negatively but they are not so likely to voice their opinions. Those who think positively, on the contrary, are likely to get in touch and express support. A lesbian woman who told her mother that she was lesbian was urged not to do anything weird (*hen na koto*), which she interpreted as an admonition not to appear in the media as lesbian. This she did not intend to do anyway because she, like many lesbian women of her generation, i.e. in their 40s, believed it to be totally impossible to come out as lesbian to the general public because life would be made impossible. They invariably referred to the case of the singer Sagara Naomi who, like Martina Navratilova, was exposed as lesbian by a lover with whom she had broken up. Sagara denied this allegation which served to increase media interest. As a result Sagara, who until then appeared regularly on NHK (Nihon Hōsō Kyoku), Japan's national broadcasting company, lost her contracts and disappeared into oblivion.

This is also said to have made Kakefuda Hiroko worried when she published her book on being lesbian in Japan (Kakefuda 1992a). Before the publication she moved and changed her phone number and I had difficulty locating her because most lesbian women could only tell that she was in hiding and the few people who knew how to contact her refused to help me to get in contact with her. Six months later, however, I met her and she said that she had not known that I was trying to contact her and if she had, she would have been happy to see me. She was dismissive when I told her what people had said six months before about her fears. In the meantime, it had become clear that the negative reactions she feared had not materialized. Her book was largely ignored by the media. Although it was sold in the larger bookstores, smaller ones usually did not stock it. The many letters she received from young lesbian women who read the book, however, indicate that at least they knew where to find it. The lack of attention to her book is also the reason why she was happy when Ueno Chizuko criticized it in an article (Ueno 1992). Although she found the contents of the criticism *bakabakashii* (silly), Ueno at least did not ignore her book. As she did not feel like discussion with Ueno, she sent Ueno a fax thanking her for the article, leaving Ueno with the assumption that she appreciated the contents.

Nowadays the media appear to take an opposite position to the times of Sagara. The popular singer, Sasano Michiru, formerly the lead singer of the successful group Tokyo Shōnen, was trying to make a comeback as a solo singer. At the same time, she said that she was eager to come out as lesbian and, according to Kakefuda Hiroko, in interviews she frequently made reference to girlfriends and to women she admired, in order to give journalists a reason to ask her whether she was lesbian. She was never asked this question, which made it difficult for her to find a natural way to come out. Two years after she had made up her mind she published a book called *Coming Out!* (Sasano 1995), which became a bestseller. She drew much media attention and gained in popularity among lesbian women and other people with an interest in the politics of sexuality.

Shortly after my relationship with Onitsuka Tetsurō started, Hirano Hiroaki from OGC was asked by a photographer whether he knew any lesbian or gay couples who were willing to appear in his photo book about unmarried couples in Japan. Hearing about this, Oni, as his friends call him, asked me, after some thought, if I wanted to appear with him. Oni's main reason for wanting to appear was that he wanted to do something together with me that would make a difference. We appeared first in the picture collection *Couple* by photographer Hashiguchi Jōji (1992) and later were asked for an interview that was published in a gay special of the youth magazine *Takarajima* (Takarajima 1993).

Oni saw my presence as a chance to come out in a natural fashion. Instead of saying that he was gay, he could say that I was his lover. This can be likened to heterosexuals introducing their partners. They do not explicitly say that they are heterosexual but show it by showing their lover who is of the other sex. If there is no lover and you want to come out, there is no choice but to say that you are gay or lesbian in so many words, which is a plight for homosexuals as opposed to heterosexuals who are assumed to be heterosexual anyway. Moreover, if there is no lover it may be difficult to make people understand what the issue is. Beforehand, Oni had come out in several circumstances and with most, if not all, of his friends, including those university colleagues with whom he had a more personal relationship. A group of students that was invited to his house for dinner was confronted with a large number of books on sexuality and especially homosexuality, which made them wonder and ask whether he was gay. At that time, Oni did not feel content about the way he handled the situation, as he merely said he was, without promoting further discussion on the subject because he felt cornered by this large group.

Our appearance in the media did not go unnoticed by most people who knew us and many old friends phoned Oni and renewed relationships. Problems in the form of negative reactions did not occur and Oni presumes that this is because people who find homosexuality *kimochiwarui* (sickening), which may be *jōshiki* among those who do not care to consider it seriously, would sooner bite off their tongues than mention it. Furthermore, he works at a university and, as in many countries, people working at universities in Japan are relatively tolerant in the sense that they have learned to act as if they were liberal and not bigoted, even if the latter is possibly closer to their actual feelings. I was surprised by a member of the office staff of my university, who on our first meeting had shocked me by referring to a mutual acquaintance as *okama,* a term for homosexual he used in a very derogatory sense, but now told me smiling in a supportive manner that he read about me in *Takarajima.*

Oni and I were neither the first to come out in the media nor the last. We were part of a growing stream which started in 1990 when members of Occur and JILGA started coming out. Early examples were the writer Fushimi Noriaki and OGC's Hirano Hiroaki, the latter of whom had previously gained fame for being a school teacher with a *Mohikan* (Mohican) haircut and alternative ways of dressing (Izumi 1990: 329–30). In the same book *Couple*, a number of members of Occur as well as an aspiring fashion designer and his lover appeared. Further, one lesbian couple is pictured in the book. After us, many more people kept appearing in magazines and on television and there was even a television programme on TBS (Tokyo Broadcasting Station) featuring a 'coming out of the week' as a set item.

It is difficult to establish whether Oni's coming out had any particular influence but among Oni's circle of friends people wanted increasingly to come out and show more personal aspects of themselves. Friends of Oni and me, the multi-media performance group Dumb Type, that performs throughout the world, decided to make a performance about sexuality and AIDS, mostly because one of its most prominent figures, Furuhashi Teiji, had developed AIDS-related illnesses. Preceding the final version, *S/N*, investigative performances called *Seminar Show for S/N*, took place in Kyoto in March 1993 and later in Fujisawa near Tokyo. Oni and I were asked to participate by talking about ourselves. Further, Matsuo Megumi, a friend who manages an art gallery, participated as a heterosexual woman coming out as divorced and having lovers. Later a journalist friend made a series of her life story in *Kyōto Shinbun* (Hayashi 1993a, b, c). As a result many old-time friends contacted her and expressed their admiration. During the performance another friend, a lesbian woman, stood up from the audience and started discussing things from her, lesbian, point of view.

A year later the performance *S/N* had its premiere in Adelaide, Australia, and now Teiji for the first time came out not only as gay but also as a person living with AIDS. Alex, which is the stage name of another friend, performed as himself, i.e. deaf and gay, and Bubu told about her experiences as a sex worker. In Tokyo, where they performed in January 1995, the line was developed further and in the spring of 1995 they toured Europe and later also Brazil, Hong Kong and various other places. For

America, it was, however, considered to be too advanced by theatre directors (Asai 1995). The last performances took place in 1996, after Teiji's death, with him appearing on video. From the same circle of friends, many people participated in the first AIDS Candlelight Parade in Kyoto in 1993 and in the first Lesbian and Gay Parade in Japan, which took place in Tokyo in August 1994. The only woman interviewed on the latter occasion by *Asahi Shinbun* and identified by her real name, Hiramatsu Miho (*Asahi Shinbun* 1994), is also part of this network of friendship and love.

On the other hand, I found a number of well-known lesbian women, who presented themselves as feminists. Since they were established media personalities, they had not considered coming out as lesbian and tended to avoid meeting me. The heterosexual feminist Uemura Kuniko said that she wanted to write a book about sex but found it impossible to write without discussing herself. This, however, she thought she could not do because the reaction (*hanpatsu*) would be insufferable. Closest to such an attempt might still be the work of women's liberationist Tanaka Mitsu, who became famous with a book she published in the 1970s (Tanaka 1975). Other feminist women, like Fukushima Mizuho or Ochiai Keiko discuss their lifestyles – Fukushima lives in *jijitsukon* and Ochiai is single – frequently in *fora* throughout Japan but, again, not their sexuality.

A heterosexual informant, who works as a day-labourer, said that he was gay at a meeting of single parents, after someone present joked that he had no objection to gay people. The man who made the joke asked what sort of man was his type, to which he reacted by saying that the joker fitted it, who thereupon was obviously embarrassed and shut up (Takehara 1993). One does not even have to be gay to come out as gay and confront people with their narrow-mindedness.

## Conclusion

There are ample opportunities for people to develop and maintain lifestyles that disagree with *jōshiki* concerning marriage in Japan. For those who are prepared to invest effort and forward planning, these lifestyles need not necessarily be characterized by marginality or poverty. Many people, however, do not plan ahead and, especially where it concerns love relationships, this may not be possible because much depends on partners. Many people run into trouble because they initially tried to follow a mainstream lifecourse, while they might have been better off developing their own alternative from the start. While women, or feminine men, may have a worse starting position economically than men, once they set out on an alternative course they are much more decided and as a result more successful. Masculine men, often tied by their occupations, have more difficulty in working out alternatives, emotionally as well as practically. As long as they can manage to *awaseru* (go along with) other people in conversations, problems can easily be avoided. This may be easier to achieve by those who are socialized in a more feminine way. It is, however, also clear that *awaseru* has its cost.

Examples of people who have come out in the media since the beginning of the 1990s have encouraged many people in many walks of life to do the same. The attitude of many young people nowadays, regardless of the question of whether they are gay, lesbian, or whether they just do not want to marry or otherwise live in agreement with *jōshiki* that seem to have become somewhat outdated, can be presented by the simple expression: '*Sore de ii n ja nai no?* (what's wrong with that?, or, so what?),' which is reminiscent of the Ejanaika movement that swept through Japan at the end of the nineteenth century and was marked by hedonism (Bornoff 1992: 307–8) and is remembered today by a magazine of that name. This attitude prevents the criticism that they are *rikutsuppoi* (know-alls). Now it is the turn for critics of alternative lifestyles to use rational argument. This is a departure from general patterns of behaviour that have governed Japanese society since the end of the Second World War and, as Benedict's work suggests, also before then (Benedict 1977). While Tsutamori teaches transvestites that nobody says that they cannot dress up in clothes of the opposite sex (Tsutamori 1991), classically trained female singer Haruka Mari, who performed at Minoya Hall in Osaka with drag queen singer Simone (Shimōne) Fukayuki,[8] said when introducing a song: 'Nowadays in Japan, anything goes.' If only people are willing to believe this, there is little to stop them.

## Notes

1 This concerns the *Kokka Kōmuin Hō*, the Civil Servant Law. It stipulates that civil servants can be dismissed if they go against the law or orders based on the law, if they go against the duties of their function, or if they do something that makes them not suitable to serve the people (*Kokka Kōmuin Hō*, art. 3, par. 82; Shiono *et al*. 1993: 139).

2 By English standards, though, these jobs are not particularly badly paid or insecure. The comparison which makes *arubaito* in Japan look as presented here, is rather with north-west continental Europe or those parts of the European Union where the Social chapter is subscribed to.

3 I think that people who read descriptions of talk about sex in, for instance, Smith and Wiswell (1982) as proof of liberal attitudes towards sexuality are mistaken. While Smith and

Wiswell may seem to imply this, the very text makes it obvious that talk about sex is limited to jokes and making fun of or criticizing other people, which, as Foucault (1978) suggested, functions to set norms which restrict sexual behaviour. As Wiswell found, it was almost totally impossible to talk with women about their actual sexual activities, even if they were the frequent subject of gossip and jokes. Comparing the people in Wiswell and Smith's work to people in my own country, I do not see a great difference in ways sex is talked about. This critique leaves intact the enormous value of the book for, while my interpretation may be at variance with theirs, the manner in which the data are presented allow me to interpret them freely.

4 The lesbian survey gives the following figures: in 35.1 per cent of the cases the reaction was one of understanding, in 21.3 per cent it was taken in a normal or natural way, 18.1 per cent felt misunderstood, in 16.0 per cent it led to surprise and in the same percentage of cases it did not lead to surprise. In 7.4 per cent of the cases distance developed (Hirosawa and Rezubian Ripōto Han 1991: 227). In the Yajima seminar survey among 77 gay, lesbian and bisexual people who came out, 48 thought that the relation did not change, 19 thought it changed and 10 were not sure. It is not made clear whether change means for better or for worse (Taniguchi 1992). In Occur's survey the reactions also were predominantly positive (Ugoku Gei. 1992: 366–8).

5 One day's results of telephone counselling on sexual harassment by a group of lawyers based in Tokyo, eventually led in 5.1 per cent of the cases to dismissal or the prospect of dismissal after complaining about the events and in 28.9 per cent of the cases to resignation or the prospect of resignation. Positive results were very few (Sugii 1990: 215).

6 In the lesbian survey 36.4 per cent showed understanding, 20.5 per cent were not surprised, 15.9 per cent became angry, and 9.1 per cent did not understand (Hirosawa and Rezubian Ripōto Han 1991: 229). The Yajima seminar survey shows that the relation remained unchanged in 23 cases and changed in 24 cases. Changes are mostly for the good. Among those who did not come out to their parents, a large majority thought that the reaction would be negative (Taniguchi 1992: 79–80).

7 As discussed in the introduction, writer Yoshiya Nobuko is the example that is always mentioned in this context. She wrote romantic girls' novels about love relationships between women, some of which are famous (e.g. Yoshiya 1924).

8 Here I write Simone Fukayuki rather than Fukayuki Simone, that is first the personal name rather than the family name, because that is how the performer does it. Both names are invented by Simone Fukayuki, Fukayuki meaning 'deep snow'.

# 7 Circles: Discussing Gender, Sex, and the Other and the Self

This chapter discusses discourses and constructions concerning gender and sex and how they affect people belonging to the various research categories. There are two main possible ways of relating to these discourses: criticizing and defying them or agreeing with them and adapting to them. Both these possibilities are prevalent in various combinations, depending on the particular topic and the circle. A third possibility is to ignore them. This is what happens with discourses on historical constructions of homosexuality in academic circles, as discussed in the introduction, which most informants did not know about or, if they did, did not regard as relevant to their situation. Therefore they are not discussed in this chapter, which is based on participant observation and contemporary writing by people belonging to my research categories. Further, this chapter discusses some features of the many circles I participated in and that were discussed with informants. A major topic is how circles and categories relate to each other.

## Sex and Gender: Female and Male, Feminine and Masculine

Three categories of people are particularly troubled by the duality of female and male: 'transgender' people, transvestites and transsexuals. The first category is called *toransu jendā* in Japan (e.g. Hashimoto and Tsutamori 1990, Tsutamori 1990a, 1993) but until very recently has not been much recognized as a category in Western academic circles. Some lesbian feminists, while basically writing on manifestations of the same phenomenon, do not mention such a word (Butler 1990, 1993, Wittig 1992, de Lauretis 1994). When the term 'transgender' or 'transgenderism' appears in Western publications, its meaning appears to be limited to transsexuality and transvestism (e.g. King 1996, Raymond 1994, 1996).[1]

Gender ambiguity, a term that is sometimes used, may be close in meaning but it is used in a more limited sense for people who are partly transformed physically (Cornwall 1994, Kandiyoti 1994) and hermaphrodites (Nanda 1990), both of whom are labelled in Japan by the same term: *jendā fukaishō* (Ishii 1991, Kuroyanagi 1992, Ino 1992). The Japanese term *toransu jendā* is a more comprehensive term, and its currency in Japan preceded that in the English language, where it still is not very widely used. It comprises all women with masculine and all men with feminine attributes, i.e. all people whose assigned gender does not wholly correspond with what they are or do. It includes for instance career women who by pursuing a career crossed the boundary enclosing female gender in relation to occupational activities. It also includes men who engage in housekeeping. It includes all my research categories and all my interviewees and ultimately probably a majority of the Japanese, or any other, people.

## Transvestism and Transsexuality

Transvestism, or cross-sex dressing, which may include wearing make-up in the case of men and moustaches in the case of women, is perhaps the clearest category of the three. Japanese words for transvestites include the Anglo-Japanese *toransubesuta-*

*ito* and the Sino-Japanese terms *isōsha* (different dresser: Ishii 1991), *iseisōsha* (different-sex dresser), *dansōsha* (male dresser) and *josōsha* (female dresser), terms that refer to women who wear men's outfits and men who wear women's outfits and make-up. There are some situations in which men are expected to dress as women, such as the *onnagata* in the Kabuki theatre, which is a man playing a female role. They may be regular superstars, who write their memoirs (Kawarasaki 1991). It is common for male students to wear women's clothes at university festivals[2] and at company parties transvestism by men is a common part of the programme, as was discussed in chapter six (p. 228). Further, there are men who work in female clothes as *gei bōi* (lit. gay boy), *okama* or *mr redii* (lit. Mr Lady) in *gei bā* or *okama bā*, which in this context are transvestite bars, and often prostitution is part of the activities engaged in. An *okama* is a cooking pot and it is said to have become a term for feminine gay men in the beginning of this century (Robertson 1992), when gay men were constructed as feminine only. In gay pornography, *okama* is often used to refer to the anus (e.g. *okama ga horareta*: his arse was dug into) and in *Kenkyūsha's New Japanese–English Dictionary* it is equated with *danshō* (male prostitute: Masuda 1988). Thus, gay men were seen as feminine male prostitutes.

In the case of women, there is Takarazuka Kagekidan, the Takarazuka Revue, in which all roles are played by women and some women specialize in playing men (Robertson 1992). There are also bars in which women work as male hosts (*Cross Dressing* 1992), *onabe bā*, some of them taking hormones to promote the growth of facial hair and the development of muscles. *Onabe* is, like *okama*, a cooking pot. *Kenkyūsha's New Japanese–English Dictionary* includes the meaning of maidservant but not that of lesbian or transvestite woman (Masuda ed. 1988), which is how most people use it.

Drag queens, men who exaggerate femininity in dressing and making-up grotesquely as women, are not very common but two groups, Takara in Tokyo and Diamond in Osaka, employ drag as part of shows they perform in clubs. One of them, Diamond from Osaka, consists mostly of women and one of their policies is to make the audience oblivious of who is female and who is male, with considerable success. A lesbian friend who often appears with Diamond participated in drag in the European Lesbian and Gay Pride Parade in Amsterdam in 1994. She was filmed many times and later she was shown in a television programme on sexual variety in the Netherlands as an example of a Dutch male drag queen. The last few years have seen an increase in the number of drag queens and their popularity at parties in Japan. Further, there are pop bands whose male members wear make-up and look very feminine, such as By-sexual (Tanaka 1991), whose name refers not to sexual preference but to looks.

There are, however, men and women who desire to cross-dress but are not actors and who do not want to do it for show but for their personal pleasure, often following compulsive inner urges. The way they dress is generally not much appreciated by people who like or are drag queens because they tend to dress like average women or men or even more conservatively than that. In the case of men, it is common to cross-dress only in closed contexts (Tsutamori 1993, *Queen*), which may be in their own house or in a transvestite club such as the Erisabesu (Elizabeth) chain with branches in Tokyo, Osaka and Nagoya (*Queen*). Outside such contexts they may limit their transvestism to wearing women's underwear. A small group, led by a man who calls himself Candy Milky, go out on the street in drag and *Himawari* (Sunflower), the magazine they produce, prints reports of transvestite men out in town or countryside, in one case of a couple attending the marriage ceremony of a friend (Kaoru 1992).

A historical example of a female transvestite, Kawashima Shigeko, who has been compared to Mata Hari, the Frisian woman who was convicted and sentenced to death for espionage in the First World War in Paris, is discussed in a recent book (Kamisaka 1992). One lesbian informant sometimes wore a complete *sarariiman* outfit in which it was hard to tell that she was not physically a man. Some early feminists, such as Hiratsuka Raichō and Ichikawa Fusae, cut their hair short and smoked cigars, which was revolutionary behaviour in the beginning of the century and led, together with their behaviour and political activities, to criticism that they were unwomanly (Robins-Mowry 1983: 68) but it is now generally acceptable, although few women, or men, smoke cigars in Japan. Interviewees who cut their hair short, sometimes shortly after being hired by a company, or wore androgynous clothes, noticed sometimes an initial shock but no long-term effects. There are also women who live in men's clothes. Underwear transvestism, although less obvious than in the case of men wearing women's lingerie, also exists with women wearing boxer shorts (Ueno 1989, Kokuhaku Rezu Kurabu 1992a).

Transsexuals change their genitals from one sex to the other with the use of surgery. These operations are generally thought to be illegal in Japan because the Eugenic Protection Law (*Yūsei Hogo Hō*) prohibits making people infertile without medical need (Sennyo 1996, Matsuo 1997). The physicians who had the expertise to carry out sex-change operations stopped doing so after the proclamation of this law in the 1960s, often urged to do so by their hospital's management that feared legal repercussions. When the law was abolished in 1996 there was a physician, however, who was trying to get permission from his hospital, the Saitama University Hospital, to carry out sex-change surgery (Sennyo 1996, Matsuo 1997). Sex-change surgery on Japanese is mostly carried out in Singapore and America, at huge cost (Torai 1992, Mika and Torai 1993a, b, Torai 1996) and often without proper counselling (Sennyo 1996, Torai 1996). Hormone treatment in order to develop a more feminine or masculine physique usually precedes surgery. A particular group in this context are what in today's Japan is called *nyū-hāfu,* literally new-half, which refers to a physical halfway status between man and woman, or *shii-mēru* (she-male). They use female hormones and sometimes silicone implants in order to acquire female breasts but, like the *travestis* of Brazil (Cornwall 1994), they do not wish to change their genitals. The risks involved led the wife of a transvestite man to demand that he refrains from using hormones (Sunaya 1992).

A person who grew up as a man but is a *ryōsei guyūsha* (hermaphrodite), which he only discovered later in life, calls himself *gei* (Hasshii 1994). To compound the general chaos about what is what, *nyō-hāfu,* as well as fully changed male-to-female transsexuals, may refer to themselves and be referred to as *gei* or *gei bōi*. It is still common for Japanese scholars who work in closely related areas of research to have difficulty understanding what I am saying because of the confusion in terminology. A Japanese sociologist I met in Oxford in 1995 asked me what I was working on and upon my mentioning the word *gei* reacted by saying that she thought that *gei* were very beautiful, often even more beautiful than women. Apparently she thought that *gei* meant male transvestite or *travesti*. Meanings of the wordings vary in accordance with the person who uses them so that one often needs to verify what is meant. The 7-year-old son of a participant at a meeting of OGC called a participant *okama,* much to the horror of his mother. When she questioned him about why he said that, it became clear that he thought that men with long hair were *okama* and that, consequently, he thought that he was an *okama* himself also, much to the hilarity of all.

Gay magazines in Japan basically present two types of men. The young and handsome and the masculine and muscled. *Adon* (after Adonis, first published in 1974), *Barazoku* (The Rose Clan, 1971) and *Badi* (Buddy, with the connotations of surfer and AIDS buddy, 1994) present both of these, while *Sabu* (slang for macho or rough, 1974) rather presents the muscular masculine type. *Za Gei* (*The Gay*, 1980) presents all sorts of men but, like the other magazines, no transvestite men or men in drag. The gay magazine *Samuson* (*Samson*, 1982) presents fat men and the newest magazine, *G-men* (1995), presents 'bear-type' men, i.e. hairy and masculine (years after Kuia Sutadiizu Hensh_ Iinkai ed. 1996a). The monthly gay magazines in 1992 had circulations from 7,000 for *Za Gei* to over 30,000 for *Adon* (Lunsing 1995) and overall sales have increased considerably lately, with the newcomer *Badi* now (1996) market leader and *Adon* having lost most of its market share after it stopped including pornographic material in order to promote a 'decent' image of homosexuality.

Transvestites and transsexuals have their own magazines, *Queen*, *Himawari* (Sun Flower) and *Cross Dressing*, the last of which ceased to appear after two issues. According to their editors, all sell about 7,000 copies bi-monthly and they thought that they were all bought by the same people. The new magazine *Nyū-hāfu Kurabu* (New-half Club) for *travestis* came to light in 1995 (Kuia Sutadiizu Henshū Iinkai ed. 1996a). While the public at large may not be much aware of it, there is a clear distinction between the world of the transvestites and transsexuals and that of gay men, the first two having different places and networks for meeting from the last. This even goes for cinemas. In the pornographic cinema Umeda Rose in Osaka, gay pornography was shown upstairs and straight pornography downstairs. The cashier downstairs said that downstairs was much more interesting because there came all sorts of people, such as *nyū-hāfu*, *josōsha* and the like, while upstairs there were only gay men.

There is much misunderstanding concerning the difference between homosexuality, transvestism and transsexuality. When I gave a talk about my research to students at my university in Japan I passed some gay magazines around. Some students were puzzled by the masculine images, which were at odds with their images of gay men. In many people's minds there is a clear link between male homosexuality and femininity in men and female homosexuality and masculinity in women. Both of these assumptions are influential for people in the process of constructing themselves in relation to their homosexual feelings. Visibility of difference plays a more important role in classifying people than their feelings or what activities they engage in, both of which are generally invisible.

The idea that someone can be gay or lesbian without any clearly visible features is for many people, including some who recognize that they themselves have homosexual feelings, difficult to perceive. While this may assist gay men and lesbian women by providing them with the privacy to investigate their feelings (Valentine 1997), it may also hinder them because they do not feel that they are, or do not wish to become, like *jōshiki* concerning homosexuality and, unless they learn of other ways of being lesbian or gay, they may have difficulty to recognize and accept their feelings. It often makes them afraid of visiting gay or lesbian places, events or groups. It also causes trouble for people who try to align themselves with constructions of masculinity or femininity.

## Femininity and Masculinity

The words *ooshii* and *memeshii* (masculine and feminine), stemming from the fauna terminology of *osu* and *mesu*, are, according to informants, presently regarded as *sabetsu yōgo* (discriminatory terms). Different from the rather rude terms *ooshii* and *memeshii* are the nowadays much-used terms *otokorashii* (manlike) and *onnarashii* (womanlike). While the former set of words refers to inalienable traits of people, the latter refers more to behavioural traits. Hence the frequent admonitions: *otokorashiku shinasai* (behave like a man) and *onnarashiku shinasai* (behave like a woman). One does not have to actually be one or the other but one has to behave like one or the other. In practice this means that those born with a vagina have to behave like a woman and those with a penis like a man. Men with feminine traits are more likely to be ridiculed than women with masculine traits, who as children may be seen as tomboys, which may be a source of pride.

The main lesbian network in Osaka even used *yancha* (tomboy) in their name, Yancha Lesbian Power (YLP), but later they changed the 'Y' into an 'O' which, according to them, may stand for *otona* (adult), *ōki na* (big), Osaka, or organization (OLP 1994). In 1996 'open' was added as a possibility to refer to the increasing openness among members about their sexuality (OLP 1997). They appear to have become ambivalent towards the childlikeness expressed by *yancha* but to be uncertain about how adult they wish to be. While women as small children may have a wider latitude of behaviour, when they start attending school femininity, expressed by demureness in attitude and speech, is expected of them (Higuchi 1986). Resistance against this seemed to be easier psychologically than in the case of men who do not wish to be masculine because the value attached to masculinity is higher than that attached to femininity.

Men who cannot manage to use masculine language and, for instance, keep referring to themselves as *watashi* instead of the more masculine *boku*, may feel uneasy about the way they are regarded (Fushimi 1991: 35). This seems to be more of a problem in Tokyo than in Osaka and Kyoto, where men in general are thought to be more feminine, while at the same time they have the aura of being romantic lovers, a difference that is similar to the difference attributed to the 'cool' northern Europeans as opposed to the 'warm' Latin lovers. Among informants from the Kansai area the use of *watashi* is quite common, among gay as well as straight men, but in Tokyo it is rare; it is only used by men when speaking to people older than themselves. Hirano Hiroaki, who grew up in Nagoya, could not make himself say the word *ore*, which is a degree more macho than *boku*, and referred to himself by the use of *boku*. He felt that as a result he was not accepted by his classmates (Hirano 1994: 182–3).

On the other hand, a lesbian interviewee avoided using *watashi* by referring to herself by her name. The popular singer Sasano Michiru writes that she uses *boku* in the lyrics of the songs she writes because she has difficulty coping with the use of *watashi*, the feminine connotation of which she finds incompatible with her desire to write from a personal and open perspective. She feels that writing from the standpoint of a woman would limit her creativity because a woman in Japanese culture is a gendered being in a manner with which her own feelings do not agree. By using *boku* she feels that she can overcome the sex divide, which obviously allows for more freedom of expression (Sasano 1995: 76–9). Of the respondents to a lesbian survey 13.1 per cent used *boku* to refer to themselves, 2.5 per cent *ore* and 15.6 per cent avoided all terms discussed here in favour of terms that have no masculine or feminine connotation, such as *uchi* (inside, often used to refer to inside groups) or *jibun* (self; Hirosawa and Rezubian Ripōto Han 1991: 171). While gay men may try to use masculine forms against their feelings, lesbian women may try to avoid using terminology that does not agree with their feelings, even though that terminology is the socially accepted one.

Among male interviewees, a considerable number had trouble during their childhood with not being as masculine as their environment expected of them. Apart from non-masculine behaviour and playing with girls, a light colour of skin, shortness and thinness were mentioned as physical features that are in conflict with masculinity. It appeared that physical features are more problematic than behavioural differences. Men who played with girls during childhood were usually not much troubled by parents and friends. Several male informants played with girls and with the support and approval of their mothers some learned to knit and to do needlework when they were children. Some interviewees who were short, thin, or had a light skin had become *ijimekko* (the victim of bullying), one saying that girls in his class had undressed him and fondled his genitals. While male homosexuality and femininity in men overlap in some cases, in many they do not and some heterosexual informants also felt that their feminine traits, which they saw as inalienable parts of themselves, caused them to be regarded as *hen* (weird). In *Barazoku* some cases were reported of gay men who were seen as *hen* at the offices where they worked and became the focus of jokes. This affected their well-being to the extent that they became mentally ill and, while one was welcomed back to his job after seeking medical care, the other had to find a different job (Itō, B. 1993, Oya Fukō 1993).

Experiences relating to masculinity at school are varied, as a discussion on a tape by Kamigata DJ Club shows. It starts with a man discussing what he calls 'overacting (*kasō ni enjiru*) masculinity', which most of his classmates did. He finds this weird (*hen*) and wonders where this image of masculinity stems from. While comparing those overacting men to *onabe*, he thinks that this overacting of masculinity may be a result of the existence of *okama*. This agrees with an explanation of the origin of homophobia: because men are afraid to recognize homosexual feelings in themselves they become uncertain when they are confronted with homosexuality in others and react in homophobic ways, which may be aggressive, ridiculing, or talkative. To counter the possibility of anyone thinking that they might be gay, they overact their masculinity (Harper 1992). The discussion on the tape continues as follows:

> A: If they sit in the company of people they always sit wide-legged. (. . .) But they don't always do that, if they return to their private rooms they'll sit like Amazons. (. . .)
> B: Really, such things must be a result of remnants of bad education: schools, in which you are taught that men should be men, that men are like that, are very common.
> C: It's tiresome, really, I hate it for being so conservative. (. . .) I became defiant (*hanpatsu shita*) because of it.
> B: I don't mean that they must behave according to the values of *okama* but why can't they act normally.
> (. . .)
> C: If they live naturally (*nachuraru ni*) straights (*nonke*) can also be my friends.
> B: Yeah, because they're natural (*shizen*). I didn't understand [what you meant] because I found people that agree with me (*jibun ni au*), people who live

> naturally. I think that that's why I lived without problems (*umaku ikita*) until now. People who are like [what you say, i.e. overacting], don't exist in my memory ( . . . ). Were there few of such [natural] people around you?
> A: I suppose you didn't look for them. At my high school there were no people with whom I got along (*mizu ga au*) in my class. If I could I was with people from other classes.
> (. . .)
> C: What a man is has been decided just like that (*katte ni*). Although we were born like we are, our environment says just like that that a man is so and so and because you have a willy (*chinchin*), you have to live so and so, that sort of thing.
> B: Yeah, that's really strong in Japan.
> C: I hate it terribly. It is not the same problem as loving men, that is another question, but I hate to be told to behave normally (*futsū ni*), to choose my clothes while keeping in mind that I am a man. (Kamigata DJ Club 1993: side one)

The last remark refers especially to the colour of clothes: colours like red, pink and purple are in general not deemed suitable for men (Lebra 1976: 78–9). Some gay men like to wear these colours because they like the colours and think they look good in them. While this discussion took place among gay men, there are also heterosexual men questioning the same matters. One interviewee took pride in being different by often wearing bright colours. Some young gay men followed Tsutamori Tatsuru's call for men to work on their beauty (Tsutamori 1990b) by shaving their legs. Body hair was generally seen as *kitanai* (dirty), even compared to that of northern Europeans, because Japanese body hair is black. Shaving legs was one way of trying to remain in the category of young and beautiful. Several men in the men's liberation group Menzu Ribu Kenkyūkai in the Kansai area explicitly stated that they participated because they felt strong disagreement with gender ascriptions and some thought that they were hampered in their possibilities because they failed to live up to general ideas of masculinity, which was mostly a problem in the workplace. Others stressed more political ideas about changing society by changing themselves and the perception of what is male and discovering ways of dealing with emotional problems, which they thought men had not been educated to do.

Within gay circles two opposing views concerning masculinity can de discerned. One is that gay men are just as masculine as heterosexual men, as presented by members of Occur from Tokyo, some of whom, like Niimi Hiroshi and Kazama Takashi, are portrayed in very masculine postures in the picture book *Couple*. They stand straddle-legged and have their arms crossed over the breast or in the pockets (Hashiguchi 1992). Niimi even said in an interview that he was 'perfectly male' (*kanzen na otoko*: Ida 1991). In Kansai groups this attitude is widely criticized. Central figures in OGC see the concept of masculinity as negative and associate it with conservative and uninteresting men, the *ossantachi* who are supposed to have the power in the Japanese establishment. The younger group Puapua, from which Gay Front Kansai has been formed, also placed gender-related problems high on the agenda (Morita 1993, 1994). A member, who is often called *obāchan* (granny) by fellow members, said he uses *onē-kotoba* (gay camp language) in order to distinguish himself from straight men (Uchikoshi 1995).

In Tokyo, at the annual national gay and lesbian groups' meeting organized by the JILGA in August 1992, the relation between discrimination against homosexuality and that against feminine men was the central theme during a plenary session. Negative attitudes towards feminine gay men were presented and a feminine man vented his anger at being discriminated against within gay circles that are supposed to further the liberation of gay men. Occur has been widely criticized for its stance that gay men are masculine because of its repressive qualities. Critics may agree that it is understandable that they wish to distance themselves from the feminine image of gay men that has often been presented in the media but that does not make it acceptable. A member of Puapua thinks that it would be good to agree that all three categories, transvestites, male-to-female transsexuals and gay men, are confronted with the derogatory term *okama*, which makes it desirable that they do not fight amongst each other but work together for improvement of their positions (Morita 1994). This idea has gained ground since then and many contacts and ways of cooperation between groups and individuals of the various categories have developed recently, evidenced by two publications in 1996 which combine all these categories and more under the heading of 'queer' (Fushimi 1996, Kuia Sutadiizu Henshū Iinkai ed. 1996b).

Within lesbian circles such problems do not play much of a role. While lesbian women of LIO (Lesbians in Occur), when appearing on television, stressed that they liked femininity in women, particularly referring to beautiful long hair, I found no antipathy towards women with masculine features among lesbian women. In LIO and other circles there are women with short hair and androgynous clothing, as well as women with feminine looks. A member of LIO said that she was shocked by a woman who called the lesbian information line and asked what they looked like. The caller seemed to think that lesbian women looked like professional wrestlers (*puro-resurā*) and all had short hair. Lesbian women of the generation that became active in relation to the *ūman ribu* (women's lib) movement in the 1970s tend to be more androgynous in their looks. Two reasons can be found for this. They are older, and older women in Japan in general use less make-up than women whose age dictates that they are in the market for marriage and from whom the environment demands more conformity to *jōshiki* concerning femininity. Further, older lesbian women are often connected to the women's liberation movement of the 1970s, which often dictated that women should not make themselves attractive to please men, in the context of which beauty contests have been much criticized (Ehara 1992c, Sechiyama 1992, Yoshizawa 1992).

A woman who was taught women's studies at a progressive university in Kyoto was not interested in feminism at all and found it apalling when a classmate said that she should not wear skirts or make-up. Later she experienced sexual harassment in her workplace and became involved in feminist activities but she continues to wear make-up. A *feminisuto* who has been important in giving feminist women back the opportunity to care about the way they look and to dress femininely is Ueno Chizuko, who described the positive feelings that can result from caring about one's looks (1988a, 1989) and even the tactical use of looks (1991c). According to some informants, she herself used to wear *bodikon* clothes, clothes that show the lines of the body to its advantage. She has cut her long hair short now but her clothes remain highly fashionable. Her sports car causes a few raised eyebrows in some feminist circles as well. She was criticized by some informants who thought that it was wrong for a woman to use her looks to further her goals.

An interviewee who was in the process of a sex change from male to female became a major topic at a party when 'he', as most people present saw her, said that she was a lesbian woman. Since most people present saw her as a man, and as regards her genitals, she still was a man at that time, she was heavily criticized for assuming this position. She had the courage to speak out because she had a lesbian girlfriend and was accepted by lesbian circles, which greatly boosted her confidence. One of the people present, a gay man, criticized her and thought that she could not appropriate the label of lesbian because she did not talk in a 'lesbian manner'. He thought that she was using 'masculine' ways of expression and gave the example of her saying that *rezu* was a wrong word to use because it was linked to pornography. While this problem had been pointed out by Kakefuda Hiroko (1992a), whose book the man liked very much, he now thought that a lesbian woman would not use such general theories (*ippanron*) but start from her personal feelings. This view stemmed from his contacts with feminist women, with whom he was involved in AIDS-related activities. In that context masculine ways of reasoning are seen as characterized by the tendency to use *ippanron* as opposed to feminine ways of reasoning that start from personal experience.

While overall in Japanese society this vision of masculinity as related to *ippanron* and femininity to personal arguments may emerge, it is not always true and both among feminist women who label themselves as *feminisuto* and among lesbian women, 'masculine' ways of reasoning are common. The case above shows that transsexuality is in Japan, as elsewhere (Bornstein 1994), one of the phenomena most likely to lead to heated discussions among people who are involved in sexual politics. If she had been born with female genitals, this discussion would not have developed, no matter how 'masculine' her reasoning was. As people involved in sexual and gender politics often divide everything into male and female, masculine and feminine, it is difficult to accommodate people who do not fit in readily.

## Talking Sex and Having Sex

Discourses concerning sex in Japan can be divided into three types, whereby I write 'can be' to indicate that there are more ways than the one employed here. One is the pornographic discourse, strongly characterized by violence, rape and sadomasochism, opposed to which there is a discourse characterized by disgust over violence and rape, pornography and prostitution, which has been a major feature of feminist constructions of sex in Japan (Ogura 1988, Minamoto 1991, Yamashita, A. 1991, Ehara 1992c, Hashizume 1992, Sechiyama 1992, Tajima 1992). Lately this discourse has come under fire from critics within feminist circles (Ōgoshi 1991) and feminists have started to discuss sex also as part of human relationships rather than only in terms of something loathsome and dirty (Uemura 1988, Kawano 1990), and to question men on their sexual activities (Onna no Sei to Sei o Kanagaeru Bunkakai 1991).

This leads the way to a third discourse, the influence of which is growing. It is characterized by a liberal attitude towards sexual activity, sometimes even including rape and violence and always including sadomasochism (Tazaki 1993a, b), which is increasingly a trendy subject to discuss. In gay pornography as well as heterosexual pornography, sadomasochism plays a major role (e.g. *Sabu*, *S & M Sunaipā* [S & M sniper], *SM Hishōsetsu* [Secret SM novels], *SM Tōkō Supesharu* [SM contributions special]). Pornography is looked at in more than one way. It is argued that gay pornography cannot be caught under the general heading of oppression of women (Fushimi 1992) and that women can also enjoy pornography (Kakefuda 1992b, 1993), culminating in the small-scale production of lesbian pornography by and for lesbian women starting in 1995 (the soft *Kusukusu* or *XX* and the hard-core *Okazu* [Side dish]), although the idea that it is incomprehensible that women may enjoy pornography in which they are victimized is still very much in evidence (Fujitani 1992).

Much is written on *hentai* sex, from anal intercourse (e.g. Ichikawa 1991, Kanezuka 1993, Tazaki 1993a) to bondage (e.g. Sawaragi 1991), fetishism (e.g. Mutsuki 1991) and sadomasochism (e.g. Kitahara 1991, Nakada 1991, Tazaki 1993a), and even people who have been convicted of murder and cannibalism may get space to vent their experience (Sagawa 1991). A persistent element in this genre is the idea that such practices are much more widespread in Europe and America (Tomonari 1991), which mirrors the writing on sexuality in Japan in the press in Western countries. This idea is supported by the existence of flourishing sadomasochist toy shops in England, whereas in Japan they hardly exist.

A male interviewee, who often talked about sadomasochism and opened a shop selling attributes for sadomasochist play, said that he did not engage in it himself with his lover. The widespread appearance of sadomasochism in pornographic videos and magazines suggests that many people are excited by it as a fantasy but not many seem to engage in it themselves. A reason why sadomasochism is so abundant in Japanese pornography can also be found in the law that prohibits showing penises and vaginas, due to which copulation scenes can not be presented without black dots or mosaic over the sex organs, making producers look for other ways to produce exciting footage. Among my lovers in Japan those who ventured to employ sadomasochist ways of pleasure pursuit limited it to the softest forms. Games in which *ijimeru* (tease, abuse) and *semeru* (tease, torture), mostly in the form of restraining the movements of the other while making him or her reach a climax, play a role are quite common.

Among lesbian informants outright sadomasochism appeared to be more popular. Several lesbian informants even came to London in order to buy toys and go to sadomasochist parties. Nevertheless, I do not believe that sadomasochist activities are more common among lesbian women than any other category in Japan. It is most likely that there was a bias among the people I met.[3] A survey among almost 1,000 university students by the Yajima seminar shows that women are less likely to want to get involved in experimenting with various ways of sexual expression than men, except when it comes to homosexual activity (Asahi 1994, Kawakoshi 1994, Miyauchi 1994, Ōshima 1994, Umeyama 1994).

Talking about sex in a personal and serious manner is largely prohibited by discourses concerning it. In general, sex is regarded as *asobi* (play) and not seen as an activity decent people discuss, including in academic contexts. *Etchi* is a word that is much used to refer to sexual activities. Explanations about its origins vary from the idea that it is the Anglo-Japanese pronunciation of the letter 'H,' said originally to stand for *hentai* or *hentaisei* (queer, abnormal or queerness, abnormality: Constantine 1992: 37–8, Tazaki 1993a: 34) to the idea of an informant that it stems from sexual activities with American GIs during the occupation, whereby the 'H' refers to the letter between the 'G' and the 'I'. Yet another informant thought it might represent the first letter of *harenchi,* which means shamelessness or impudence. I initially thought that it stemmed from *erochikku* (erotic) because that comprises most of the meanings in which it is used. In a gay *manga,* for example, a man asks his lover not to undress because he finds his *sarariiman* suit so *etchi* (Yamazaki 1993). *Etchi* is also used to refer to sexual activity and anything that is sexually exciting. A young gay informant, for instance, said that he had done *sukoshi etchi* (a bit of *etchi*) with a former teacher, which referred to mutual masturbation. When watching pornographic videos at a clandestine video shop in Osaka, people used *etchi* to refer to scenes and actors they found particularly exciting.

This attitude was widespread among men but among women talk of sex often produced a more serious mood. A lesbian interviewee thought that women could not discuss sex because they lacked the words for it, but this seems to have changed considerably lately and, increasingly, informants showed no sign of lacking words for discussing sex in ways similar to men. A *feminisuto* thought that she had a very good relationship with a close friend because they could talk about everything, even about sex, which suggests that discussing sex is very uncommon in her environment. The tendency not to talk about sex in a personal way by and among *feminisuto* might be a result of their marginality within the academic world in which sex is not considered to be a proper subject for discussion, unless it is in terms of syndromes and illnesses and only in terms of 'other people' or 'research populations'.

Female informants were often little concerned with finding lust in sex. An interviewee called me to ask advice about how to react towards the advances of a married man at her job. She wondered whether it was morally wrong for her to comply. Her main concern was whether she was wronging someone else, i.e. his wife, not whether she wished to have sex with him or what was in her own interest. Indeed, few female informants seemed to care much about themselves when it concerned sex. One was shocked after she had sex with a member of a foreign pop group and her boyfriend dumped her saying that she was stupid because she had expected him to accept her escapade like she had accepted his before. Another informant tries to enjoy sex but has difficulty finding men who are not boring. She wrote about her experiences and ideas, concluding that in general her feelings with regard to sex are characterized by a feeling of prostituting herself (Shibuya 1990). Similarly, Dumb Type's Bubu, who works as a prostitute or sex worker (*sekkusu wākā*), as she prefers to refer to herself, felt that having sex with her ex-husband was at times not essentially different. Similarly, Fukushima Mizuho as a teenager, thinking that for a women there was only the choice between housewife and prostitute, thought that it would be preferable to be a prostitute to devoting all her life to one man because being a prostitute gives more freedom (Fukushima 1991b: 95). She found a third option, though, and became a career woman instead.

At a discussion with the performance group Dumb Type in preparation for the *Seminar Show for S/N* performance staged in March 1993 in Kyoto, a woman said that she did not wish to have sex because she could not stand the idea of lying underneath a man. In her eyes, heterosexual sex meant that a man was lying on top of her grinding his penis inside her vagina. This, indeed, seems to be the general picture people in Japan have of sex that is not *hentai*. Hirano Hiroaki of OGC wrote an essay concerning the way sex is constructed around the penis and that sex in the minds of most people seems to consist of sticking the penis into one orifice or another: the mouth, the vagina, or the anus (Hirano 1994: 184–207). The typical pattern of heterosexual sex in pornography as well as in heterosexual relationships is that the woman resists weakly and says things like: 'Please stop', only to gradually become excited and overcome by her feelings of lust. The English writer John David Morley also describes heterosexual sex in Japan in this vein (Morley 1985).

Many women are not very pleased with this pattern of heterosexual sex and grow tired of pleasing men without having much pleasure themselves and resort to masturbation (Baba 1988, Moa Ripōto Han ed. 1983). This attitude has been linked to the so-called 'second virgin syndrome', i.e. women who decide to return to celibacy after having been sexually active for a while. This is again an example of the liberal use of the word 'syndrome'. Most women interviewed for a book on it did not have sex for one or two years after separating from boyfriends (Mizuno 1992). Not having sex for a while hardly warrants the label of 'syndrome', unless one should regard the commonplace as illness. Others put up with their husbands' and boyfriends' desires because 'it can't be helped', or 'because he will become aggressive otherwise' (Moa Ripōto Han ed. 1983: 512–13). Among 34 feminist women who were asked how they thought about love with men, 12 thought that love with men was possible, one that it was impossible, 11 that love was not something to strive for, that it was a mere illusion, and 10 had opinions at odds with this division, one of them, Fujieda Mioko, criticizing it for its heterosexist implications: love as presented in the survey questions was heterosexual love (Ueno ed. 1990).

Similarly, in a book on the history of sexuality in Japan, sexuality appears to mean heterosexuality: homosexuality is wholly ignored (Teruoka 1992). Large-scale research has been conducted on sexuality but it invariably ignores the possibility of homosexuality (Moa Ripōto Han ed. 1983, Kyōdō Tsūshin. 1984, Baba 1988, Munakata and Tajima eds 1992). In Ueno Chizuko's work the existence of homosexuality is not ignored but the contents deal only with homosexuality in America and in its most visible forms in Japan, both of which are not very informative about homosexuality in Japan in general (Ueno 1988a, 1989, 1991a, 1992). Female sexuality is mostly discussed in terms of men who do not please and how to find satisfactory relationships (Uemura 1988, Kawano 1990, Tajima 1992). Discussed least seriously of all is the sexuality of heterosexual men. Very little material exists on men who visit prostitutes (Fukushima 1991b), which is a feature also present in Western discourses (Hart 1994).

Two male informants were raped when they were children, one by a neighbour when he was 8 years old, twenty-five years before he told me, and the other as a 13-year-old. The latter said during the interview that he was raped when in boarding school by classmates and used it to explain further developments in his life. Women who were raped usually saw it as part of an abusive relationship and did not stress the rape itself as being of any particular significance. In the weekly magazine *Asahi Journal* a discussion developed after Matsuura Rieko, who has been raped herself, said that *feminisuto* should not get so upset about rape and that it was not really of great importance (Andachi and Matsuura 1992). This was strongly criticized by women who felt that such pronouncements hurt rape victims (e.g. Murayama 1992). Among female informants rape appeared to be taken as an extreme form of sexual harassment when it concerned relationships at work. Sexual harassment itself has only recently become recognized as a problem. Until then it was standard for victims to 'cry themselves to sleep (*nakineiri*)', a common attitude also among other victims, such as those of industrial pollution (Kawamura 1994: 131).

The construction of sex as sticking a penis into an orifice makes it plausible that most people think that homosexual activity between men consists of anal intercourse, which within a gay context may be represented by the chrysanthemum and the sword (*kiku to katana*). Ruth Benedict probably did not know this when she used the symbols to represent Japanese culture (Benedict 1977). Hashimoto Osamu complained because she robbed him of a book title that would have fitted his book on Japanese gay men (Hashimoto 1986: 55). A gay informant even bought Benedict's *Kiku to Katana* in the 1960s because he expected it to be on homosexuality. Hashimoto resorted to using the lotus (*hasu*) instead of the chrysanthemum, which he uses to represent what he calls *gokuraku chinko* (happy-go-lucky willy). In this book, *Hasu to Katana* (The lotus and the sword), Hashimoto, like Hirano, criticizes the simplistic focus on anal intercourse and advocates other ways of reaching sexual satisfaction (Hashimoto 1986, Hirano 1994). My own experience with Japanese, interview results and written sources such as personal advertisements in gay magazines, indicate that ways of having sex other than anal intercourse are common among gay Japanese men. Many informants explicitly stated that they 'cannot have anal sex', usually referring to the inability to receive a penis but sometimes also the inability to penetrate. In addition there are many who do not like anal sex.

The construction of sex as sticking a penis into an orifice also denies the possibility of sex between women. Non-lesbian informants, indeed, wondered how on earth women could have sex with each other, '*penisu ga nai no ni* (even though they have no penis)'. While in more streetwise circles possibilities such as rubbing clitorises against each other and oral sex may be known (Constantine 1992: 140), many people seem not to be able to imagine such possibilities. Lesbian pornography, made for men, is the form of pornography that is most under fire from those who want to protect youth from 'bad influences'. For example, the Osaka prefectural government established a local ruling (*jōrei*) which made it illegal to sell lesbian pornographic cartoons and picture collections in shops where minors go. They called this 'homosexual pornography', which gave rise to complaints from gay groups in the area, who felt that their freedom of information was endangered. Some gay magazines are important sources of information on what is happening in Japan and abroad (*Adon*, *Barazoku*, *Badi*) and they and the others are important for making contact with other gay men (Morita 1992b, Dōseiai Kaihō Undō Dantai Puapua 1992). Gay groups' complaints made the Osaka prefectural government see that this ruling was discriminatory and it was amended (Hattori 1996). In lesbian circles *minikomi* are the major means of spreading information and keeping contact, and until recently in the above-mentioned *XX* and *Okazu*, these *minikomi* contained no pornography.

An important and influential discourse concerning homosexuality has been developed since the mid-1970s by authors of *shōjo manga* (girls' comics), who describe homosexual relationships between boys or men. The presentation of homosexual relationships in them is very romantic and the protagonists are invariably beautiful. Japanese scholars discuss gay *shōjo manga* addressing the question of why they are popular among young women (Aoyama 1988, Ogura 1991, Fujimoto 1991, Matsui 1993, Tanigawa 1993) and ignoring the fact that many of them are bought by boys and men. Apart from reading the *manga*, they do little research into the question of why young women like them but merely philosophize, wondering, for instance, whether girls find it easier to read about sex in which no women are involved and such. Many gay informants read these *manga* when they were at high school and later, which leads me to believe that at least part of their success is due to the fact that men read them. *June*, a magazine that based itself on the genre, increasingly leans towards gay magazines, including drawings by Kimura Ben, who also draws for the gay magazine *Sabu*.

Women who read gay *shōjo manga* said that they thought that the drawings of the boys, who often are very androgynous or feminine, were *suteki* (attractive) and that they felt attracted by the romantic stories, which is what male informants also said. They are said to be stories to dream away from daily reality, even if they are increasingly realistic. Often they are set in future or past times and/or in foreign countries. The gay writer Fushimi Noriaki recognizes that the presentation of homosexuality in *shōjo manga* is at variance with reality but since his childhood days he has enjoyed reading them and he could reassure *manga* writer Yoshida Akemi that he does not feel that she is hurting gay men (Yoshida and Fushimi 1992, Fushimi 1993). Satō Masaki, however, sees the explicit depiction of gay sex in *yaoi*, which is a hard-core pornographic sub-genre of these *manga*, as homophobic, which led to a lengthy discussion between him and women who enjoy reading and drawing such material. While Satō maintains that a false image of gay men is being misused for the pleasure of women (e.g. Satō 1996), his opponents maintain that *yaoi* has no relation to male homosexuality as it actually exists and is only part of a world of fantasy which should be allowed freedom of expression (e.g. Tanigawa 1995).[4]

While readers of *manga* are of course aware that they do not depict reality and idealize and romanticize homosexual relationships to a great extent, I found several women who referred to them as a reason why they became interested in meeting gay men in real life. For young gay men they were supportive in the sense that they provide something positive to identify with and especially since some of the newest publications often deal with problems with family and colleagues or classmates in contemporary situations (Akisato 1986, 1992, Takaguchi 1991, 1993),[5] they give them something to compare themselves to. I found that young gay men who dislike the gay magazines for their pornographic character often like *shōjo manga*.

*Shōjo manga* most likely have contributed to positive attitudes towards homosexuality among women and gay men. Some gay bars nowadays are frequented by heterosexual women who like to be with gay men. They are called *okoge* (fag hags), after the burnt residue that sticks to the *okama* (cooking pot). It is this phenomenon that is discussed in the special feature in *Crea* on homosexuality that marked the start of what came to be called the *gei būmu* (gay boom) in the mass media (*Crea* 1991) and it is also the theme of a book, *Okoge*, later made into a film, which toured Japan with considerable success in 1992 (Nakajima, T. 1992). At a workshop someone suggested that the popularity of films about gay men among young women in Japan is due to the fact that they are filmed from a female viewpoint. This may be true for some Japanese films but the explanation does not agree with the fact that the English film *Maurice* or the Canadian film *No Skin off my Ass*, in which women hardly play a role, are equally popular. *Shōjo manga* on gay men also often feature very few women playing an active part. It appears that the aesthetics of male homosexuality, combined with the socially subversive aspect of their love, which makes it the quintessence of true love, are what draw women towards them.

In contrast to the often positive depictions in *shōjo manga*, homosexuality is in Japan widely seen as *iyarashii* (disgusting) or *kimochiwarui* (sickening), as a result of which many gay men and lesbian women think of it as *hazukashii* (shameful). These labels are methods of dismissing a phenomenon, rather than being related to strong feelings and in that sense they are rather superficial. They are *jōshiki* which keep order in a system of thought that does not consider homosexuality seriously (Shibatani 1990: 129). If people are confronted by someone who presents her or himself as lesbian or gay they may not see that person as *iyarashii* or *kimochiwarui*, which in general refers rather to activities than states of being. Sex as such is often seen as *iyarashii* and many gay men think of it as such as well, although they do not often think that they themselves are particularly *iyarashii*. They may think that certain sexual activities are and that sex for the pursuit of lust and unrelated to love is *iyarashii*. *Hazukashii* is anything concerning sex when it becomes known or visible. As long as no one knows, there is nothing to be ashamed about. An interviewee at whose house I stayed brought me to the station because I had much luggage and he wanted to help me carry it. He thought it was *hazukashii* to walk next to me because people would know that he was gay. This did not concern people who actually knew him, because they know that he is gay, but rather people who do not know him. At a Christmas party with a gay circle participants were asked to bring underpants for a gift exchange. Those who received sexy and scanty briefs like G-strings and Y-fronts screamed: '*hazukashii*', while many others had bought large boxer shorts, which are seen as erotically neutral. Notwithstanding Ueno Chizuko's idea that single men wear boxer shorts because they can wear them longer than briefs so that they have less laundry (Ueno 1989), I believe that they wear them because briefs come only in two varieties, the traditional large ones their fathers wear and the new sexy ones, which only became generally available in the 1990s and may be seen as making sex objects of those who wear them. Especially in the case of students who often bathe at public baths (*sentō*), where their underwear is exposed, the type of underwear they wear may be subject to much consideration.

Words like *iyarashii* can be used in a positive sense. In pornography the words *iyarashii*, *kimochiwarui* and especially *hazukashii* are frequently used to add to the excitement. Sex is all these things and it seems that the subversive character attributed to it is what makes it interesting to many people. An outright sadist lover used these words frequently when we played, referring to various poses and activities.

## Circles: Discussing the Self and the Other

Rather than giving an outline of all the various circles and discussing their activities in detail, this section intends to describe some of the debates that exist within categories and between them. Reasons for joining circles are often multiple. Making friends can be more important than a political goal. This is especially true for people engaging in gay and lesbian circles, some of which are solely oriented towards leisure. However, women may also engage in politically oriented groups because they like the atmosphere rather than because they subscribe to the political aims. The function of some gay circles was explicitly to provide a *yasuragi no ba* (a place to feel at ease, to relax), where stress could be released. This suggests that they may be seen as replacing a function of the *uchi* (home), which according to *jōshiki* is the place where men can release their tensions and feel at ease.

### Feminist Women

Most feminist informants in their 40s started their feminist activities in the 1970s under the banner of *ūman ribu* (women's lib), which is a word some still use. They do not call themselves *ūman ribā* (women's libber) and they rarely call themselves *feminisuto*, which according to them refers to women working at universities and engaging in and writing books in the area of women's studies, or, as one of them said, is widely understood in Japan to mean a gallant man. Women engaged in *ūman ribu* said that they are different from the academic, well-known *feminisuto* because they engage in grassroots activities and often do not follow the intellectual debates of *feminisuto*, although they enjoy seeing *feminisuto* like Ueno Chizuko or Tajima Yōko win an argument in live and televised debates.

Ueno Chizuko has been criticized for using male language, for ignoring the realities in the dreary lives of poor women (Yamashita, E. 1991) and for riding on the waves of popularity and thereby creating distance from women who might otherwise become interested in feminism (Ehara 1992a). These critiques partly seem to be the result of Ueno's very popularity, and also of the fact that she transcends norms concerning the behaviour of feminist scholars. To the critique that she uses men's language, Ueno replied that she, indeed, is a 'freak' who does not fit neatly into the gender patterns of Japan. She is neither fully woman nor fully man and there is nothing wrong with that (Ueno 1993: 124–7). Nobody can ignore the fact that Ueno has brought growing attention to feminist ideas, which was most likely greatly helped by the fact that her language is understood by many men. Among my informants it appeared that Ueno is read more by men, while women prefer Ogura Chikako's work, which they see as more personal and direct but which is less liked by men because they think that she is too negative about men (Ogura 1988, 1989, 1991).

The generation of women around 30 years old or younger who engage in feminist grassroots activities feel they do not have much in common with *ūman ribu*, which in their way of thinking seems to be represented by Chūpiren, a group that had a brief but loud history in the 1970s and aimed at legalizing the contraceptive pill. This group split off from the group that set up Shinjuku Ribu Sentā, a centre in Tokyo where feminist activities were organized, after Chūpiren's founder, Enoki Misako, wrote a report on the use of the pill which blatantly ignored the disadvantages the other women wanted to be included. Enoki has even been accused of being an agent for the pharmaceutical industry because of her uncritical advocacy of the pill and because she disappeared after her movement's failure (Akiyama 1991). The group's activities were characterized by storming on to stages and making their claims – a lesbian interviewee remembered that they once stormed the stage at the yearly New Year's Eve television show *Kōhaku Uta Gassen*, in which the male singers, dressed in white, compete with female singers, dressed in red – and the ensuing press coverage gave the whole *ūman ribu* movement a bad name that still resonates.

Nevertheless, feminists who do not label themselves as such but engage in grassroots activities are the successors to the *ūman ribu* movement of the 1970s, even if they do not ascribe to it. Some of them can be found in groups like Pāpuru: Sei Bōryoku o Yurusanai Onnatachi no Kai (Purple: Women's Group against Sexual Violence), which fights sexual harassment and is one of the most radical feminist groups in Japan. Pāpuru split off from Onnatachi no Rōdō Kumiai (Women's Labour Union) after an internal fight over a case in which a member was sexually harassed by a man from a labour union with which they collaborated. While the women of Pāpuru wanted to take on the case and sue the man in question, the others felt sorry for his wife and wanted to keep things quiet. An interviewee of Onnatachi no Rōdō Kumiai said that they should not be too radical because that would only serve to make them inaccessible to women caught up in labour disputes. This is also a reason why they do not use words like *feminisuto* or *ūman ribu* to refer to themselves.

Feminist women may participate in meetings like those of the gay circle OGC and many were present at the Onna no Fesutibaru (Women's Festival), which is held every year in Kyoto in relation to International Women's Day in March. This festival is an *ūman ribu* type of happening rather than one dominated by *feminisuto*, who tend to meet more in *kenkyūkai* or *gakkai* (study meetings / seminars or conferences). The difference between *feminisuto* and other women's liberationists may be somewhat overconstructed because there are also academics engaging in grassroots activities and because the large majority of women's liberationists do not label themselves at all. The majority of women described above just do what they feel they should do, a trend that can be seen in many places in the Japan of the early 1990s. Working without labels seems to be more effective because most labels have negative connotations attached to them.

*Feminisuto* in their 40s have shown prejudice towards homosexuality, such as Ueno Chizuko who wrote that gay men are women-haters and lesbian women men-haters (Ueno 1991a: 13–14) but also others who tended to be prejudiced about lesbian women and had concluded from some rare meetings that they are man-hating. While, as discussed in the introduction (p. 25), there has been a group of lesbian feminists who wanted to have nothing to do with men and there probably still are lesbian women who hate men, I did not meet lesbian women who were against men only because they were men, even among informants who are radically feminist. The idea of gay men and lesbian women as hating the other sex was in all cases caused by basing a judgement on apparently fragmentary knowledge.

This could be called homophobia but in all cases the informants changed their positions after I commented that I knew many lesbian women in Japan who do not hate men or, in the case of Ueno, after gay men and lesbian women in Japan criticized her and provided the information to prove that she was wrong. Thus, prejudice can easily be replaced by providing proper knowledge, which makes this 'homophobia' seem far less deeply rooted than that one may find in Western countries, where offered information is often not listened to. A feminist woman who herself was described by *feminisuto* as the prime example of a *sōsharu rezubian* (social lesbian) thought that women become lesbian because they find men unlikeable. I did not meet any *rezubian* who thought that and such reasoning is refuted by most lesbian women who, like gay men, generally maintain that their homosexuality is part of their inner most being.

## Lesbian Women

Lesbian women have been among the most radical feminist women in Japan but the fact that those who brought this contribution to feminism are lesbian women is hardly recognized. Some ten years ago Ueno Chizuko even wrote that, unlike in America, lesbian women had little influence within the women's movement in Japan (Ueno 1991a: 120–3). Lesbian women who are active in feminist groups said that they did not think that others knew that they were lesbian and that they thought it did not really matter because it was more important to share feminist activities in sisterhood (*shisutāfuddo*). As a result, lesbian women are often not recognized as such within feminist circles and sexuality is not discussed. An interviewee from Pāpuru said that she did not know what the sexual preference of most of the group members was and some time after the interview commented that she had been investigating her own feelings, which led her to wonder whether she was lesbian herself.

In 1984 the lesbian group Regumi (Le Group, whereby 'Le' stands for 'lesbian') was founded by women who came together from feminist scenes and from the lesbian bar scene in Shinjuku (Hisada 1991). Some years later Regumi Sutajio (Studio) was founded. This is an office space where meetings can be held, where a telephone line is set up for people seeking contact and which is the base where *Regumi Tsūshin*, the newsletter of

Regumi, is produced. Interviewees who are active in Regumi said that this space, which is located in a building where feminist organizations are assembled, is surrounded by heterosexual women who do not know very well how to deal with the presence of a lesbian organization in their midst. Lesbian circles are loosely organized and tend to place much stress on talking or partying together. Regumi is not really a group but rather a loose network which offers the possibility for women to use a space and a name under which to develop activities.

Not until the early 1990s did lesbian women start to discuss being lesbian at major women's conferences in Japan. The first time was at the Asian Women's Conference in Tokyo in the spring of 1992, which was repeated two weeks later in Osaka. In the plenary session a lesbian woman from Thailand spoke about lesbian women in Asia, stressing the need for an economic base for a woman to be able to maintain a lesbian lifestyle, that is to be able to remain unmarried and to take care of her own financial needs. This is endorsed by the case of a women's community in Kwangtung (Guangdong) in southern China, where women could live independently from men because they had the power to earn an income through a particular form of agriculture that did not exist elsewhere in China (Sankar 1986).

At the same conferences lesbian women held workshops about being lesbian, which lesbian women I spoke with afterwards found unsatisfying because heterosexual feminists attending were only interested in the question of how they have sex, which was not a topic the lesbian women wished to discuss. They felt that demands by heterosexual feminists of lesbian women that they reveal their sexual activities, while heterosexual feminists remain silent about their own, was a form of unwarranted curiosity.

Ueno Chizuko was widely attacked for her critique of Kakefuda's book, in which she states that Kakefuda writes about many things but omits discussing her (Ueno's) point of interest: lesbian sex (Kakefuda 1992a, Ueno 1992). Her critics read in her article a confirmation of what they perceive as her insensitivity concerning homosexuality (Asakura 1992, Irokawa 1992, Hirano 1993).[6] While such critics have a point, it must be remembered that Ueno wrote about homosexuality at a time when most scholars wholly neglected it, and thereby helped to pave the way for more discussion. In March 1993 lesbian mothers were the theme of a workshop at the Women's Festival in Kyoto, which led to a more satisfactory discussion, according to lesbian informants. Grassroots feminists in general seemed to be more open towards lesbian women than *feminisuto,* who tended to draw conclusions after hearing very little instead of questioning their own beliefs and feelings.

Constructions of lesbian women often follow American constructions and the influence of international feminist contacts is clearly present, although the meanings may vary somewhat. They include *sōsharu rezubian* (social lesbian), which refers to close female friendships, *chotto rezu* (a bit lesbian), which refers to women who are dissatisfied with having sex with men and may try lesbian sex, political lesbian, which refers to lesbian women who say that they are lesbian for feminist reasons and *rezubian separetisuto,* lesbian separatist, which was explained by a woman who labelled herself as such as lesbian women who want to have meetings and *gasshuku* without women who are not sure what their sexual preference is or who say that they are bisexual.

Political lesbians, i.e. women who say that they became lesbian for political reasons, exist in the generation of *ūman ribu* who became active in the 1970s but Kakefuda Hiroko thought that this construction was nonsensical (Kakefuda 1992a). When I interviewed her, she explained that she understood that people may explain their sexual preference in that manner but that she thought that it was an explanation developed after the fact. Many younger lesbian women thought that the labels above were superfluous constructions and that women who use them, mostly lesbian and heterosexual feminists, were *katai* (tough, difficult) and had irrelevant theoretical discussions. Calling themselves *rezubian* was quite enough and they did not need all these different labels. In 1995 a new trend developed to use *bian*, the last part of *rezubian*, developed, which seems to suggest that the word *rezubian* is still one found difficult to take in one's mouth by many of the women in question, which may have to do with the difference in perception of the scope of feelings of women for women in a Western and in a Japanese context, as Kakefuda said.

## Gay Men

Liberal people are sometimes at a loss as to what word to use to describe gay men because they all have negative connotations. There may even be a danger that people start to avoid discussing homosexuality for fear of unintentionally discriminating against gay men, as happened with the *burakumin*, a 'special status group' or outcastes (Ohnuki-Tierney 1987), the discussion of whom is taboo in many contexts (Pharr 1990). *Homo* is most widely understood to have the same meaning as 'gay' in English – which is one of the reasons why I agreed to use it in the title of a Japanese publication on homosexuality in the Netherlands, the other being that *homo* is also the common and most neutral Dutch word for gay (Lunsing 1994c) – but in some gay activist circles it is attacked because it is an abbreviation of *homosekushuaru*, and 'abbreviations are derogatory', which seems to be an idea imported from America (Lunsing 1996b).

The word *gei*, which is their choice, obviously based on the homophony with the English gay, meant at the time of my fieldwork to most other Japanese, including sociologists and the like, transvestite or transsexual. When I used it in an essay, the liberal Buddhist monk who reviewed it thought that it was *sabetsu yōgo* (discriminatory terminology) until I clarified that gay activists advocate its use. Since they have been very tenacious in using *gei*, it has become a common term in the media and for the first time gay men in Japan appear to have succeeded in influencing the wording used to speak of them. Lately, however, words like *homo* and *okama* are once again increasingly used for self-labelling and there are even people who see the use of *gei* as homophobic because of its trendy connotations and because negative Japanese connotations accompanying *homo* and *okama* are thus avoided instead of being dealt with (Onitsuka 1996).

Many gay men call the world of gay bars and other localities *kono sekai* (this world), which clearly refers to otherworldliness. Terms for becoming involved in gay scenes include *kono sekai ni hairu* and *kono michi ni hairu* (to enter this world and to enter this way) and the more negative *kono michi/sekai ni ochiiru* (to fall down to this way/world). These terms are still much in use and to those who use them in relation to themselves they have no negative connotation. The world of gay bars is, however, patronized by only a minority of gay men. While it is well-known that one of the largest concentrations of gay bars in numbers in the world exists in Tokyo, these numbers may be misleading because most of them are very tiny, some seating no more than a maximum of eight persons (Lunsing 1994a).

Some nights the bars remain virtually empty – I once spent the night on my own with a waiter until five o'clock in the morning without any other customer arriving – and on other nights there may be but a small number of customers. All in all, about ten customers might be the average number of customers per gay bar per night at most, which means that no more than 2,000 gay men visit Shinjuku's over 200 gay bars (Lunsing 1994a) on average nights. Adding to this the gay bars in Ueno and other areas of Tokyo, the number still remains well below 5,000, compared to a population of 30 million in the area. Occur's survey shows that many gay men do not go to bars, whether for lack of money or for lack of interest (Ugoku Gei. 1992). Occur maintains that gay bars are not sufficient for living a gay lifestyle. They want to be gay for twenty-four hours a day, not for a couple of hours in the evening (ibid.). Like many other circles, they organize events like hiking in the mountains, picnics, sports events or visits to temples, shrines and other tourist spots to further the goal of being gay the whole day, besides their political activities.

In 1986 Occur split off from JILGA, which was founded in 1984 when the Swedish president of the ILGA (International Lesbian and Gay Organization) came to Japan and visited Minami Teishirō (Minami 1990). Foreign influence is thus undeniably present in the formation of gay movements in Japan. Minami succeeded in setting up branches of JILGA in Osaka, Nagoya and Sapporo, but the Osaka branch, of which Hirano Hiroaki is a central figure, soon severed relations with him because he was too authoritarian. A later attempt to establish a group in Kobe to combat AIDS ended in disruption at the first meeting. Some participants, however, set up a gay group, Ru Kurabu Asshu (Le Club H), which I shall discuss below. Osaka groups have very little contact with foreign organizations but I felt that they were ideologically closer to groups in Western countries because they stressed equality and the importance of everyone being able to have his or her say, as opposed to Occur and JILGA, which in comparison are quite hierarchical. Other groups have developed unrelated to JILGA, many at universities but in one case based on a religion.

A man who lost his second lover decided that he should try and find a lover from his own background. Being a member of the new religion Sōka Gakkai,[7] he placed an advertisement in the gay magazine *Barazoku* using wording that he knew would be understood as related to Sōka Gakkai by other members. He received many replies from gay Sōka Gakkai members and some others but found no lover. Nevertheless, he met most of these people and they decided to start a gay network for members of Sōka Gakkai and what they call 'friends': people who are not members of Sōka Gakkai but may nevertheless participate. They asked Ikeda Daisaku, the honorary president of the sect, whether it was all right for them to start a gay network and received a positive reply, which greatly enhanced their zeal. Contrary to my information on other new religions, such as Tenrikyō (The Tenri Teachings), Seichō no Ie (The House of Growth) and Tōitsu Kyōkai (The Unification Church), which prohibit homosexuality,[8] Sōka Gakkai's stress on the growth of the individual, which means that anything that comes from the inside of a person is good and deserves to be developed, according to Ikeda appears to include homosexuality. Placing additional advertisements in gay magazines, the network, called B-Netto, for Buddhist Network, grew within a year to 100 members with several chapters throughout Japan. After the founder of the group exposed as gay another member in a local young men's chapter of Sōka Gakkai, he was ostracized and the Tokyo branch changed its name to Kokoro no Nettowāku: Network of the Heart.

In the Kansai area five gay circles were closely related and have enormous overlaps in participants. They were Ru Kurabu Asshu (Le Club H), mentioned above, which rather unsuccessfully tried to combine leisure with political activism,

DON! (Do Over Naturally!), which is a leisure circle engaging in outdoor activities and sports, Sākuru T (Circle T), which engaged in personal discussion, Puapua, which engaged in political activities, and Kamigata DJ Club, which made cassette tapes with discussions and music that are sent to hundreds of gay men throughout Japan. The last three have combined to form Gay Front Kansai in 1994 so that activities could be streamlined and office space could be rented.

DON! evolved from Ru Kurabu Asshu and from DON! the group Fain Kurabu (Fine Club), later renamed Puraimu Kurabu (Prime Club), was formed. It wanted to be a group of more mature gay men, as DON! members who were close to their 30s felt that they could not relate well to those in their teens or early 20s. In their first advertisement they invited people not to be alone with their *nayami* concerning marriage but to come and share their worries. Many people reacted, some of whom had been isolated as gay men until then. One of them, a 28-year-old man from a small town, said that he had been afraid to come but that the men were not as scary and weird as he had always imagined other gay men to be and that he made many friends. He was, however, disappointed in the lack of discussion of *nayami*, although he understood that they first should get to know each other by engaging in various activities.

This necessity to get to know each other before engaging in more serious matters, seemed to be a problem in most gay circles that intend to do more than engage in leisure activities (*asobu*). OGC meetings are characterized by undirected discussions about anything that is brought up, often centring around people who are participating for the first time. Puapua's meetings were characterized by lengthy discussions about how they should operate as a group before activities finally started. Since new members or participants continually join these groups, trying to keep everyone in place would mean that nothing could be done. The solutions vary. OGC makes decisions in an informal way and people usually agree that any activity undertaken is all right, following a proposal by those who intend to undertake it, usually some of OGC's central figures. Puapua has combined with other groups to form Gay Front Kansai and they established a special group to welcome newcomers. Occur is hierarchically organized and newcomers have to express their adherence to a set of rules and to the leadership (Akā 1992). For reasons unknown to me, Occur often refuses people who wish to participate, especially when they are from Western Japan.[9]

In Tokyo contacts between lesbian and gay groups are mostly limited to contacts between individuals. JILGA has very few lesbian members and while Occur claims that about half of its members are lesbian, in practice LIO is a separate organization that does very little together with the male members. Lesbian women related to Regumi often felt that Occur's men as well as Minami were too macho and too little interested in women to warrant efforts to cooperate, but lesbian circles around Kakefuda Hiroko, who herself has many male gay friends, cooperated with JILGA on many occasions, not least the first Lesbian and Gay Parade, held in August 1994 after the annual JILGA conference. Later, however, this cooperation broke up and support for JILGA greatly diminished, most of its members leaving out of displeasure over Minami's authoritarianism.

In Osaka lesbian women and gay men work together at times, especially OGC and YLP or OLP, who held a session together questioning feminism in relation to homosexuality at the Women's Festival in Kyoto in 1988 and in 1995 had a shared New Year's party. In 1996 OLP women combined with a newly founded mixed group, based at Kyoto University, Project P, the 'P' of which refers to people, to question how the Lesbian and

Gay Parade in Tokyo was organized in 1996. Lesbian women and gay men are in general quite positive about each other, unless they know no gay men or lesbian women respectively, in which case their ideas may be based on general prejudiced ideas about the other, in ways comparable to feminist women's prejudices towards homosexuality.

Among gay men a form of sexism was prevalent in some circles, especially those who frequent gay bars and saunas and those who are more advanced in age. One interviewee, who had lived in France for a long time, thought that French feminists were quite all right but hated (*daikirai*) Japanese *feminisuto*, whom he found dogmatic and homophobic. When I asked him to elaborate, however, he seemed not to be too sure what he meant. Among his friends he counted many lesbian women. Young gay men often have very good relationships with women, whether they are heterosexual or lesbian, and OGC is even criticized by Occur for not being a gay group but a feminist group because they are strongly oriented towards feminist ideology (Miller 1992), which is largely attributable to Hirano Hiroaki's influence.

OGC worked together with feminist groups, such as Pāpuru, in a demonstration against a violent rape that occurred on a platform of the Midōsujisen, the central underground line that runs between north and south in Osaka, while people walked by acting as if they did not notice. Further, OGC members work in a crèche for children at the yearly Women's Festival in Kyoto. Nevertheless, their activities are increasingly focused on informing people about homosexuality, something that has been furthered strongly by appearances in the media, following which people of various organizations contacted OGC to ask them to come and give information. Hirano Hiroaki was asked to give a presentation at a meeting of the singles' network, after which a member of that network started coming to OGC meetings. Similarly, members of the men's liberation group Menzu Ribu Kenkyūkai may turn up at meetings of the singles' network and at meetings of OGC. Some people spend nearly every Sunday with one group or another.

The threshold for participation in almost all these groups is low. One can just turn up and participate. The only problem consists of the psychological threshold. Many people have images of gay men and lesbian women influenced by media depictions and therefore they are afraid to meet them. Once they do, they are usually relieved to find that gay and lesbian people are often quite 'normal' in their eyes. While their ideas may be very different from mainstream thought, these ideas are important features for which participants appreciate the meetings. Ideas different from *jōshiki* is more often than not what people seek, for *jōshiki* concerning their sexual preferences can often not be combined with a lifestyle and a self-image they wish to have. Thanks to publications that were part of the gay boom, many people who remained isolated have come into contact with these groups (Lunsing 1997).

## Conclusion

In this chapter I hope to have given some idea about the problems concerning the establishment and acceptance by members of my research categories of their feelings or ideas and the discussions surrounding them within their own circles. Apart from the themes discussed here, such as discourses on sex and gender, there are others that I could have included, but this field is so wide that I had to limit myself to themes that pushed themselves to the fore throughout the research and while writing. Debates in and between circles and categories are lively and often emotionally loaded because they often border on discussing each other's most personal feelings. I witnessed and heard of many more debates than described here but I hope the description here suffices to provide some insight into the environment in which many people come to assert themselves as feminist, gay, or lesbian, also if they do not label themselves accordingly.

## Notes

1 Janice Raymond defines 'transgenderism' as follows: 'The term transgenderism covers pre-operative and post-operative transsexuals, transvestites, drag queens, cross-dressers, gays and lesbians, bisexuals and straights who exhibit any kind of dress and/or behaviour interpreted as "transgressing" gender-roles' (Raymond 1996: 215) but then writes that the majority of transgenderists are men who 'rather than transcending, i.e., dismantling and going beyond gender-roles, seek to combine aspects of traditional femininity with aspects of traditional masculinity' (ibid.), which suggests that what she herself designates as transgender is rather more limited than her definition. The transgendered men concerned may be the most visible but there is no way of establishing that they are the most numerous, let alone that they form the majority of transgenderists. Her statement that they are, has obviously to do with her argument against transgendered men, which, as Whittle (1996) made clear, also lacks empirical basis. Raymond occupied herself merely with the most visible transgender phenomena that fitted a stereotype she sees as harmful to women's emancipation.

2 See for instance a report on such a happening in *Queen* (Tsuru and Kame 1993).

3 This bias appears to be partly due to the fact that I have been presented as an expert in the field of sadomasochism in a lesbian publication (LIB 1994: 40), which can be attributed to the fact that I spoke of sadomasochism with one or more of the compilers.

4 Articles of the *yaoi ronsō* have been assembled in four specials of the *minikomishi Choisir*, in which much of the discussion was printed (Satō 1996).

5 An early and very famous example of the genre is Takemiya Keiko's *Kaze to Ki no Uta* (Poem of the wind and the trees), a very complex story set in nineteenth-century France. The main protagonists are two boarding school boys, one of whom, Gilbert, is intially portrayed as bad and working his way through school by offering sexual services but whose character later is elaborated in long flashbacks. The other, Serge, who comes to love him, is virtuous but his mother was a gypsy, as a result of which he is discriminated against from the beginning. Eventually they have to run away from the boarding school in order to escape the evil uncle of the bad one and make a living in poverty. Finally Gilbert is run over by a carriage and dies and Serge returns home to assume his title of marquis (Takemiya 1977–84, 17 volumes, originally published from 1976). Another example is Yamagishi Ryōko, whose *Hiizuredokoro no Tenshi* (The angel from the sun) liberally describes the life of Shōtoku Taishi, the promulgator of Buddhism in the Nara period, who is believed to have lived in the seventh century and is described in this *manga* as an extremely beautiful and feminine homosexual man. His love for a friend, however, does not materialize (Yamagishi 1991–2, 8 volumes). One example, which gay men advised me to read, was a story about a young man who leaves his

parents to go and work as a female, or transvestite, prostitute in the city. Later he returns home dressed as a woman but his parents want him not to be seen by the neighbours and ask him to leave and not return (Ōshima 1992), which seems to be a quite plausible story in present-day Japan. More recently *shōjo manga* of the genre show even more reality, for instance Akisato Wakuni's *Nemureru Mori no Binan* (The beautiful sleeping man in the woods) and *Tomoi* (name of the main character), together telling the story of Tomoi's unhappy love life. His first lover develops AIDS-related illnesses and leaves him to return to his native Germany and his second lover is killed by his jealous wife, when he tries to prevent her from killing Tomoi. Disillusioned, Tomoi goes to meet his death in Afghanistan (Akisato 1986, 1992). Another example is a story by Takaguchi Satosumi, whose heroes fall in love with each other and defy their classmates after their father and mother move in together. In this case one of the protagonists dies in a traffic accident, leaving the other in loneliness (Takaguchi 1991, 1993).

6 Ueno Chizuko became a major example in this chapter for a number of reasons. She was my supervisor and therefore I learned to know her well. Further, she has a high profile, which added to the tendency among informants to want to talk about her. Finally she is one of very few *feminisuto* who have written about homosexuality, which has been picked up by gay and lesbian writers, as discussed. Other *feminisuto* often had similar opinions but did not put them into writing and thereby avoided the critique Ueno received.

7 See Earhart (1974), Metraux (1988) or White (1970) for more information on Sōka Gakkai. Members of Sōka Gakkai I spoke with said that Sōka Gakkai was a philosophy of life,

not a religion, but their practices include chanting at meetings and other behaviour that is similar to that in other sects.

8 My information on this is purely verbal. One informant had been a member of the Tōitsu Kyōkai (The Unification Church) and at a discussion it appeared that it was general knowledge that the Tōitsu Kyōkai saw homosexuality as a sin. Other informants provided similar information about Tenrikyō, Seichō no Ie and some other new religions. They tend to be conservative in the sense that they usually ardently support marriage and parenthood against divorce and anything else that is not in line with the continuation of a heterosexual lifestyle. See Hardacre (1986) or Earhart (1974) for more information about new religions.

9 One interviewee who called Occur's helpline felt rebuked by them after he tried to talk about his personal problems, another informant was told that they would call him back, which they never did and a man with cerebral palsy wrote that he was dexterously (*migoto ni*) refused (Hanada 1994), something that was not much different from the reaction of the cerebral palsy society when he tried to discuss homosexuality there. Occur, however, seems to have changed its policy in that it referred Hanada to Osaka-based groups, something which they did not do previously.

# 8 Conclusion

> Marriage is a reprehensible institution. Stuck to a partner until your spirit is broken, you resign yourself to your fate and trudge on to death. For the survivor an afterbloom is possible but usually the good years are gone. In the period you should deliver important work you are a burden to each other. (Warren 1991: 85)

This quote is translated from the diaries of the Dutch gay writer Hans Warren who, like most Dutch gay men of his generation, has been married. It was originally written in the early 1970s, when lifestyles other than heterosexual marriage became gradually possible in the Netherlands. There are very few Dutch gay men or lesbian women over 50 years old who have not been married; many, indeed, still are married. In Japan the situation is similar, albeit that younger generations also often have been or are married, a phenomenon that in the Netherlands declined considerably after the 1960s. This quote indicates the extent to which a social institution can be a burden on people's lives, if that institution does not agree with their feelings. Much of anthropology occupies itself with describing social institutions and social constructions, while ignoring the people for whom these things are a burden. Throughout this investigation I have focused precisely on those people for whom the social system is a burden, and their lives, rather than anything else.

Above all, this book provides ethnographic descriptions of

topics and features that have been under-reported and, in my opinion, will remain under-reported even after this work. I have discussed the life of a large variety of people from several angles. I started from the angle of marriage as it is generally viewed and political discussions relating to it in chapter three, continued from the angle of those who try to comply with the idea that marriage is the only proper way to live in chapter four, subsequently wrote from the angle of how people live who do not comply with this idea in chapter five and from the angle of how people cope with an environment that does not readily accept their ways of living and thinking in chapter six. In chapter seven discussions people have in various circles were presented in order to provide a picture of how their participants think about particular themes and see each other and themselves.

Using these different angles, even though presented in a linear way, I have tried to preserve some of the many-sided chaos that constitutes life. Much more work needs to be done in this field and therefore I do not believe it to be sensible to draw it too much into a theoretical framework. I believe that, especially in the case of homosexuality, there is already an imbalance between relatively little credible empirical data and an over-abundance of theoretical insights. I do not believe that such insights are always to the benefit of lesbian women and gay men or anyone else, as I discuss below.

In this chapter, I draw out four themes. Three of these were discussed in the introduction and one concerns changes, that occurred while I was in the field and afterwards, from which I draw some ideas of what the future might bring. Since these themes underpinned the thesis throughout, I intend to use this final chapter to make their roles explicit. They are: (1) space, gender and sexuality, (2) constructions of homosexuality, (3) selves and (4) changes and developments, in the last of which possible future developments are investigated. Since these themes were not discussed separately in the previous chapters, at times I introduce material that has not been presented previously, in order to promote clarity.

## Space, Sexuality and Gender

Japanese society has long provided niches for those who feel that they cannot live like everyone else. As discussed in chapters six (pp. 215-6) and seven (pp. 263-4), for single women, gay men and other transgender people there are the roles of prostitute or the role of entertainer, in shows and in clubs as well as on television, whereby the latter is reminiscent of the role of 'special status people', who were itinerant performers (Ohnuki-Tierney 1987). The *geinōkai* (show-business world) is cast as outside 'normal' society. Until recently it was not felt to be possible to maintain a single or gay lifestyle apart from such contexts and therefore those who desire to live outside of them often feel that they have to suppress their homosexuality, or any gender attribute that does not agree with *jōshiki*, not only in public but also in private contexts. The existence of a gay shadow world in which gay men can have their moments of pleasure may function as a safety valve for gay men's feelings of stress produced by the suppression of their feelings for men. It is, however, a limited world in which they cannot live entirely, unless they bid farewell to their life in the mainstream world: for instance, men who work in gay bars on a more permanent basis rarely maintain much contact with relatives.

Gay groups and networks typically try to construct a base different from this world, culminating in Occur's wish to build a 'gay community' by asking members to move to Nakano-*ku*, a ward in Tokyo (Ugoku Gei. 1992: 270). Other groups and networks do not entertain such ideas and are more directed towards changing society as a whole in order to accommodate the possibility of gay men and lesbian women living anywhere without suppressing their homosexuality. In a critique of Occur's idea of building a community in a geographical sense, even the term 'gay ghetto' has been mentioned (Onitsuka 1993). As discussed in chapter seven (pp. 300–1), in the Kansai area relations between gay and other groups relevant to this book are well developed, which makes the idea of a community in which only gay men and lesbian women are concentrated less appealing: they have many heterosexual friends. As discussed in chapter six (p. 232), Furukawa Kei from Tokyo also found that his wish not to live entirely in gay contexts made him want to come out as gay to heterosexual friends.

As discussed in the introduction (p. 14) and in chapter three (p. 74), any man who is not married lacks credibility as a fully adult person. A single man is seen as in a state of incompleteness and, unless he can make people believe that he is not entirely single, for instance, by making people believe that he has a girlfriend, this implies that he is not taken as a serious and reliable person. While single heterosexual men, like gay men, may find relief from the stress produced by their status by visiting bars and drinking, unlike the case of gay men there are no bars that cater specifically for them. Staff in regular bars are not likely to harass them much, but the question of whether they are married is likely to be asked and may increasingly lead to embarrassment. Even in a bar run by two single women a single elderly woman and I were cautioned to be careful not to chase other customers away, when we were loudly saying that people should not marry and that single life is much more enjoyable.

Showing that one is happy to be single may be seen as offensive, which makes it impossible for single men to be happily single in most bars. Even though in Japan it is usual for men to go out without their wives, a wife is assumed to be present in the background and waiting at home to assist her husband.

For lesbian women the picture looks somewhat less daunting. As discussed in chapter three (p. 75) and seven (p. 270), their sex implies that they are not seen as fully adult persons in the sense of ungendered fully adult persons to start with and therefore women who decide that they do not wish to live like anyone else may feel less mental stress if they decide not to marry. As they are usually not part of the mainstream male lifestyle, they may perceive that they have less to lose than men, especially if they come into contact with women's networks, within which it may even be possible to find employment. The chances are also that, unlike in the case of men, not being married may enhance their career prospects because companies generally think that married women are not worth investing in, as was suggested by the case of a woman, discussed in chapter six (p. 241), whose divorce was warmly approved of by her company because it meant that she would not have children and quit work.

If a woman marries, her existence is seen as being dependent on another person's, her husband's; if she does not marry, it is seen as being dependent on parents or other family. The latter case, whether it concerns lesbian or heterosexual single women, implies that they have failed to accomplish their assigned gender roles as daughter, wife and mother, which implies that they are even less of a person than women who live in accordance with *jōshiki* concerning their gender role. Among my informants, women mostly had low-paid insecure jobs. Those who worked at universities felt that they had been discriminated against: it was much more difficult for them than for men to get hired as full-time staff. Often they were temporary lecturers on hourly contracts, and hourly wages are typically hardly enough to live on. Nevertheless, money and the status it may bring was often not considered to be all that important, as long as there was enough to get by.

Space in Japanese society may be seen as neatly divided into women's space and men's space. Women's space is inside the house and men's outside. Where they meet, roles are clearly defined and leave little room for people to behave differently. In bars as well as in the household, women are expected to serve, although there are exceptions to the rule, such as clubs where women are served by male hosts (Lunsing forthcoming). These exceptions are, however, like the gay bars, part of another world, in which one cannot live entirely. Feminist groups are an example of women's space that is different from other women's spaces in the sense that ideally men have no influence on it. Men cannot enter this space unless they behave in a manner that denies some of the gender attributes which *jōshiki* assigns to their sex. Other networks, such as the singles' network and the men's liberation group, similarly demand of participants that they distance themselves from part of the gender attributes as they are assigned to their sex according to *jōshiki*. Single heterosexual men have the least space of all specifically dedicated to them, the irony being that by marrying they can become the fully adult persons around whom Japanese society at large is organized.

In interaction, the social status of a person matters more than his or her feelings and status is measured in clear-cut ways such as marital status and occupation. The concept of compulsory heterosexuality was proposed by Adrienne Rich to refer to the force used to make people, in particular women, adapt to heterosexual lifestyles, which may culminate in rape if they do not comply (Rich 1993). People are expected to marry and therefore to be heterosexual and heterosexual sex may be forced upon women. In Japan many people feel a strong compulsion to at least appear to live in accordance with the marriage system but because there is not much need to present a spouse, or to act out feelings of affection in public, the contents are less important. *Kateinai rikon* (divorce within the household), as discussed in chapters three (p. 96) and four (p. 150), is the clearest example of a marriage that is not what it may seem. As long as people appear to be 'properly (*chan to, kichin to*)' married, they can do whatever they like. The greatest problems are encountered by those who are not married and cannot pass themselves off as being part of a heterosexual couple. Unless they agree that they would rather be married and thereby deny the validity of their own lifestyle, their unmarried status implicitly questions part of the very basis of society, even if they do not make pronouncements against marriage.

Japanese society provides for some contexts in which women can present male gender attributes and men female, most notably the theatre and company parties at which wearing drag is a common part of the programme, as discussed in chapters six (p. 229) and seven (p. 264). These places and spaces are, like the areas where men can be gay and women can be lesbian, very restricted. Nevertheless, I found people who live their lives in ways that defy the gender boundaries. Tsutamori Tatsuru, discussed in chapter five (pp. 204–6), was during my fieldwork period from 1991 to 1993 probably the most famous example and one of the most extreme because he does not simply cross over to female gender but appropriates and discards attributes of both female and male gender as he wishes. I found many informants who do similar things, albeit in less extreme ways and often more limited in time and space.

This defies the traditional view of gender as two large wholes opposing each other, in contrast to my personal view of gender, which I set out in the introduction (p. 12–3), as opposing sets of attributes from which people may compose their own selection, if they can find the freedom to do so. In Japan this freedom is there to be used by anyone who dares to defy *jōshiki*, and people increasingly seem to do this. Badinter wrote about young upper-class people in France, that there is little left to distinguish men from women (Badinter 1986), and in Japan too, in some circles, the overlap of the divisions of gender and sex is disappearing. Women are men and men are women, or more simply: people are people. Differences remain but not in accordance with the division of the sexes. As stated in the introduction (p. 12–3), this allows also for labelling attributes 'feminine' and 'masculine' without a sexist connotation: what is feminine is not bound to women, as what is masculine is not bound to men. As long as we disregard social structure, we can be anything we want, the only limits are set by our creativity and our capability to acquire space.

## Constructions of Homosexuality

As discussed in the introduction (p. 25), there are many historical constructions of male homosexuality in Japan in contrast to a relatively small number of constructions concerning female homosexuality[1] and feminist women. Sex was a man's world. This does not, however, necessarily give men an advantage over women in achieving alternative lifestyles: constructions may be a burden rather than offering support. As noted in chapter seven (p. 261), I found no male homosexual informants who related historical constructions to their own situation. This may be due to two possible causes: either a large change took place somewhere between the Meiji era and the end of the Second World War, or the historical constructions were never of much relevance to the majority of Japanese men engaging in homosexuality. While changes most likely have occurred, I believe that Watanabe exaggerates when he writes that all men could engage in pederasty, as he translates *danshoku,* before the Meiji era and that this system was lost when modern homosexuality surfaced in the 1960s (Watanabe and Iwata 1987: 127). Today all men have easy access to sex with young men but many do not care for it, which most likely was no different in earlier times.

The construction of homosexuality in historical periods as pederasty is related to ancient Greek constructions (Greenberg 1988), which have been transplanted to Japan, as evidenced by the translation of the word *danshoku* into pederasty. Why love of older men for younger men needs a special label, whereas the more widespread love of older men for younger women is hardly ever discussed as something of particular interest, is never explicated and the only explanation I can think of is that heterosexual thought dominated most discourses throughout time and therefore homosexuality was an area that was more subject to scrutiny than heterosexuality. In Japan this may seem to be less the case, given the parallel terms *danshoku* and *joshoku,* but this leaves the mainstay of structured heterosexuality in marriage equally untouched because *joshoku* is the love of young women outside marriage.

Foucault's writings suggest that pederastic activities gradually became less acceptable in ancient Greece as a result of discourses concerning it (Foucault 1978, 1988a, b). Foucault has been criticized for constructing the whole from the part because he constructed Greek sexuality from debates among free male citizens, who made up but a small minority of those living in Athens, where his work is set (Foxhall 1994). This critique is, however, based upon a misreading. Foucault is very clear that he is not constructing a whole but only a part. The critique should not be aimed at Foucault but at readers who mistook Foucault's intentions and treat his constructions as if they are more than constructions particular to a small group in ancient Greece. As Foucault writes, the major function of constructions is to constrain behaviour.

In *The History of Sexuality* the most revealing episode might be the one where the question of whether love of boys or love of women is morally superior leads to a discussion between Charides, whose stance is that the love of women is superior because it is nature, and Callicratides who argues that the love of boys is superior because it is better than nature: it is culture (Foucault 1988b: 214–24). The arbiter Lycinus declares that Callicratides is the winner of the argument because of the purity accorded to the love of boys which is cast as platonic (ibid.: 226). Theomnestus, however, disagrees:

> Whereas, in order to link together pleasure and virtue, the advocates of boys stressed the absence of any sexual act, he [i.e. Theomnestus] reinstates the physical contacts that one enjoys, the kisses, the caresses, and the gratification, as the real reason for the existence of his love. Seriously, he says, they can't make us believe that the whole pleasure of this relationship is in looking into each other's eyes and in being enchanted by friendly conversation. Looking is

> agreeable, certainly, but it is only the first stage. After that comes touching, which thrills the whole body. Then kissing, which is timid at first but soon becomes eager. The hand does not remain idle during this time; it glides down under the clothing, squeezes the breasts for a moment, descends the length of the firm belly, reaches the 'flower of pubity' and finally strikes the target. (Foucault 1988b: 227, referring to Plutarch)

Foucault interprets this as a reminder that 'it is not possible (. . .) to keep the *aphrodisia* outside the domain of love and its justifications' (ibid.), thereby suggesting that an obligation was felt to deny what was really important in the love of boys, i.e. sexual gratification, in order to keep it acceptable. While this kept pederasty in ancient Greece acceptable among free men, sex between two adult men met with strong disapproval but nevertheless occurred (Foucault 1978, 1988b).

Constructions of homosexuality as pederasty also exist in China (Furth 1993, Hinsch 1990, Xiao 1984) and in Islamic countries (Chebel 1988, Schmitt 1992), where recent research has shown that adult men also engage in homosexual activities with adult men and that the roles of the insertor and insertee are not necessarily always clearly separated (see Xiao 1984 and McGough 1981 on China; see Khan 1992, Reed 1992, Sofer 1992, Tapinc 1992, McDonald 1992 and the novelist Busi 1993 on Islamic countries). This also holds for the construction of homosexuality as sex between a passive, feminine man and an active, masculine man. This construction can be related to a debate concerning male homosexuality in Mexico and among Latin Americans in North America. In Mexico and among Latin Americans homosexuality meets with strong disapproval but bisexuality is acceptable, whereby it is assumed that the bisexual man is sexually dominant. Therefore, especially middle-class men who prefer sex with men but can manage sex with women often have a heterosexual lifestyle publicly, while calling themselves bisexual and feeling strong attraction towards men, which leaves their male sexual partners to bear the brunt of discrimination against homosexuality. This construction is criticized because it is not actually always true that the 'bisexual' man is active and the other passive (Taylor 1986, Lumsden 1991, Murray 1992b, Almaguer 1993).

The Native American *berdache,* who was a man who dressed like a woman, did women's work and often had ritual functions, was common in many Native North American tribes. The *berdache* has been constructed as a prototype of institutionalized homosexuality. *Berdaches* have been thought to be hermaphrodites and sodomites (Whitehead 1981). *Berdaches* did not, however, necessarily engage in homosexuality. Among Native Americans homosexual activity was not necessarily related to gender, and homosexual activity between men who otherwise had male gender attributes also has been reported. In some tribes people did not mind if male men engaged in homosexual activities, in others it met with negative sanctions (ibid.). This suggests that the categorization of the *berdache* as homosexual and the view of the institution of the *berdache* as a niche for homosexual men was a result of constructions concerning homosexuality prevalent among Western scholars. In reality there was no direct relation between the gender-crossing activities of the *berdache* and male homosexual activities.

Among the Sambia of Papua New Guinea there exists a

famous example of ritualized homosexuality. Boys become men by fellating older men and later are fellated themselves by boys (Herdt 1987). As Greenberg (1996), referring to Herdt, points out, there is a large variation in the amount of pleasure men derive from the practice, some being very enthusiastic, others limiting it as much as possible. There are also men who persist in homosexual activities beyond ritual and refuse to marry. They are regarded as 'rubbish men', men who failed to become 'proper' adult men (Herdt 1987). What Herdt's work suggests is that any man can engage in homosexual activity if it is culturally constructed as necessary. This, however, does not show that homosexuality is determined by culture. The existence of gay 'rubbish men' suggests rather the contrary, which supports Whitehead's tentative conclusion that in any culture, regardless of its constructions of homosexuality, there are men who prefer to engage in homosexual activity (Whitehead 1981), which also is the only explanation for men risking death penalties for their love of men, as happens in Iran today. Hirschfeld's stress on the similarity of homosexuality throughout the world (Hirschfeld 1914: 528), although it may have been partly for political motives, seems not to be all that far from the mark.

In the Japanese situation it is plausible that pederasty, better translated into *shōnenai* (lit. love of boys) than *danshoku* which, as discussed in the introduction (pp. 27–8), was also used to refer to sexual activity between adult men (Hirschfeld 1914: 618, Ihara 1990: 180–3, Dunn and Torigoe eds, transl. 1969: 41–4, Leupp 1995: 137–44), was more readily accepted by Japanese than homosexual activity between adult men (Benedict 1977: 131) and that even if the younger one was actually adult he might have presented himself as a minor or adolescent. In Japan sex is, as discussed in chapter seven (pp. 279–85), seen as an activity taking place between an active and a passive person, characterized by an imbalance of power, which makes it difficult to perceive that two adult men, between whom an imbalance in power may not be evident, might engage in sex. Many gay men and lesbian women call their lovers *ko* (boy or girl, chapter six, pp. 240, 248) but this does not mean that they are minors or even necessarily younger than themselves. It is a way of referring to someone other than the person one addresses in an intimate and tender way.

A general contention among scholars I know is that modern homosexuality, that is a homosexual relationship between adult men who are gay rather than men who engage in gay sex (Greenberg 1988: 484–6), did not come into existence in Japan until after the Second World War (e.g. Furukawa, M. 1992, 1993, Watanabe and Iwata 1987). While this may be true in the sense of modern homosexuality becoming a widely held construction, which however still has its limitations, as discussed above, Japanese history knows examples of long-term homosexual relationships between adult men, similar to the construction of modern homosexuality. The neglect of them may be a result of a zealous following of Western constructions concerning changes in homosexuality that led people to turn a blind eye to evidence that did not fit.

It seems that, apart from its recently having become a construction that is widely adhered to, there is nothing modern about modern homosexuality as an activity, or, indeed, as a way to view oneself, as Greenberg also suggests with his writing on European men who saw themselves as gay in past centuries (Greenberg 1988: 484). Just as the present day *shōjo manga* (girls' comics), as discussed in chapter seven (pp. 286–8), often do not present homosexuality in a realistic way and, just as the mass media have until recently persisted in depicting gay men only as prostitutes and transvestites, neglecting the majority, earlier writings are unlikely to provide a representative picture of homosexual activities in Japanese history.

Women may be constructed as weak and dependent, as incapable of taking care of themselves and living on their own. Japanese history provides examples of women who lived independently and exercised great power, as discussed in the introduction (p. 19–20). They have been picked up by feminist women to defy constructions of women as weak and dependent. I believe there are two reasons why gay scholars have not done the same thing. One is that there were, until very recently, no gay scholars in Japan working in this field, and the second is that foreign, mostly American, gay scholars have chosen to deal with Japan as something otherworldly, something that they could use to their own advantage. It seems that, rather than consider the relation of widely held constructions to actual behaviour, they were content with finding constructions that did not wholly deny homosexuality its right to exist, as widely held constructions in their own culture do.

Given the prevalence of homophobia in America, it should come as no surprise that American gay and lesbian scholars may overemphasize positive features of homosexuality elsewhere in order to provide a mirror to criticize their own culture. Pat Caplan's remark that homosexuality is of particular interest for investigating the relation between gender and sexuality (Caplan 1987, referred to in the introduction, p. 13) can also be seen in this light. The only reason why homosexuality may be of particular interest is that, as a result of the homophobia that prevented scholars from investigating it, few actual facts are known about it, while at the same time it has been more subject to moralistic scrutiny than heterosexuality in Western contexts.

While gay movements in Western countries, and most notably in America, try hard to dispel the construction of gay men as pederasts or men who love boys, scholars have accepted similar constructions about other cultures in history as well as in present times, without asking gay people in the cultures concerned about their activities, which, when it concerns historical data, is unfortunately impossible. Many Anglo-American lesbian and gay scholars appear to have tried to present a construction of homosexuality in their own culture that they expected to be least offensive to people having difficulty accepting anything different from a heterosexual norm. This led to the construction of homosexual relationships as relationships between two consenting adults who love and respect each other and, apart from the fact that they are both of the same sex, are in any other respect similar to some idealized type of heterosexual relationships (Kitzinger and Coyle 1995), even though, if they looked around, they would notice that equality in relations is not common in heterosexual any more than homosexual contexts.

Politics seem to have had a rather deplorable influence on gay studies in Anglo-American contexts. Perhaps lesbian women are not that unfortunate in having fewer historical constructions to deal with. Notwithstanding lesbian and gay historians' efforts to reclaim a past, it is the present that matters most and a past can be as much of a burden as anything else. I do not understand why it should be of importance to me to know that Tchaikowsky was a gay man who felt compelled to marry, unless I should be struggling with accepting my own homosexuality because of internalized homophobia and find in him an example of someone who never overcame that struggle. Even then, I fail to see how knowing it could take me any further. Many informants, lesbian women as well as gay men, were little concerned with the past or the not-so-near future: they live today and are quite happy to construct their own sexuality without reference to history. Foucault said many years ago, when he spoke at New

York University, that what was thought one way can be thought another (Greenberg, referring to Foucault, 1988: 489) and therefore, I would suggest, what was thought one way can be made irrelevant by thinking another way.

The idea, prevalent among anthropologists specializing in Japan but not in sexuality, that married men can unproblematically have gay sex on the side (verbal communication) is in Japan generally thought to be very strange (Hikage 1987, and many informants). The only Japanese who were said by informants to think that gay men could marry unproblematically were parents of gay sons and lesbian daughters and other significant others. In this context, however, the belief that once the children are married they may become 'normal' or that if they marry at least the family's honour is protected by this ostentatious adaptation to social norms, suggests that homosexuality is not taken very seriously. In addition, the stress on the outwardly directed side of marriage suggests that such friends and parents do not regard the contents of marriage as of much importance either. While bisexuality can be found in literature (e.g. Oe 1989) and may be discussed as a possibility within gay and lesbian contexts, I found that there is nothing remarkable about the prevalence of men who see themselves as bisexual in Japan, compared to the European countries where I have lived.[2]

The prevalence of the use of the term *nōmaru* (normal) for heterosexual suggests that people have only begun to consider heterosexuality as something particular after they came to know gay men or lesbian women in their daily life. Until then they may see homosexuality as an *asobi* some weird people may engage in, as something that exists on television, or as an interesting topic to philosophize about in academic ways. When they are made to consider the existence of homosexuality right beside them in their daily lives, in their families or in their workplaces, the meaning of homosexuality changes in the sense that it may become something anyone might be, which may produce the recognition of their own sexuality as *hetero* instead of *nōmaru*. Many Japanese have not hitherto realized this, but the numbers who now have are growing. While Ueno wrote that homosexuality can only exist by the grace of heterosexuality, as a counter-value (Ueno 1992), it seems to be the other way around: heterosexuality only exists by the grace of homosexuality. If the existence of homosexuality is not recognized as a legitimate possibility, heterosexuality is merely 'normal', an aspect of everyone and as such does not require a label. Homosexuality can change 'normal' heterosexuality.

## Selves

Among feminist women there were three major themes related to asserting their emancipatory and feminist ideas. First, there are women who think that they were born feminist or, more precisely, with egalitarian ideas. Already as children they felt strong disagreement with roles and patterns of behaviour assigned to them, and their childhood was in many cases characterized by conflicts with parents who wanted them to be *onnarashii*. Second, causes for embracing feminist ideas have been experiences like sexual harassment or forms of discrimination in the workplace, such as the expectation that women serve tea, problems in marital relationships and problems with parents relating to matters such as a choice not to marry legally or a choice to pursue higher education. Third, it was important that they established contact with other feminist women or organizations.

Among heterosexual singles things are similar. While some feel that they were born with ideas against *jōshiki* concerning marriage and many other realms of life in Japan and hated the *wan patān* (one pattern) lifestyle that they felt was forced upon Japanese, others asserted themselves only after they saw themselves confronted with the fact that they might never marry. Likewise, contact with singles' networks or feminist groups was often a condition for heterosexual singles to regard being single positively.

Among lesbian women and gay men, a major problem concerns the fact that asserting oneself as gay or lesbian may mean that one cannot maintain a mainstream lifestyle. Unlike feminist women and assertive singles, who do not wish to have a mainstream lifestyle, many gay men and lesbian women are quite conservative, which may prohibit them from accepting their homosexuality. One young man said that he was heterosexual but contradicted this by seeking sex with men. He was young, inexperienced and insecure and said that he was heterosexual while actively courting men. Most men of his age who say that they are gay are afraid to visit the gay-bar area where I met him. In a gay bar where we sat later that night the bartender told him that he could not be heterosexual and seek sex with men: he must at least be bisexual. On a later meeting it appeared that he felt he could not be bisexual or gay because he was supposed to return to the countryside to take on his parents' farm after completing his studies. He would have to marry. Therefore he insisted on calling himself heterosexual, even though he was solely attracted to men and when he had sex with a woman he felt that something was 'not quite right (*nanka hen*)'.

Some liberal heterosexual men gave the explanation that all people are born with the possibility of having sex with both sexes, which is an idea that was also popular in gay circles in some Western countries (Duberman 1977), but they had never experienced sex with men themselves. In the men's liberation network in Osaka I suggested that they could try and have sex with men, without success. They were mostly involved in long-term relationships with women and thought it wrong to 'deceive' them and, probably more importantly, they simply could not imagine it to be pleasant. Feminist women who like to use the term 'sisterhood' to refer to intimate relationships with women similarly do not extend this to having sex with women, even if they say that they might prefer to share their life with a woman. Gay men, on the contrary, often have sexual experiences with women and they seldom produce explanations such as that everyone has the possibility to have sex with both men and women. While physically they can have sex with women, it is not what they prefer. They feel attracted to men and trapped in situations where they cannot avoid having sex with women. The only place where I found it to be common for heterosexual men to have sex with men is in prostitution, in which case money is their motive (Lunsing forthcoming).

Bisexuality is often seen as a manifestation of homophobia. The reasoning is that people say that they are bisexual because they have difficulty accepting their homosexuality. This may be partly a reason why many women are vague about the question of whether they are lesbian or not. It appears, however, that the more time people spend in gay or lesbian environments the more likely they are not to call themselves bisexual but homosexual or to become accepted as bisexual. In my experience, younger heterosexual men in particular are more open towards experimenting with homosexuality than in Western countries and, as mentioned in chapter seven (p. 280, Asahi 1994, Kawakoshi 1994, Miyauchi 1994, Ōshima 1994, Umeyama 1994), female students are more open towards experimenting with homosexuality than male students. This of course blurs the dividing line between homosexual and heterosexual, but in most cases homosexual activity by the uncommitted is incidental, because if one does not actively seek homosexual experience one is not likely to find much of it.

The philosopher Asada Akira wrote in support of homosexuality (Asada 1991, 1992) but remained vague about his own sexual preference. At a panel discussion in 1994 he was asked about it and answered that he was 30–40 per cent gay and 60–70 per cent straight (Asada and Hirano 1995). According to informants, on later occasions the gay percentage rose at the expense of the heterosexual. The influence of the Kinsey scale[3] may be present here, as is the influence of Foucault and possibly also queer theory. The late Terayama Shūji and Nakazawa Shinichi said that they were gay in their mind but did not desire to engage in homosexual activities (Terayama according to informants, Nakazawa and Yōrō 1992). This position is generally not taken seriously in gay circles. Asada maintains that it is not interesting to come out as gay because it does not question the categories society constructs to divide people (Asada and Hirano 1995). Unfortunately, he does not progress much beyond giving percentages to split his sexuality and saying that coming out as gay is limiting oneself to a social construction that never can be entirely what one is.

A more developed stance is that of Hibino Makoto who said in 1996 that he was 'just a beautiful-skin fetishist (*tada no kirei na hada fetchi*)' to indicate his attraction towards young men with a smooth skin. This does not mean, however, that he does not use the word *gei* for himself in contexts where people appear to be prejudiced about homosexuality or in contexts where this can help him find a lover (Hibino 1996), i.e. for political purposes or for personal benefit. While Hibino also points at the problem of people who say that they are bisexual because they find it difficult to assert themselves as gay, he himself appears to have progressed beyond presenting oneself as one thing. He is already thinking of what to call himself next, when the beautiful-skin fetishist becomes boring or outdated for him. His strategy of playing around with labels new and old was very well received, especially among lesbian women and women who decline to say that they are lesbian but definitely are not straight. While Asada's position is still open to criticism for being homophobic and not accepting his homosexuality, which is a common critique of women and men who want to have something to do with homosexuality but are unclear about their own sexuality, Hibino's position overcomes such criticism.

Within gay groups I witnessed some debates on the question of why people become gay, where the entire gamut from Freud's Oedipus complex, via behaviourism, to the latest genetic and biological explanations are presented merely to conclude that all explanations, which they investigated seriously, lack credibility. None of the explanations can possibly cover all cases of homosexuality, manifestations of which are very varied. Like many feminist women who thought that they were born feminist, most gay men thought that they were born gay and found the question of why irrelevant. Lesbian women added to this that all these explanations are about gay men and leave lesbian women largely untouched.

One way of dealing with constructions is to adapt the view of the self to them. Even if constructions are stigmatizing, people may find it easier to behave in accordance with them because they feel that is what is expected of them (Goffman 1980). The construction of gay men as transvestites and transsexuals leads to suicides by gay men who later come to regret having taken hormones to grow breasts or sometimes even having had a sex-change operation in order to fit the construction (Kuroyanagi 1992).

The hypothesis, discussed in the introduction (p. 17), that the fact that Japanese are taught to switch between role performances from one context to another may make it relatively easy for them to cope with certain parts of themselves that they prefer to keep to themselves, needs some qualification. While it may be easier in the sense that they have to make less effort to switch in accordance with contexts, this does not make people's feelings less problematic. It is a *nayami* (trouble, worry) to feel compelled to cover up part of one's being by switching role behaviour. While the idea of 'multiple selves' (Kondo 1992) could very well fit in with being gay in one context and 'normal' in another on the level of the 'interactional self' (Lebra 1992), I found that in the end most Japanese gay men see themselves as gay and lesbian women see themselves as lesbian, both in quite an essentialist manner. This does not prohibit them from not presenting themselves explicitly as gay or lesbian, especially in contexts where sexuality is not of much importance.

Therefore, I believe that Kondo's idea of multiple selves is rather superficial. She seems to discuss not selves but presentations of selves, which is not all that surprising because her research took place with people in the contexts of work and the family (Kondo 1990, 1992, 1994), contexts where people may not show their inner selves. Japanese, indeed, seem to be relatively sophisticated in dealing with varying presentations of themselves in a variety of contexts and do not allow themselves to be led astray by the idea that they have to present unchangeable selves regardless of contexts. Their inner selves appear rather to be stronger precisely because they feel less of a need for confirmation by others, unlike for instance Americans who tend to present their selves all the time as if they were unchangeable and essential to their personhood, adhering to some identity or other. This seems to suggest that they are insecure about what they are and therefore seek confirmation from others continually.

The idea that companies may be seen as families represented in the title of a paper of Dorinne Kondo (1994) by '*uchi no kaisha* (my company)' may be right in many cases but the use of *uchi* does not necessarily indicate any particular adherence to a group. *Uchi* may have the connotation of a close-knit group in many cases, but not always. It is also one of the words lesbian women use to refer to themselves if they wish to avoid the use of *watashi* with its feminine connotation (Hirosawa and Rezubian Ripōto Han 1991: 172). In this case, *uchi* simply means 'I' or 'my', as also seemed to be the case with an interviewee who used the term *uchi no haha*, which referred to a mother who lived alone, not to a group member. In addition to this, the facts that single women have difficulty living together and that efforts at living in groups in Japan are seldom successful, as discussed in chapter five (pp. 177–9), suggest that feelings of belonging to families and companies are rather the result of pressure and the feeling that there is no choice but to belong, than that it actually is what people would choose if they felt they had a choice. My informants typically felt a strong aversion to the invasion of their privacy by the felt need, be it economic or emotional, to be part of a company or their family to an extent they clearly did not choose themselves. Perhaps Japanese are much more individualist than they have always been presented.

Informants who were closeted felt that their *tatemae* behaviour was not their real self and that even what some people perceived as expressions of their *honne* was not either. Their view is that homosexuality is an inalienable part of themselves. Regardless of the question whether it is expressed on the interactional level or not, to their inner selves it is highly important. In some cases it could be seen as part of the non-self, the *muga*, which is raw nature (Lebra 1992), and, when seen as the source of homosexuality, agrees very well with the ideas Japanese have of why they prefer same-sex relationships. A man who forsook having sex with men in favour of marriage even wrote that his *honnō* (instinct) was homosexual (Yukio 1992). Following the idea of *muga*, homosexual activities can be engaged in without the inner self of the person in question recognizing it as part of his or her being: the young man who said he was heterosexual while seeking sex with men can be seen as having been interactional in words while *muga* in deeds, as was the woman, discussed in chapter four (pp. 146), who said she was bisexual while clearly being more interested in women. The feelings located in the *hara* (the belly), which Lebra calls *muga*, may be denied but they do not go away. Both people feel that they cannot be homosexual because of their duty to continue the *ie* (household) they were born into.

Lebra's non-self can, perhaps, be found in sexual activity. Gay men sometimes describe sex as losing themselves. In gay magazines many men describe sexual adventures in which they were made *mechakucha* (incoherent, confused), which means that the partner did whatever he wished with them, without giving them much of a chance to influence the course of events, as a result of which they ultimately become nothing but feelings. They lose themselves in this play that seemingly has no boundaries and, indeed, may in extreme cases actually have none. Ultimately, murder may be part of the game, which clearly indicates that *muga* is not the same as the Sanskrit *anatma*, as was suggested in the introduction (p. 18). Whereas Indian Buddhism generally held that *anatma* was nature itself and nature was good (Carrithers 1985: 254), as Sōka Gakkai's Ikeda Daisaku also believes as discussed in chapter seven (p. 233–4), a critique of Buddhism from the Trika Kaula sect of Kashmir as well as my findings suggest that *muga* is nature and nature itself is without value: neither good nor bad (Anderson 1985: 203). In the Japanese context, harmony combines good and bad: good and bad are indivisible (e.g. Okano 1991). Nature can be anything. The term *muga* was, however, never mentioned by any of my informants and when I asked about it nobody thought that she or he had such a thing. The essentialist view of homosexuality most Japanese adhere to, however, suggests clearly that they construct it as nature, as does the remark by the man, mentioned above, who called it his instinct.

Japanese society is not different from most other societies in that in general homosexuality is viewed in ways that are difficult to accept for those it directly concerns. Typically it is 'other' and the idea that one might actually meet someone who is gay or lesbian in one's daily life is alien to many people, as expressed by a woman who said that her mother saw her as ET, the extra-terrestrial from the American film of the same title, when she told her she was lesbian. ET is also a term that pops up in the lesbian writer Izumo Marō's book on her personal experiences (Izumo 1993: 103). Homosexuality being generally quite incomprehensible, as for instance Rich (1993) has pointed out and as has also been clarified in recent Japanese lesbian and gay publications (Kakefuda 1992a, Ugoku Gei. 1992, Itō S. 1993), often makes it difficult for people to express their attraction to persons of their own sex. ET is, however, a rather likeable creature, which suggests that even if one is not readily understood, one does not necessarily encounter negative reactions.

While many Japanese are unclear about their own sexual preference, acceptance of one's own feelings appears to be less problematic than in many Western countries. The problem is rather how and whether to express them. Fear of encountering homophobia in others seems to play a lesser role than internalized homophobia or the fear of being different which is then attributed to an environment that is supposed to be hostile towards homosexuality. This fear of being different, however, is instilled in Japanese from the earliest days of education, in which ostracism, or being shut out of the group, forms the major sanction against unwarranted behaviour (Hendry 1986a). Harmony and cooperation are key words in schools, thus the stress on not being too different is further intensified (White 1987). While this is not in particular directed at homosexuality, many people who see themselves as gay or lesbian think that they cannot let this be known to people outside gay or lesbian contexts.

Opposed to shame, which is felt when other people become aware of one's homosexuality, guilt about homosexuality is seldom felt because usually people believe that it is not something they have any influence over. Guilt only comes into play when a person has wronged someone, such as a spouse who has been kept in the dark about their partner's homosexuality, and even that seems to be a novel development. Guilt towards parents was expressed by only one interviewee (chapter six, p. 225). Empathy with parents' worries about having a child who does not live up to their hopes was common but this could not be helped. The problems expressed by *nayami* relating to homosexuality are located in the interactional self, the self that deals with society (Lebra 1992), where the question of revealing one's feelings or hiding them is constantly present.

Feminists were ridiculed in the 1970s. Although feminism may be the word to describe how some women think and act, *feminizumu* is not the word most feminists identify themselves with. As in the case of lesbian women and gay men, the activities and the ideology are not so much the problem as the label. For coming out in America and England labels are extremely important. However, rather than what one actually does or feels, it is the label that is mentioned. Labels are short and seemingly comprehensive. Rather than acknowledging and identifying with a label, people may act and identify with the activity as long as they are engaged in it. This seems to be more characteristic of Japanese ways of management of self-image than in most Western societies. When a major activity is uncontested and valued as positive, people may use it to construct their interactional self, which is of fundamental importance in work or family situations (Kondo 1990, 1992), but otherwise it may remain in their inner self (Lebra 1992). Work and family situations were usually of little importance to how people see themselves in relation to their sexuality, regardless of the question of whether these situations were supportive or not.

Coming out towards oneself in this relation is an acknowledgement that the role of feminist or gay, lesbian or single is a role that fits one, rather than determining one's whole identity, as is often the case in Western countries. This acknowledgement is, however, important. Although it may not seem much, it is a large step away from not recognizing a possibility people encompass in themselves. It is a step away from seeing oneself as the same as anyone else. It is taking a little distance from *jōshiki* of what men and women are, a step away from the assigned gender roles and, in that sense, a revolutionary deed in a culture where the idea that a man naturally marries a woman and vice versa is very strong and omnipresent. One identifies not directly with some particular label that is generally regarded as deviant but one does acknowledge that one is different and at odds with the surrounding *jōshiki* concerning what people are.

## Changes and Developments

One of my major questions was whether it is possible to live an openly gay, lesbian, feminist, or single lifestyle in Japan. This question I can answer with yes, it is. That I can answer affirmatively has much to do with the political and economic climate of today's Japan. The political climate is very liberal, which is by some informants partly attributed to the demise of the Liberal Democratic Party which in 1993 ended the situation of one-party rule in Japan that had lasted for over forty years. The demise of the Liberal Democratic Party has, according to them, led to a climate in which no group clearly holds power.

However, it might just as well be that the emergence of gay and lesbian movements and the diversification of lifestyles coincided with the change in the political status quo in what is a larger socio-cultural change taking place in Japanese society, which seems to be a move towards greater individuality. When looking at the time gay and lesbian people started to make themselves heard, it is obvious that it cannot be true that the one followed the other. Nevertheless, the volatile political situation is likely to have increased the fear of being accused of discriminatory activities or pronouncements and the negative media attention that could bring, which makes politicians and bureaucrats more likely to listen carefully to lobbyists and people with complaints in order to acquire some proper knowledge before divulging opinions about matters of sexuality and gender.

When in 1993 I went with a group of gay men to complain about the AIDS policy of the Osaka city and prefectural governments, the functionaries demanded that we did not record anything that was being said in order to keep a friendly atmosphere. Nevertheless, the talks were written about by Hirano Hiroaki in OGC's *minikomishi*, *Musubikko*, and by others and the local government was criticized, but this did not lead to any change in their attitude: the talks continued. Initially the officials showed surprise that there was something like a gay network in Osaka, which led to severe criticism of their ignorance of what is happening in the area they are supposed to govern. Publications and television programmes in which gay individuals and networks appeared had become quite abundant by then. Not much was done, however, with the knowledge we offered, for example that HIV-testing facilities were insufficient and should be open at times other than office hours because a working man is not likely to ask his boss for time off to have an HIV-test, something that was not heeded until more than two years later.

Nevertheless, the fact that the talks continue indicates that the officials are willing to listen and this, combined with the increasing numbers of organized gay men and lesbian women, makes it most likely that their influence will grow. As discussed in chapter seven (p. 286), the rulings on pornography have already been adapted to demands of Gay Front Kansai. In the end it is in the interest of Japanese society as a whole to take AIDS seriously and there is no category which has as many well-informed members as gay men, something that is also true in Western countries or other Asian countries, such as Thailand, Hong Kong, the Philippines and Singapore (verbal information from personal contacts and television). In Tokyo the groups AIDS Action and Occur have become discussion partners of the metropolitan government and of the national government of Japan in the development of AIDS policies. AIDS-related activities led to the AIDS Candlelight Parades in Tokyo and Kyoto in which a majority of participants were lesbian and gay (Lunsing 1994b, 1999b). This certainly helped to build up the momentum for the first successful Lesbian and Gay Parade, which is a development that seems also to be occurring in many other Asian countries. AIDS brought together gay men and other people in their environment for reasons other than to have sex, and once they are together it is likely that they will develop more activities.

Another reason why I believe that lesbian, gay, single and feminist lifestyles are more feasible in Japan today than, for instance, twenty years ago concerns economics. A growing demand for workers has made it possible for many women to find jobs and, even if they are still underpaid and insecure compared to men's jobs, they make it possible for women to live independently of men, which also makes it possible to engage in feminism openly, without hiding their activities from husbands and fathers, or to maintain lesbian lifestyles. The increase in the sheer numbers of unmarried men makes it increasingly difficult and unprofitable for companies to base their hiring and promotion policies on marital status. If they do, they are bound to lose out with regard to the quality of their personnel because their choice is more limited than that of companies who do not select on such criteria. The recent increase in unemployment seems to have had mixed effects. While some informants had difficulty finding a suitable job after they returned to Japan from a period of studying abroad, others were quite happy to be unemployed (in popular slang: *pū o yaru*) while receiving social benefits so that they could devote their time to interesting activities in gay, lesbian or feminist areas. Money is still sufficiently obtainable, as long as one does not place one's demands too high.

Applying the argument that basing hiring and promotion policies on sexual preference harms companies to a debate in two NATO countries, England and the US, which refused access to openly gay men and lesbian women to the army, I would suggest that their army personnel is less highly qualified than that of other nations. Asked about the Japanese army's (euphemistically called self-defence forces, *jieitai*) policy concerning homosexuality, the public relations bureau of the defence agency answered that there was no problem and that they were not planning to formulate a policy on it. In cases where people turned out to be gay or lesbian after having joined the forces there also was no reason to dismiss them (Ikeda 1993). The fact that this was discussed at all in Japan is entirely due to its having been a major theme in America.

Foreign influence clearly played a role in getting homosexuality into the newspapers, magazines and on television. The situation in Japan, however, appears to be very different from that in, for instance, America. Once homosexuality became openly discussed it did not meet with vehement opposition. At worst it meets with indifference but more likely it meets with interest. As noted in chapter seven (p. 288), much of what may seem to be homophobic attitudes can be attributed to a lack of knowledge. Once proper knowledge is provided many Japanese have no qualms about accepting homosexuality as a fact of life that is neither good nor bad but just is. Japan has no Jesse Helms, no Pope, or any person who is clearly homophobic and has the power to harm the rights of gay men and lesbian women.

The only serious discussion in which homosexuality is questioned alongside transsexuality is in relation to marriage. As noted in chapter three (p. 99), Ninomiya Shūhei wrote about the marriage law and pleaded that same-sex marriages should also become possible (1991). Years later a professor of Tokyo University wrote two articles criticizing this, mainly because marriage according to him is supposed to be an institution to produce children and because it would confuse parental rights, basing his notions largely on the French marriage laws (Ōmura 1995a, b). The interesting thing about this discussion is that it is one between heterosexual scholars, who apparently are quite Western-oriented. Among gay and lesbian people in Japan I found that there was next to no discussion about same-sex marriage, except for interested questions about the situation in the Netherlands and Denmark. Striving towards making same-sex marriage possible was typically seen as a goal that was far beyond reach in the present situation, and those advocating it are usually people of or close to the movements that strive to change the laws to allow spouses to both keep their own names in marriage.

At least in theory, human rights are quite well regulated and the Japanese constitution clearly states that no discrimination can be made against adult citizens, where the term adult is not related to the marital status but to the age of the person. If one demands one's constitutional rights they seem to be granted usually, although it may take a long time. The outcome of Occur's court case against the metropolitan government of Tokyo about a youth hostel under its administration that refused them lodgings because they were openly gay, was positive for Occur. The metropolitan government had to pay compensation for having disregarded the human rights of members of Occur. It also lost its appeal against this court ruling (*Japan Times* 1997). A legal framework supporting the equality of gay, lesbian, single and feminist people already exists, although not much use is made of it and it may take a long time before legal precedents will be established that recognizes our rights. There are lately also voices that say that legal action may not be to the benefit of lesbian and gay people because by it they become legally defined and thus the manifestation of homosexuality is limited to boundaries. In this view, expounded by Hino Masaaki at the gay studies seminar at the University of Tokyo in February 1996, not having legal precedents offers more freedom for sexual variety.

Foreign influence is very noticeable in the import of terminology. As we have seen in chapter seven, however, the meanings of the wordings may be different in Japanese than in the language of origin. 'Lesbian separatist' in English means a woman who does not want to have anything to do with men, in Japanese it is a woman who wants to have occasional overnight trips with groups of only lesbian women. As Kakefuda Hiroko made explicit when she saw me write *rezubian* instead of lesbian in an English text (chapter two, p. 50), *rezubian* can be seen as inclusive of women with intimate friendships with women, which would be excluded by the English term, unless one uses it in the sense of Rich's lesbian continuum (Rich 1993), which few people do. *Gei* to many Japanese still means transvestite man or male-to-female transsexual.

Another example is the term *kuia* (queer). In Japan it translates perfectly as *hentai*, which was used in publications long before the concept came into use in America in its present meaning of non-straight (Lunsing 1995). The idea existed prior to usage in America. And whereas it can be seen that 'queer' in America has been used to denote nothing other than homosexual (Signorile 1994), in Japan, where it came to be used from 1995 onwards, it is clearly understood to include the whole gamut of non-straight people, from transsexuals to transvestites, homosexuals, bisexuals, handicapped homosexuals, self-confessed masturbators, hermaphrodites, a large variety of transgenderists or even 'over-genderists' and fag hags (all interviewed in Fushimi 1996). Ueno Chizuko called herself a 'freak' (Ueno 1993 [1990]) before the idea of queer arrived in Japan, and made a good case for the inclusion of at least a proportion of feminists under the term.

A current trend is not to use words like *gei* or *kuia*, but instead to return to indigenous terms like *okama* or *hentai*. The idea behind this is that the imported terms seem trendy and classy and using them is a form of homophobia, fear of being different, or not really accepting oneself for what one is in a Japanese context (Onitsuka 1996). This goes against the American trend of using 'gay' instead of 'homosexual' and now 'queer' instead of 'gay' as if changing wording changes society. The indigenous terms have stronger meanings that are more widely understood or misunderstood and thereby provide greater possibility for really making people understand what their prejudices are and thereby changing not only one's perception of self by accepting them but also Japanese *jōshiki*. In addition to this, many people appear to enjoy using the indigenous terms and to have overcome their qualms about the negative connotations they may have.

For feminists, gay men and lesbian women, the early 1990s were a most interesting period. Japan made great strides on the way to the improvement of their social positions, so much so that an informant who was awarded a fellowship to conduct research abroad decided to stay in Japan in order not to miss out on the developments. He simply thought it more interesting to be in Japan than elsewhere. If this momentum keeps up at the pace it has been since 1990, Japan may soon become one of the most liberal countries with regard to sexuality and possibly gender.

Famous feminists increasingly let their voices be heard and they are increasingly taken seriously by the media, even leading to attempts at serious criticism (e.g. Sawada 1992), whereas formerly they used to be laughed at. On the grassroots level many young women who are not particularly interested in feminism are fending for themselves and questioning the gender roles assigned to them. While many still will marry and be housewives, others will find alternative ways of living their lives. Being single may still not generally be seen as 'normal' but the diversification of Japanese society has allowed for the establishment of circles, networks, neighbourhoods and other surroundings, where it is not considered to be weird (*hen*).

When I conducted my fieldwork, already many students had decided to write dissertations on homosexuality, even if their supervisors did not know what to think of it. In only a few cases was it refused by superiors because it was not an appropriate theme, a position that with the increase in lesbian and gay studies throughout the world will probably become less tenable in the future. Lesbian and gay circles are appearing all over the country, many at universities but also outside them, with the latest news (1995) of new lesbian groups in Okayama, Takamatsu and Hiroshima, members of which have been brought together by way of Kakefuda Hiroko's *minikomishi, Labrys*. While most of these groups initially are social rather than political, from them political ones tend to develop, as I witnessed in the Kansai area during my fieldwork period. The increase in sales of gay magazines and in coverage of homosexual matters in the mass media also suggests that the climate is speedily improving not only for gay men and lesbian women but also for transvestites, transsexuals, and all other people who do not fit heterosexual marriage, to establish their own lifestyles in an infinite variety. Many people are still kept from this but, as discussed above, this can be largely attributed to their fear of showing themselves to be different. Due to the presence of an increasing number of people who came out and met with little adverse reaction, many are likely to follow in their footsteps. The Japanese establishment is advised to take them seriously because they are not likely to disappear.

Since Japan, unlike many Western countries, has no clear-cut national moral system based on religion, it should be relatively easy to adapt smoothly to the needs of people with alternative lifestyles. The major change needed is a change in common sense, that makes alternative lifestyles acceptable to the majority of Japanese people. This work has only just begun but it appears to be much easier than, for instance, in England where, as mentioned in the introduction (p. 4), open discussion seems to be difficult to achieve, and without that nothing works. Japan knows a tradition of listening to the other carefully if the other has enough power to make herself or himself heard. This power gay men, lesbian women, singles, feminists, people in common-law marriages, single parents, transvestites and transsexuals increasingly appear to have. In fact, they may have had it all along but not realized that they had it or not have known ways of putting it to good use.

Some Japanese gay and lesbian activists and colleagues criticized me when in 1996 I spoke at the gay studies seminar at Tokyo University in this positive manner about the Japanese situation. They stressed that there are still many problems with companies and with the bureaucracy and that prejudice is still widespread. Of course they are right but, compared to most other countries in the world, it appears that in Japan much is possible once people start doing something about changing society and, in the few years in which gay and lesbian groups and individuals have started to make their voices heard, much has been achieved. While efforts at change in America and England have been mostly directed towards changes in laws, leaving the common sense of the majority of the population untouched, in Japan much effort goes into educating people about sexuality and gender and changing *jōshiki*, which means changing society as a whole. This is of course time-consuming but Japan is moving in the right direction and as long as that continues I remain positive.

People have started to live their lives the way they want to, without trying always to comply with the demands of family and society at large. At times they will come across a boundary but at least then they will know where the boundary is. If Kakefuda Hiroko had not decided to come out as lesbian, lesbian women in Japan might still have thought that such an action would lead to powerful negative reactions. This did not happen, nor did it in any other recent case I know of. Negative reactions were typically of little importance to the person receiving them. Only in cases of people who did not come out themselves but were found out, which weakens one's position considerably, did they have much influence. Boundaries are being explored and, it seems, most of them have not yet been reached. Where the permitted space ends is not clear but it appears to be much larger than anyone expected.

## Notes

1 Jennifer Robertson writes that there is much historical evidence of female homosexuality in Japanese history, without indicating what she is referring to (Robertson 1992), but I assume that much of it is covered by the evidence I found and discussed in the introduction. This evidence does

not point at widely held constructions and it has hardly been picked up and discussed by Western, or Japanese, scholars, as Robertson notes.

2 The Netherlands, Austria and England.

3 The Kinsey scale divides people along a scale from fully homosexual via dominantly homosexual, bisexual, dominantly heterosexual to fully heterosexual, based on people's sexual experience. On this scale, any variation is possible between the two extremes (Kinsey *et al.* 1948).

# Appendix A: Glossary

In the glossary Japanese words and their translations are given. Rather than meanings in dictionaries I present meanings as I perceived them to be present in the field.

**ai**: tender love, stable affection
**aijin**: lover, mistress or its male counterpart
**aijō**: tender love, stable affection, especially between spouses
**aijō kankei**: love relationship, especially between spouses
**akiramegata**: give-up type, refers to giving up trying to find the ideal spouse and settling for someone less
**ama**: female diver
**amae**: emotional dependence
**aniki**: older brother
**arubaito**: low-paid, unstable jobs
**asai**: thin, light
**asobi**: play, not serious activity
**asobu, asonde ru**: play, have fun, enjoy oneself, engaging oneself in not serious activities
**asshu**: gay, Franco-Japanese pronunciation of 'H', referring to *homo*, used among gay groups in Osaka
**atarimae**: a matter of course, self-evident
**atatakai**: warm in both meanings
**atatakai katei**: warm home

**awase, awaseru**: go along, adapt to
**baisekushuariti**: bisexuality
**baisekushuaru**: bisexual
**bakabakashii**: silly, stupid, ridiculous
**bankonka**: marrying later in life
**barashita**: have been found out, past tense of verb *barasu*: be found out
**bekkyo jijitsukon**: living-apart common-law marriage
**bekkyo kekkon**: living-apart marriage
**besshi undō**: movements for obtaining the right for spouses to keep their different names in marriage
**bian**: new term for lesbian
**bodikon**: clothes that show the lines of the body to its advantage, often short, tight, skirts
**boku**: I, polite masculine, may be avoided when speaking to superiors, but not necessarily
**boshi katei**: single-mother household
**buraku**: area where outcastes (*burakumin*) live or used to live
**burakumin**: outcastes
**burikkoburi**: acting the *ingénue*, a *burikko* is a woman who keeps presenting herself as a naive girl
**burujoa feminizumu**: bourgeois feminism
**chan to**: properly
**chichinashi ko**: fatherless child
**chigo**: Buddhist novice engaging in sexual activities with adult monks
**chinchin**: willy
**chinko**: willy
**chitsu**: vagina
**chōjo**: eldest daughter

**chōkōgakurekigata**: high-educational-record type, referring to marriages taking place at relatively advanced age because high education was pursued
**chotto rezu**: a little bit lesbian, used for women who are predominantly heterosexual but may engage in lesbian sex occasionally out of curiosity or for want of agreeable men
**daikirai**: hate
**daitokai**: metropolis
**daiku**: dyke
**danchi**: public or company housing complex with high-rise buildings, similar to a housing estate in England
**danka seido**: system of registration of households in Buddhist temples, prevalent in the Tokugawa period (1603–1868)
**danshō**: male prostitute
**danshoku, nanshoku**: homosexuality, or love of men, often translated as pederasty, opposite of *joshoku*
**dansōsha**: male dresser, female transvestite
**de aru**: be
**debusen bā**: gay bar specializing in fat men and those who seek fat men
**dokushin**: single
**donkan**: insensitive, blunt
**dōseiaisha**: homosexual
**dōsei suru**: live together, cohabit
**enkai**: company or other group parties with food and drink
**enmusubi**: tying a bond, referring to marriage
**erochikku**: erotic
**etchi**: Anglo-Japanese pronunciation of 'H', queer, abnormal, refers often to sexual activity and what is found erotic or exciting

**feminisuto**: feminist, mostly understood as a feminist scholar but also as a gallant man

**feminizumu**: feminism

**fūfu yōshi**: adoption of a married couple that becomes successor to the household

**fukesen bā**: gay bar specializing in older men and thosewho seek older men

**furin**: illegitimate sex, extra-marital sex, immorality, unethical

**fushi katei**: single-father household

**fushizen**: unnatural

**futokutei tasū**: indefinite number

**futsū**: ordinary, normal, common, heterosexual

**futsū ni**: normally

**futsū no otokō**: ordinary, normal, common or heterosexual man

**fozoku sangyū**: the pleasure industry

**gakkai**: conference

**gakusei undō**: student movement

**gaman suru**: endure

**gasshuku**: overnight group trip

**gei**: gay, often understood as transvestite or transsexual, but by gay movement presented as politically correct

**gei bā**: gay bar, male transvestite bar

**gei bōi**: gay boy, occupational transvestite, male prostitute

**gei būmu**: gay boom, media hype concerning malehomosexuality

**geinōkai**: world of show business

**gei ojisan**: a gay old man

**gisō kekkon**: camouflage marriage

**gokuraku**: happy-go-lucky, nirvana, paradise, bliss

**gomakasu**: evade giving answer to a question

**haigūsha**: spouse
**haipuri**: pretty high-school boy, used among gay groups in Osaka
**hanamuko gakkō**: bridal school for men, school where men are taught how to present themselves in order to make a woman wish to marry them
**hanninmae**: half a person, see also *ichininmae*
**hanpatsu**: adverse, defiant reaction
**harenchi**: shamelessness, impudence
**harigata**: dildo
**hasu**: lotus flower
**hazukashii**: shameful
**hen**: weird, strange, anomalous, abnormal
**hentai**: weird, queer, anomalous, abnormal
**hentaisei**: queerness, abnormality, anomaly
**hetero**: heterosexual
**hichakushutsushi**: illegitimate child, legal term
**hikon**: unmarried
**hishinzoku setai**: non-family household
**hiyatoi rōdōsha:** day labourer
**hōkenteki**: feudal
**homo**: gay, homo, in some circles seen as derogatory, abbreviation of *homosekushuaru*
**homosekushuaru**: gay, homosexual
**honne**: real feelings, opposite of *tatemae*
**honnō**: instinct
**hōritsukon**: legal marriage
**ichininmae**: adult or adult married couple
**ichininmae no onna**: fully adult women, i.e. a fully adult gendered being
**ichininmae no shakaijin**: a fully adult person
**ie**: household, continued through generations

**ie seido**: household system
**ijimekko**: the victim of bullying
**ijimeru**: tease, abuse
**ikebana**: flower arranging
**ima**: living room
**inaka**: countryside, also used to refer to the town one is born, if that is not Osaka or Tokyo and one lives in one of these towns
**ippan jōshiki**: general *jōshiki*, general common sense
**ippanron**: general theory
**ippan tsūkan**: general feelings
**ippan tsūnen**: general concepts
**ippu ippu sei**: one-man–one-woman-system, monogamy, in gay and lesbian context also one-man–one-man-system and one-woman–one-woman-system
**ippu tasai sei**: one-man–several-women-system, system in which a man has sexual relationships with several women or several wives simultaneously
**isharyō**: compensation money
**iseisōsha**: different sex dresser
**isōsha**: different dresser
**ittaika**: physical unity
**ittaiteki**: unified, united, in one body
**iya na me**: nasty eyes, negative reactions
**iyarashii**: disgusting, distasteful
**izakaya**: Japanese-style drinking and eating place
**jān**: exclamation used in a particular network to express shock
**jei**: good, Franco-Japanese pronunciation of 'G', referring to desirable men among some gay men, used among gay groups in Osaka
**jendā fukaishō**: gender ambiguity

**jibun ni au**: agree with oneself
**jieitai**: self-defence forces, euphemism for army
**jijitsukon**: common-law marriage
**jinruigaku**: anthropology
**jōrei**: local regulation
**jōshiki**: common sense
**joshoku, nyosoku**: heterosexuality, or love of women, opposite of *danshoku*
**josōsha**: female dresser, male transvestite
**jūminhyō**: official address register
**jūmin todoke**: registration of official address
**kabuki**: type of theatre
**kafū**: culture of the house
**kafuchōsei**: patriarchate
**kagema yarō**: young actor being taught to become *onnagata* and often expected to engage in prostitution
**kakkō ii**: handsome, good-looking, stylish
**kamingu auto suru**: coming out
**kamu auto suru**: coming out
**kanojo**: she, girlfriend, female partner
**kanri shakai**: the administration society, used in left-wing circles to refer to the power of the bureaucracy, which is presented as all-mighty
**kanshō suru**: interfere
**kanzen na hetero**: fully or perfectly heterosexual
**kanzen na homo**: fully or perfectly homosexual
**kanzen na otoko**: fully or perfectly male
**kareshi**: he, boyfriend, male partner
**kasō ni enjiru**: overact
**katai**: difficult, hard, tough, inaccessible
**katana**: sword, also symbol for penis
**kateinai rikon**: divorce within the household

**katte ni**: just like that
**kawaisō**: pathetic, sad
**kayoi jijitsukon**: commuting common-law marriage
**kayoi kekkon**: commuting marriage
**keishiki kekkon**: marriage in form
**keiyaku kekkon**: contract marriage, marriage whereby a contract is signed to establish the date of divorce
**kejime**: ability to distinguish
**kekkon**: marriage
**kekkonshiki**: marriage ceremony
**kekkon tekireiki**: the proper age to marry
**kekkon todoke**: marriage registration
**kenkyūkai**: study group, study group meeting, seminar
**ketsuen kankei**: blood relationship
**kichin to**: properly, neatly
**kiku**: chrysanthemum, symbol of the imperial house, also symbol for anus in gay contexts
**kimochiwarui**: sickening, sick, distasteful
**kirai**: dislike, hate
**kitanai**: dirty, filthy
**ko**: door, household
**ko**: boy
**koi**: passion, romantic love
**koibito**: lover, the one and only love
**kojin**: individual
**kokka**: state
**kokorogurushi**: pain in the heart
**kōmuin**: civil servant
**kongaishi**: extra-marital child
**konin**: marriage, legal term
**konin seido**: marriage system
**kono michi**: this way, see *kono sekai*

**kono sekai**: this world, used to refer to gay world or gay bar circuit
**koseki**: household register
**koseki seido**: household registration system
**kowai**: frightening, frightened, among some informants used to express shock, see also *jān*
**kuia**: queer
**Kurisumasu kēki**: Christmas cake, also used to refer to women who remain unmarried after having become 25 years of age
**kyariā ūman**: career woman, career women
**kyōdō seikatsu**: living together
**kyōmei kekkon**: brother–sister marriage, marriage in which the relationship between the spouses is likened to that of a brother and sister
**manga**: comics
**manshon**: concrete apartment, high-class, expensive housing in cities
**masutō**: bartender
**marijji**: marriage, romantically used Anglo-Japanese term
**mechakucha**: incoherent, confused, messed around
**meiwaku**: trouble
**meiwaku o kakeru**: cause trouble
**memeshii**: feminine, derogatory when used for men
**mesu**: female, biological terminology
**miai**: meeting a prospective marriage candidate, also *omiai*
**migoto ni**: dexterously
**mikon**: not yet married, single
**minikomi, minikomishi**: small-scale publications or magazines, mostly produced by politically oriented groups and organizations but also by individuals and non-politically oriented organizations

**miryokuteki**: charming
**mizu ga au**: the water meets, get along with
**mr redii**: Mr Lady, occupational transvestite
**muga**: non-self
**muko yōshi**: adopted husband, refers to type of marriage in which the husband adopts the name of the house he marries into and eventually becomes the successor to the head of household
**muko yōshi kekkon**: marriage in which the husband is adopted into a household, see also *muko yōshi*
**mura hachibu**: ostracism
**nachuraru ni**: naturally
**naien**: common-law marriage with the intention of legal marriage
**nakineiri**: crying oneself to sleep
**nakōdo**: marriage go-between
**namakemono**: sluggard
**nanka chigau**: something's not quite right
**nanka hen**: something's not quite right, same as *nanka chigau*
**nanshoku**: see *danshoku*
**nayami, nayamu**: worry, trouble, be troubled
**nayanda**: past tense of *nayamu*
**nazo**: riddle, enigma
**niisan**: older brother, polite way of addressing young and middle-aged men
**ninchi suru**: recognize
**nōmaru**: normal
**nonke**: straights, used in gay circles
**nyoshoku**: see *joshoku*

**nyū hāfu**: new half, half man, half woman, man who uses hormones and/or silicone transplants to have breasts and look feminine
**nyūseki**: entering the register, i.e. *koseki*
**nyū ūman**: new women, new woman
**obāchan**: granny
**obasan**: aunt, way of addressing middle-aged women
**okaeri**: welcome back
**okama**: cooking pot, often derogatory; feminine gay man, transvestite man, male prostitute
**okama bā**: male transvestite bar
**okashii**: weird, funny, strange
**ōki na**: big
**okoge**: residue that sticks to cooking pot (*okama*), hence fag hag
**OL**: Office Lady, female clerical worker
**omocha**: toy, play-thing
**omoiyari**: empathy
**omiai**: see *miai*
**onabe**: cooking pot, lesbian, masculine woman, transvestite woman
**onabe bā**: female transvestite bar
**onē kotoba**: gay camp speech, effeminate speech used by men
**onnagata**: men who play female parts in *kabuki* theatre
**onna no ko**: girl
**onna no shiawase**: women's happiness, i.e. marriage
**onnarashii**: womanlike
**ooshii**: masculine, derogatory when used for women
**ore**: I, masculine, not polite
**ossan**: derogatory for *ojisan*, middle-aged man, older man
**ossantachi**: plural of *ossan*

**osu**: male, biological terminology
**otoko asobi**: playing with men, male homosexual activities
**otoko no ko**: boy
**otoko pettogata**: man-as-pet type, referring to marriage in which the woman is older or has a higher position in society than the man
**otokorashii**: manlike
**otona**: adult
**otōto**: younger brother
**penisu**: penis
**pū o yaru**: slang for being unemployed
**puro-resurā**: professional wrestler
**rabu chairudo**: love child
**rankōgata**: promiscuity
**renai**: love
**renai kankei**: love relationship
**renai kekkon**: love marriage
**renjō**: passionate, romantic love
**rezu**: lesbian, often derogatory, abbreviation of *rezubian*
**rezubian**: lesbian
**rezubian būmu**: lesbian boom, media hype concerning lesbian women
**rezubian no obasan**: elderly lesbian woman
**rezubian separetisuto**: lesbian separatist
**rikai dekinai**: cannot understand, incapable of understanding
**rikon**: divorce
**rikutsuppoi**: argumentative, know-all
**ryōsei guyū**: hermaphrodite
**ryōtō**: double-sworded, bisexual
**S**: short for sisterhood or *shisutāfuddo*
**sabetsu yōgo**: discriminatory term

**samurai**: warrior
**san**: Mr, Ms, Mrs
**san K**: three K, three highs, referring to height, educational record and occupational position of men
**sarariiman**: salaried worker, company employee
**sei ippai**: fully, to the full, to the utmost
**seken**: the surrounding world, the outside world, the surrounding people, the neighbourhood, other people
**sekentei**: public face
**sekkusu wākā**: sex worker
**semeru**: tease, torture
**sentō**: public bath
**shakai byōri**: social pathology
**shakaigakusha**: sociologist
**shigusa**: manner of movement
**shimin undō**: citizen's movement
**shindoi**: tiresome
**shinguru**: single
**shinrai dekiru**: trustworthy
**shinzoku setai**: family household
**shiseiji**: illegitimate child
**shisutāfuddo**: sisterhood, referring to a bond between women as opposed to men, also *S*
**shitsurei**: impolite
**shizen**: nature, natural
**shōgatsu**: New Year, usually three days, but *shōgatsu* parties may be held weeks later
**shōjo manga**: girls' comics
**shōkōgun**: syndrome
**shōnenai**: love of boys, pederasty
**shufu ronsō**: discussions about the housewife
**shūi**: environment, surrounding people

**sōsharu rezubian**: social lesbian, used to refer to women who live with women or prefer to be with women without being sexually engaged
**sono koto**: that, used to refer to homosexuality in order to avoid the word homosexuality
**soto**: outside, opposite of *uchi*
**suru**: do
**suteki**: stylish, fashionable
**tada no sukebe**: just lewd, just a lecher
**tada no tomodachi**: just friends
**tanshin funin**: one spouse temporarily living elsewhere for the sake of work
**tarento**: talent, television personality without apparent talents
**tatemae**: face behaviour, opposite of *honne*
**tekitō ni awaseru**: go along as fits the situation, adapt to the situation
**tennōsei**: emperor system
**tokutei no**: steady, definite
**tomodachi**: friend
**tomodachi kekkon**: friendship marriage
**toransubesutaito**: transvestite
**toransu jendā**: transgender, referring to people who have attributes that are generally assigned to the opposite sex
**tsukiai**: personal relationships
**tsurai**: painful, bitter, hard to bear
**uchi**: inside, opposite of *soto*
**ukiyoe**: picture of the floating world
**ūman ribā**: women's libber
**ūman ribu**: women's lib
**urusai**: troublesome
**usotsuku**: lie

**wagamama**: selfish, self-centred, egoistic, but also used proudly and positively to discern oneself from people with not much will of their own

**wakasen bā**: gay bar specializing in young men and those who seek young men

**wakashu**: young actor being taught to become *onnagata* and often expected to engage in prostitution

**wan patān**: one pattern, the same as everyone

**watashi**: I, polite

**yakuza**: Japanese mafia

**yancha**: tomboy

**yaoi**: explicit pornographic genre of girls' comics describing male homosexuality

**yasashii**: kind, friendly

**yasuragi no ba**: a place to be at ease, to relieve stress

**yogoresen**: dirt lovers, men who like to have sex with day labourers

**yome**: bride, also *yome-san*

**yome o morau**: receiving a bride, marrying for man

**yome-san**: bride, also *yome*

**Zainichi Kankoku-/Chōsen-jin**: Koreans living in Japan, respectively aligned to South (Kankokujin) and North (Chōsenjin) Korea

# Appendix B: Research Groups

This list includes groups participant observation was conducted with, indicated by P.O., as well as groups on which data were sought through interviewing members, reading their writings, and writings about them. Pol. stands for political, soc. for social, and stud. for study oriented.

## Feminist Groups

**Pāpuru: Sei Bōryoku o Yurusanai Onnatachi no Kai**: Purple: Women's Group against Sexual Violence, pol.
**Onnatachi no Rōdō Kumiai**: Women's Labour Union, pol.

## Other Emancipatory Groups

**Menzu Ribu Kenkyūkai**: Men's Liberation Study Group, P.O., stud., soc.
**Kakushinhan?: Shinguru**: Crime of Conviction?: Single, also **Shinguruzu Netto**: Singles' Network, P.O., stud., soc.
**Dokushin Fujin Renmei**: Single Women's League, pol., stud., soc.
**Onna no Ishibumi no Kai**: Women's Group of the Memorial Stone, P.O., soc.

**Hitori Aruki no Kai**: Group of People who Walk Alone, P.O., stud.

**Fūfu Besshi no Hoseika o Jitsugen suru Kai**: Group for the Realization of Legalization of Separate Names for Spouses, pol.

**Fūfu Bessei Sentakusei o Susumeru Kai**: Group for the Promotion of Free Choice of Separate Names for Spouses, pol.

**Shussei Sabetsu no Kaihō o Motomeru Onnatachi no Kai**: Women's Group that Seeks Liberation from Birth Discrimination, pol.

## Gay and Lesbian and Gay Groups

**JILGA**: International Lesbian and Gay Association Japan, P.O.

**Akā: Ugoku Gei to Rezubian no Kai**: Occur: Group of Moving Gays and Lesbians, P.O., pol., soc., stud.

**OGC: Osaka Gei Konmyūniti**: Osaka Gay Community, P.O., pol., stud., soc.

**Ru Kurabu Asshu**: Le Club H, P.O., soc., stud., pol.

**DON!** (Do Over Naturally!): P.O., soc.

**Puapua: Sekushuariti to Jendā Kaihō Dantai**: Puapua: Group for the Liberation of Sexuality and Gender, P.O., pol., stud., soc.

**Kamigata DJ Kurabu**: Kamigata DJ Club, P.O., soc., stud.

**Sākuru T**: Circle T, stud., soc.

**Gay Front Kansai**, pol. soc., stud.

**Fain Kurabu**, later **Puraimu Kurabu**: Fine Club, Prime Club, P.O., soc.

**B-nettowāku (B-netto)**, in Osaka **B-nettowāku (B-netto)**

**Kansai**, later in Tokyo **Kokoro no Nettowāku**: B (Buddhist) Network, Network of the Heart, P.O., soc., stud.

**Out & About**, international lesbian and gay leisure circle, P.O., soc.

## Lesbian Groups

**Regumi**: Lesbian Group, soc., stud., pol.

**LIO**: Lesbians in Occur, soc., pol., stud.

**YLP**, later **OLP**: **Yancha Rezubian Pawā, Osaka Rezubian Pawā**: Tomboy's Lesbian Power, Osaka Lesbian Power, also Adult (*Otona no*) Lesbian Power and Open Lesbian Power, P.O., pol., soc., stud.

Kakefuda Hiroko's Lesbian Network, P.O., soc., stud., pol.

## Miscellaneous Groups and Circles

**Renai no Tatsujin Kōza**: Course for Becoming an Achiever in Love, P.O., stud., soc.

**Ueno Chizuko Zemi**: Ueno Chizuko's Seminar, P.O., stud., soc.

**KKSK: Kansai Kazoku Shakaigaku Kenkyūkai**: Kansai Sociology of the Family Seminar, P.O., stud.

**Toshi Minzokugaku Kenkyūkai**: Urban Ethnology Seminar, P.O., stud.

**Umechika Fōramu**: Umechika Forum, political grassroots group, P.O., pol., stud., soc.

**Damu Taipu: Dumb Type**, theatre performance group, P.O., soc., pol. stud.

**Diamond**, **Shanghai Love Theater**, drag performance group, P.O., soc.

Kyoto-based private network of people involved in activities concerning gender, sexuality and AIDS, P.O., soc., pol.

Osaka-based private network of people involved in traditional left-wing activities and feminist activities, P.O., soc., pol.

Tokyo-based private networks similar to the two above., P.O., soc., pol.

# References


Abramson, Allen (1993) Between autobiography and method: Being male, seeing myth and the analysis of structures of gender and sexuality in the eastern interior of Fiji, in *Gendered fields: Women, men and ethnography*, Diane Bell, Pat Caplan and Wazir Jahan Karim eds, London and New York: Routledge, pp. 63–77

Agar, Michael H. (1980) *The professional stranger: An informal introduction to ethnography*, New York: Academic Press

Aide Suisse Contre le Sida (1992) Eizu yobō no tame no sēfu sekkusu (Safe sex for the prevention of AIDS), translation of a Swiss pamphlet, in *Za Gei* (The Gay) No. 126, November, pp. 40–8

Akā (1992) Kaiin kenshō, Kiyaku zenbun, Kiyaku (Member's charter, Preamble to the contract, The contract), in *Dōseiai kenkyū josetsu: Dōseiaisha to iseiaisha no hikaku chōsa yori* (An introduction to the study of homosexuality:From a comparative investigation of homosexuals and heterosexuals), Yajima Zemi ed., Uhauha Hakusho '91, Tokyo: Chūō Daigaku Bungakubu Shakaigakka, pp. 164–71

Akisato, Wakuni (1986) *Nemureru mori no binan* (The beautiful man in the sleeping forest), Tokyo: Shōgakukan

Akisato, Wakuni (1992) *Tomoi*, Tokyo: Shōgakukan (first print 1987)

Akiyama, Yōko (1991) Enoki Misako to Chūpiren: 'Ribu shishi nōto' yori (Enoki Misako and Chūpiren: From 'Lib epic notes'), in *Joseigaku Nenpō* (Chronicle of Women's Studies) No. 12, pp. 109–15

Akiyama, Yōko (1992) Urufu no Kai no koto: 'Ribu shishi nōto' yori (About the Wolf Group: From 'Lib epic notes'), in *Impaction* No. 73, Tokushū: Ribu 20nen (Special: 20 years of liberation), pp. 30–7

Almaguer, Tomas (1993) Chicano men: A cartography of homosexual identity and behavior, in *The lesbian and gay studies reader*, Henry Abelove, Michèle Aina Barale and David M. Halperin eds, London and New York: Routledge, pp. 255–73

Amadiume, Ifi (1987) *Male daughters, female husbands: Gender and sex in an African society*, London and New Jersey: Zed Books

Andachi, Akira and Matsuura, Rieko (1992) Sore de mo onna wa kudaranai (Even then women are insignificant), in *Asahi Jānaru* (Asahi Journal) Vol. 34 No. 11, March 13

Anderson, Alexis (1985) Purity and power among the Brahmans of Kashmir, in *The category of the person: Anthropology, philosophy, history*, Michael Carrithers, Steven Collins and Steven Lukes eds, Cambridge: Cambridge University Press, pp. 190–216

Angrosino, Michael V. (1986) Son and lover: The anthropologist as non-threatening male, in *Self, sex and gender in cross-cultural fieldwork*, Tony Larry Whitehead and Mary Ellen Conaway eds, Urbana and Chicago: University of Illinois Press, pp. 64–83

Anonymous (1991) Ā, kekkon: Isshō dokushin de sugosubeki ka o kangaeru!! (Oh, marriage: Thinking of whether I should remain alone my whole life!!), in *Sabu*, September, pp. 92–4

Aoki, Yayoi (1987) *Shinguru karuchā: Posuto kazoku no yukue* (Single culture: Tracing what comes after the family), Tokyo: Yūhikaku

Aoyama, Tomoko (1988) Male homosexuality as treated by Japanese writers, in *The Japanese trajectory: Modernisation and beyond*, Gavan McCormack and Yoshio Sugimoto eds, Cambridge: Cambridge University Press, pp. 186–204

Arahata, Kanson (1978) Blutbefleckte freie Liebe (Bloodstained free love), in *Frauen in der Revolution: Wilde Blumen auf unfreiem Feld* (Women in the revolution: Wild flowers in an unfree field), Terasaki Akiko and Ilse Lenz eds, transl., Berlin: Karin Kramer Verlag, pp. 103–7

Ardener, Shirley (1978) Introduction: The nature of women in society, in *Defining females: The nature of women in society*, Shirley Ardener ed., London: Croom Helm, pp. 9–48

Asada, Akira (1991) Gei mūbumento no tame ni (For a gay movement), in *Impaction* No. 71: Gei riberēshon (Gay liberation), Inpakuto Shuppankai, August, pp. 72–80

Asada, Akira (1992) Anata e no tegami: Jobun ni kaete (A letter to you: A preface), in *Gei ripōto: Dōseiaisha wa kōgen suru* (Gay report: Homosexuals speak out), Ugoku Gei to Rezubian no Kai (Occur) eds, Tokyo: Tottori Shinsha, pp. 3–7

Asada, Akira and Hirano, Hiroaki (1995) Asada-Hirano tōkusesshon: Gei akutibizumu no kanōsei: Hetero shakai e no teigen (The Asada / Hirano talk session: Proposals to the heterosexual society), in *Gei no 11 gatsusai tengoku hōkokushū* (Report collection of the celestial gay November festival), Kyōdai 11Gatsusai Gei Purojekuto Jikkō Iinkai ed., Kyoto, pp. 25–69.

Asahi, Miwa (1994) Sie taikenbetsu bunseki (Analysis according to sexual experience), in *Sei kōi ni taisuru daigakusei no ishiki* (The consciousness of sexual activity of university students), Yajima Zemi, Seiai Chōsa Kenkyūkai ed., Tokyo: Chūō Daigaku Bungakubu Shakaigakka, March, pp. 80–9

*Asahi Shinbun* (1992) Kekkon shinai otokotachi: 10nen de baizō, Seiō ni chikazuku (Men who do not marry: Doubled in ten years: Closing in on

Western Europe), in *Asahi Shinbun*, Osaka evening edition, 18 July

*Asahi Shinbun* (1994) Dōseiaisha no jinsei wakatte: Hatsu no rezubian-gei-parēdo Tokyo de (Understanding the life of homosexuals: The first lesbian and gay parade in Tokyo), in *Asahi Shinbun*, Osaka morning edition, 8 August

Asai, Takeshi (1995) Teiji Furuhashi: Furuhashi Teiji Interview, in *Dice* (Daishi) No. 8, February, pp. 14–17

Asakura, Fumi (1992) 'Iseiaisha no feminisuto?' ga yomu *Sekushuariti wa shizen ka* ('A heterosexual feminist' reads *Is sexuality nature?*), in *Yagō* (Illicit Affairs), No. 29, October, pp. 3–5

Baba, Megumi (1988) Fujin Kōron ripōto: Dokusha 2200nin no seiteki yokkyū chōsa (Fujin Kōron report: Research into the sexual desires of 2,200 readers), in *Fujin Kōron* (Public Discussion of Women), December, pp. 279–340

Bachnik, Jane (1983) Recruitment strategies for household succession: Rethinking Japanese household organization, in *Man* Vol. 18, pp. 160–82

Bachnik, Jane (1992) *Kejime*: Defining a shifting self in multiple organizational modes, in *Japanese sense of self*, Nancy R. Rosenberger ed., Cambridge: Cambridge University Press, pp. 152–72

Bachnik, Jane (1994) Introduction: *uchi/soto*: Challenging our conceptualizations of self, social order, and language, in *Situated meaning: Inside and Outside in Japanese self, society, and language*, Jane Bachnik and Charles Quinn Jr eds, Princeton: Princeton University Press, pp. 3–37

Bachnik, Jane and Quinn, Charles Jr eds (1994) *Situated meaning: Inside and outside in Japanese self, society and language*, Princeton: Princeton University Press

Back, Les (1993) Gendered participation: Masculinity and fieldwork in a south London adolescent community, in *Gendered fields: Women, men and ethnography*, Diane Bell, Pat Caplan and Wazir Jahan Karim eds, London: Routledge, pp. 215–33

Badinter, Elisabeth (1986) *L'un est l'autre: Des relations entre hommes et femmes* (The one is the other: Relations between men and women), Paris: Editions Odile Jacob, Paris

Barnlund, Dean C. (1975) *Public and private self in Japan and the U.S.: Communicative styles of two cultures*, Tokyo: The Simul Press

Benedict, Ruth (1977) *The chrysanthemum and the sword: Patterns of Japanese culture*, London: Routledge Kegan Paul (first publication 1946)

Bessatsu Takarajima (1991) *Onna o aisuru onnatachi no monogatari* (Stories of women who love women), Bessatsu Takarajima No. 64, Tokyo: JICC Shuppan (first print 1987)

Bethel, Diana Lynn (1992) Life on Obasuteyama, or, inside a Japanese institution for the elderly, in *Japanese social organization*, Takie Sugiyama Lebra ed., Honolulu: University of Hawaii Press, pp. 109–34

Blackwood, Evelyn (1995) Falling in love with an-Other lesbian: Reflections on identity in fieldwork, in *Taboo: Sex, identity and erotic subjectivity in anthropological fieldwork*, Don Kulick and Margaret Willson eds, London and New York: Routlegde, pp. 51–75

Bloch, Maurice (1991) Language, anthropology and cognitive science, in *Man* Vol. 21 No. 2, pp. 183–98

Bolton, Ralph (1995) Tricks, friends, and lovers: Erotic dimensions of the fieldwork experience, in *Taboo: Sex, identity and erotic subjectivity in anthropological fieldwork*, Don Kulick and Margaret Willson eds, London and New York: Routledge, pp. 140–67

Bornoff, Nicholas (1992) *Pink samurai: An erotic exploration of Japanese society*, London: Grafton (first print 1991)

Bornstein, Kate (1994) *Gender outlaw: On men, women, and the rest of us*, London and New York: Routledge

Bosse, Frederike (1994) Keine Arbeitslosen in Japan?: Ein Versuch, die japanische Arbeitsmarktstatistik 'richtig' zu lesen (No unemployed in Japan?: An attempt to read the Japanese labour market statistics 'correctly', in *Japan: Wirtschaft, Politik, Gesellschaft* (Japan: Economy, Politics, Society), April, pp. 181–7

Brinton, Mary C. (1992) Christmas cakes and wedding cakes: The social organization of Japanese women's lifecourse, in *Japanese social organization*, Takie Sugiyama Lebra ed., Honolulu: University of Hawaii Press, pp. 79–107

Burgess, Robert G. (1984) *In the field: An introduction to field research*, London, Boston and Sydney: Allen & Unwin

Busi, Aldo (1989) *Seminar on youth*, London and Boston: Faber & Faber

Busi, Aldo (1990) *The standard life of a temporary pantyhose salesman*, London and Boston: Faber & Faber

Busi, Aldo (1993) *Sodomies in elevenpoint*, London and Boston: Faber & Faber

Butler, Judith (1990) *Gender trouble: Feminism and the subversion of identity*, London and New York: Routledge

Butler, Judith (1991) Imitation and gender subordination, in *Inside/out: Lesbian theories, gay theories*, Diana Fuss ed., New York and London: Routledge, pp. 13–31

Butler, Judith (1993) *Bodies that matter: On the discursive limits of 'sex'*, London and New York: Routledge

Califia, Pat (1988) *Macho sluts*, Boston: Alyson Publications Inc.

Callaway, Helen (1993) 'The most essentially female function of all': Giving birth, in *Defining females: The nature of women in society*, Shirley Ardener ed., Providence and Oxford: Berg, pp. 146–67

Caplan, Pat (1987) Introduction, in *The cultural construction of sexuality*, Pat Caplan ed., London and New York: Routledge, pp. 1–30

Carrithers, Michael (1985) An alternative history of the self, in *The category of the person: Anthropology, philosophy, history*, Michael Carrithers,

Steven Collins and Steven Lukes eds, Cambridge: Cambridge University Press, pp. 234–56

Carter, Rose and Dilatush, Lois (1977) Office Ladies, in *Women in changing Japan*, Joyce Lebra, Joy Paulson and Elizabeth Powers eds, Boulder: Westview Press, pp. 75–88

Cecchini, Rose Marie (1977) Women and suicide, in *Women in changing Japan*, Joyce Lebra, Joy Paulson and Elizabeth Powers eds, Boulder: Westview Press, pp. 263–96

Cesara, Manda (1982) *Reflections of a woman anthropologist: No hiding place*, London: Academic Press

Chebel, Malek (1988) *L'Esprit du sérail: Perversions et marginalités au Maghreb* (The spirit of the harem: Perversions and marginalities in the Maghreb), Paris: Lieu Commun

Childs, Margaret H. (1980) Chigo monogatari: Love stories or Buddhist sermons? in *Monumenta Nipponica* Vol. 35 No. 2, Summer, pp. 127–31

Chō, Shinya (1992) Koibito to no seikatsu, kekkon ni tsuite no ishiki (Life with a lover, the consciousness of marriage), in *Dōseiai kenkyū josetsu: Dōseiaisha to iseiaisha no hikaku chōsa yori* (An introduction to the study of homosexuality: From comparative research on homosexuals and heterosexuals), Yajima Zemi ed., Uhauha Hakusho '91, Tokyo: Chūō Daigaku Bungakubu Shakaigakka, October, pp. 111–19

Clifford, James (1986) On ethnographic allegory, in *Writing culture: The poetics and politics of ethnography*, James Clifford and George E. Marcus eds, Berkeley, Los Angeles and London: University of California Press, pp. 98–121

Cohen, Anthony P. (1994) *Self consciousness: An alternative anthropology of identity*, London and New York: Routledge

Condon, Jane (1986) *A half step behind: Japanese women of the 80s*, New York: Dodd Mead

Constantine, Peter (1992) *Japanese street slang*, New York and Tokyo: Tengu Books

Cornwall, Andrea (1994) Gendered identities and gender ambiguity among *travestis* in Salvador, Brazil, in *Dislocating masculinities: Comparative ethnographies*, Andrea Cornwall and Nancy Lindisfarne eds, London and New York: Routledge, pp. 111–32

Cornwall, Andrea and Lindisfarne, Nancy (1994) Dislocating masculinity: Gender, power and anthropology, in *Dislocating masculinity:Comparative ethnographies*, Andrea Cornwall and Nancy Lindisfarne eds, London and New York: Routledge, pp. 11–47

*Crea* (1991) Tokushō: Gei no runessansu '91 (Special feature: Gay renaissance '91), in *Crea*, February, pp. 63–109

Creet, Julia (1995) Anxieties of identity: Coming out and coming undone, in *Negotiating lesbian and gay subjects*, Monica Dorenkamp and Richard Henke eds, New York and London: Routledge, pp. 179–99

Cross Dressing (1992) Dansō kurabu sennyū shuzai: Shinya no reijintachi (Depth investigation into a female transvestite club: Midnight's young women in men's clothes), in *Cross Dressing* No. 2, April, pp. 64–6

Davies, Peter (1992) The role of disclosure in coming out among gay men, in *Modern homosexualities: Fragments of lesbian and gay experience*, Ken Plummer ed., London and New York: Routledge, pp. 75–83

Davis, Nanette J. (1977) Feminism, deviance and social change, in *Deviance and the problem of social change*, Edward Sagarin ed., Beverly Hills and London: Sage Publications, pp. 247–76

de Beauvoir, Simone (1976a) *Le deuxième sexe I: Les faits et les mythes* (The second sex I: The facts and the myths), Paris: Folio (first edition 1949)

de Beauvoir, Simone (1976b) *Le deuxième sexe II: L'expérience vécue* (The second sex II: The experience lived), Paris: Folio (first edition 1949)

de Lauretis, Teresa (1994) *The practice of love: Lesbian sexuality and perverse desire*, Bloomington and Indianapolis: Indiana University Press

DeVos, George A. (1985) Dimensions of self in Japanese culture, in *Culture and self: Asian and Western perspectives*, Anthony J. Marsella, George A. DeVos and Francis L.K. Hsu eds, New York and London: Tavistock Publications, pp. 141–84

DeVos, George A. (1986a) The relation of guilt towards parents to achievement and arranged marriage in Japan, in *Japanese patterns of behavior: Selected readings*, Takie Sugiyama Lebra and William P. Lebra eds, Honolulu: University of Hawaii Press (revised version of first 1974 edition) pp. 80–101

DeVos, George A. (1986b) Religion and the family: Structural and motivational relationships, in *Religion and the family in East Asia*, George A. DeVos and Takao Sofue eds, Berkeley: University of California Press, pp. 3–34

Doi, Takeo (1975) *The anatomy of dependence*, Tokyo: Kōdansha

Doi, Takeo (1985) *Omote to ura* (Front and back), Tokyo: Kōbundō

Doi, Takeo (1986) *The anatomy of self: The individual versus society*, Tokyo: Kōdansha

Dokushin Fujin Renmei Kinenshi Henshū Iinkai ed. (1977) *Wadatsumi no koe o towa ni: Dokushin Fujin Renmei jūnen no ayumi* (Voices of the ocean for eternity: Ten years of the Single Women's League), Tokyo: Dokushin Fujin Renmei

Dokushin Fujin Renmei 20nenshi Henshū Iinkai ed. (1987) *Hanayaka ni shinguru raifu: 20nen o kinen shite* (A bright single life: Remembering 20 years), Tokyo: Dokushin Fujin Renmei

Domenig, Roland (1991) Aids in Japan (AIDS in Japan), in *Beiträge zur Japanologie* (Contributions to Japanese Studies) Band 29–II: *Japan von AIDS bis Zen* (Japan from AIDS to Zen), Eva Bachmayer, Wolfgang Herbert and Sepp Linhart eds, Vienna: Institut für Japanologie der Universität Wien, pp. 506–25

Dōseiai Kaihō Undō Dantai Puapua (1992) Kōgibun (Open letter [to the Secretary of Osaka prefecture, Nakagawa Yasuo]) in *Dōseiai o kangaeyō: Ittai gei tte, nan ya nen* (Let's think about homosexuality: What on earth is gay?), at Osaka Daigaku Gakuensai, Sekushuariti and Jendā Kaihō Dantai Puapua ed., Osaka, 1–3 November

Douglas, Mary (1992) *Purity and danger: An analysis of the concepts of pollution and taboo*, London and New York: Routledge (first publication 1966)

Duberman, Martin (1977) The bisexual debate, in *Marriage and alternatives: Exploring intimate relationships*, Roger W. Libby and Robert N. Whitehurst eds, Glenview: Scott, Foresman & Company, pp. 241–56

Dubisch, Jill (1995) Lovers in the field: Sex, dominance, and the female anthropologist, in *Taboo: Sex, identity and erotic subjectivity in anthropological fieldwork*, Don Kulick and Margaret Willson eds, London and New York: Routledge, pp. 29–50

Duelli Klein, Renate (1983) How to do what we want to do: Thoughts about feminist methodology, in *Theories of women's studies*, Gloria Bowles and Renate Duelli Klein eds, London and New York: Routledge, pp. 88–104

Dunn, Charles J. and Torigoe, Bunzō, eds, transl. (1969) *The actor's analects* (*Yakusha rongo*), Tokyo: University of Tokyo Press

Durkheim, Emile (1964) *The rules of sociological method*, Sarah A. Solovay and John H. Mueller transl., George E.G. Catlin ed., New York: The Free Press

Earhart, H. Byron (1974) *Religion in the Japanese experience: Sources and interpretations*, Belmont: Wadsworth Publishing Company

Ebisaka, Takeshi (1986) *Shinguru raifu: Onna to otoko no kaihōgaku* (Single life: Teachings on the liberation of women and men), Tokyo: Chūō Kōronsha

Edwards, Tim (1994) *Erotics and politics: Gay male sexuality, masculinity and feminism*, London and New York: Routledge

Edwards, Walter (1989) *Modern Japan through its weddings: Gender, person, and society in ritual portrayal*, Stanford: Stanford University Press

Ehara, Yumiko (1992a) Feminizumu no nanajū nendai to hachijū nendai (The seventies and eighties of feminism), in *Feminizumu ronsō: Nanajū nendai kara kyūjū nendai e* (Feminist controversies: From the seventies to the nineties), Tokyo: Keisō Shobō, pp. 1–46 (first print 1990)

Ehara, Yumiko (1992b) Feminizumu riron e no shōtai: Burujoateki feminizumu kara posutomodan feminizumu made (An invitation to feminist theory: From bourgeois feminism to postmodern feminism), in *Wakaritai anata no tame no feminizumu nyūmon* (An introduction to feminism for those who want to understand), Bessatsu Takarajima No. 85, Tokyo: JICC Shuppan, pp. 10–24 (first print 1988)

Ehara, Yumiko (1992c) Feminizumu mondai e no shōtai (An invitation to feminist questions), in *Feminizumu no shuchō* (Assertions of feminism), Ehara Yumiko ed., Tokyo: Keisō Shobō, pp. 263–310

Ekuni, Kaori (1992) *Kirakira hikaru* (Twinkle), Tokyo: Shinchōsha

Essed, Philomena (1984) *Alledaags racisme* (Everyday racism), Amsterdam: Feministische Uitgeverij Sarah

Evans, David T. (1993) *Sexual citizenship: The material construction of sexuality*, London and New York: Routledge

Faludi, Susan (1992) *Backlash: The undeclared war against women*, London: Chatto & Windus

Foucault, Michel (1978) *An introduction: The history of sexuality 1*, Harmondsworth: Penguin Books (first publication in French in 1976)

Foucault, Michel (1988a) *The use of pleasure: The history of sexuality 2*, Harmondsworth: Penguin Books (first publication in French in 1984)

Foucault, Michel (1988b) *The care of the self: The history of sexuality 3*, Harmondsworth: Penguin Books (first publication in French in 1984)

Foxhall, Lin (1994) Pandora unbound: A feminist critique of Foucault's *History of sexuality*, in *Dislocating masculinity: Comparative ethnographies*, Andrea Cornwall and Nancy Lindisfarne eds, London and New York: Routledge, pp. 133–46

French, Marilyn (1992) *The war against women*, New York: Ballantine Books

Fujieda, Mioko (1983) The women's studies movement in Japan, in *The Japan Christian Quarterly* Vol. 49 No. 2, Spring

Fujieda, Mioko (1990) Nihon no josei undō: Ribu saikō (Japan's women's movement: The revival of liberationism), in *Joseigaku Nenpō* (Chronicle of Women's Studies) No. 11, pp. 1–8

Fujimoto, Yoshiko (1982) Kazoku o koeta hirogari o motomete (In search of expanses beyond the family), in Ikegami Chizuko ed., *Shinguru mazā: Kekkon o erabanakatta onnatachi no sei to sei* (Single mothers: The life and sex of women who did not choose marriage), Tokyo: Gakuyō Shobō, pp. 33–48

Fujimoto, Yukari (1991) Shōjo manga ni okeru 'shōnenai' no imi (The meaning of 'paedophilia' in girls' comics), in *Nyū Feminizumu Rebyū* (New Feminism Review) No. 2: Onna to hyōgen: Feminizumu hihyō no genzai (Women and expression: Contemporary feminist critique), Mizuta Noriko ed., May, pp. 280–4

Fujitani, Yukari (1992) Onna no yokubō da kara: Rediisu komikku ni miru onna no sei gensō (Because it is women's desire: Women's sexual illusions in ladies' comics), in *Nyū Feminizumu Rebyū* (New Feminism Review) No. 3: Porunogurafii: Yureru shisen no seijigaku (Pornography: The politicology of the swaying gaze), Shirofuji Kayako ed., pp. 70–90

Fujiwara, Akira (1972) *Kokumin no rekishi: Taiheyō sensō* (The history of the nation: The Pacific War), Tokyo: Eibundō (third print)

Fukae, Masako (1988), Fūfu bessei (Different names for spouses), in *Kazoku* (Family), Kanei Sodeko ed., Tokyo: Shinyōsha, pp. 114–27

Fukushima, Mizuho (1991a) *Rabu chairudo: Kongaishi sabetsu o koete* (Love child: Overcoming discrimination against illegitimate children), Tokyo: Aki Shobō

Fukushima, Mizuho (1991b) Uru sei, kau sei (The sex that sells, the sex that buys), in *Sekushuariti to kazoku* (Sexuality and family), Henbō suru kazoku (Family in transformation) series No. 2, Tokyo: Iwanami Shoten, pp. 95–111

Furth, Charlotte (1993) Androgynous males and deficient females: Biology and gender boundaries in sixteenth- and seventeenth-century China, in *The lesbian and gay studies reader*, Henry Abelove, Michèle Aina Bairale and David M. Halperin eds, London and New York: Routledge, pp. 479–97

Furukawa, Kei (1993) Taka ga gei saredo gei (It may be insignificant but I am still gay), in *Kick Out*, No. 7, October, p. 23

Furukawa, Makoto (1992) Kindai Nihon ni okeru d_seiai no shakaishi (A social history of homosexuality in modern Japan), in *Za Gei* (The Gay), May, pp. 24–60

Furukawa, Makoto (1993) Sekushuariti no shakaigaku: Dōseiaisha no shakaishi (The sociology of sexuality: A social history of sexuality), in *Wakaritai anata no tame no shakaigaku nyūmon* (An introduction to sociology for those who want to understand), Bessatsu Takarajima No. 176, Tokyo: JICC Shuppan, May, pp. 218–22

Furukawa, Makoto (1994) Sekushuariti no henyō: Kindai Nihon ni okeru dōseiai o meguru mittsu no kōdō, in *Nichibei Josei Jānaru* No. 17, pp. 29–55, published in English as: The changing nature of sexuality: The three codes framing homosexuality in modern Japan, in *US/Japan Women's Journal* (English supplement) No. 7, pp. 98–127

Furukawa, Makoto (1996) Dōseiai no hikaku shakaigaku: Rezubian, gei sutadiizu no tenkai to danshoku gainen (A comparative sociology of homosexuality: The development of lesbian and gay studies and the concept of pederasty), in *Sekushuariti to shakaigaku* (The sociology of sexuality), Inoue Toshi, Ueno Chizuko *et al.* eds, Tokyo: Iwanami Shoten, pp. 113–30

Fuse, Akiko (1984) The Japanese family in transition, parts I and II, in *The Japan Foundation Newsletter* Vol. 12, nos 3 and 4, pp. 1–11 and 1–11

Fushimi, Noriaki (1990) Aisarenu riyū: Otoko to otoko no renaigaku (Why they are not loved: The science of love between men and men), in *Nyū Feminizumu Rebyū* (New Feminism Revue) No. 1: Renai tekunorojii (Love technology), Ueno Chizuko ed., pp. 242–54

Fushimi, Noriaki (1991) *Puraibēto gei raifu: Posuto renairon* (Private gay life: Post-love theory), Tokyo: Gakuyō Shobō

Fushimi, Noriaki (1992) Gei poruno e yōkoso (An invitation to gay pornography), in *Nyū Feminizumu Rebyū* (New Feminism Revue) No. 3: Porunogurafii: Yureru shisen no seijigaku (Pornography: The politicology of the swaying gaze), Shirofuji Kayako ed., pp. 212–17

Fushimi, Noriaki (1993) Kondo umarekawattara gei ni naritai (If I am born again I want to become gay), in *Tanbi shōsetsu, gei bungaku bukku gaido*

(Aesthetic novels: A gay culture book guide), Kakinuma Eiko and Kurihara Chiyo eds, Tokyo: Byakuya Shobō, pp. 229–31

Fushimi, Noriaki (1996) *Kuia Paradaisu: 'Sei' no meikyū e yōkoso* (Queer Paradise: An invitation to the labyrinth of 'sex'), Tokyo: Shōheisha

Gebhard, Paul H. and Johnson, Alan B. (1979) *The Kinsey data: Marginal tabulations of the 1938-1963 interviews conducted by the Institute of Sex Research*, Philadelphia: Saunders

Geddes, Margaret (1970) The status of women in postwar Japan: A critical examination of the contribution of the occupation authorities toward raising the status of women in Japan, in *Australian Outlook* Vol. 31, No. 3, pp. 439–52

Geertz, Clifford (1983) *Local knowledge: Further essays in interpretive anthropology*, New York: Basic Books Inc. Publishers

Geertz, Clifford (1988) *Works and lives: The anthropologist as author*, Oxford: Polity Press

Geertz, Clifford (1993) *The interpretation of culture*, London: Fontana Press (first print 1973)

Genet, Jean (1977) *Miracle de la rose* (Miracle of the rose), Paris: Folio (first print 1946)

Genet, Jean (1978) *Notre-Dame-des-Fleurs* (Our lady of the flowers), Paris: Folio (first print 1948)

Genshi Shuzaihan ed. (1991) *Kekkon dekinai otokotachi?: Otoko no iibun* (Men who cannot marry?: What men have to say), Tokyo: Suna Shobō

Gochros, Jean Schaar (1989) *When husbands come out of the closets*, New York and London: Harrington Park Press

Goffman, Erving (1980) *Stigma: Aantekeningen over het omgaan met een geschonden identiteit* (Stigma: Notes on the management of spoiled identity), Utrecht: Bijleveld (original publication in English 1963)

Goffman, Erving (1987) *The presentation of self in everyday life*, Harmondsworth: Penguin

Goode, William J. (1960) A theory of role strain, in *American Sociological Review* Vol. 24, August, pp. 483–96

Gōssmann, Elisabeth (1990) Am Anfang war die Frau die Sonne (In the beginning woman was the sun), in *Nippons neue Frauen* (Japan's new women), Ruth Linhart and Fleur Wōss eds, Reinbeck: Rohwolt, pp. 14–31

Greenberg, David F. (1988) *The construction of homosexuality*, Chicago and London: University of Chicago Press

Greenberg, David F. (1996) The pleasures of homosexuality, in *Sexual nature, sexual culture*, Paul R. Abramson and Steven N. Pinkerton eds, Chicago: University of Chicago Press, pp. 223–56

Gudykunst, William B. and Ting-Toomy, Stella (1988) *Culture and interpersonal communication*, Newbury Park: Sage Publications Inc.

Hamabata, Matthews Masayuki (1990) *Crested kimono: Power and love in the*

*Japanese business family*, Ithaca: Cornell University Press

Hanada, Minoru (1994) Shōgaisha to shite, gei to shite (As a handicapped person, as a gay person), in Poko a Poko (Little by Little) Vol. 3, November, pp. 39–50

Hane, Mikiso transl., ed., intr. (1988) *Reflections on the way to the gallows: Voices of Japanese rebel women*, New York: Pantheon Books

Hannay, M. ed. (1993) *Van Dale handwoordenboek Nederlands-Engels* (Van Dale concise dictionary Dutch/English), Utrecht and Antwerp: Van Dale Lexicografie

Haraven, Tamara T. (1992) Between craft and industry: The subjective reconstruction of the life course of Kyoto's traditional weavers, in *Japanese biographies: Life histories, life cycles, life stages*, Susanne Formanek and Sepp Linhart eds, Vienna: Verlag der ōsterreichischen Akademie fūr Wisschenschaften, pp. 197–207

Hardacre, Helen (1986) *Kurozumikyō and the new religions of Japan*, Princeton: Princeton University Press

Harper, Phillip Brian (1992) Racism and homophobia as reflections on their perpetrators, in *Homophobia: How we all pay the price*, Warren J. Blumenfeld ed., Boston: Beacon Press, pp. 57–66

Hart, Angie (1994) Missing masculinity?: Prostitutes' clients in Alicante, Spain, in *Dislocating masculinity: Comparative ethnographies*, Andrea Cornwall and Nancy Lindisfarne eds, London and New York: Routledge, pp. 48–65

Hashiguchi, Jōji (George) (1992) *Couple (Kappuru)*, Tokyo: Bungei Shunju

Hashimoto, Osamu (1986) *Hasu to katana: Dō shite otoko wa 'otoko' o kowagaru no ka?* (The lotus and the sword: Why are men afraid of 'men'?), Tokyo: Kawade Bunko

Hashimoto, Osamu (1987) *Ai no yagurumasō* (A cornflower of love), Tokyo: Shinchō Bunko

Hashimoto, Osamu (1988) *Fūga no tora no maki* (Secrets of elegance), Tokyo: Sakuhinsha

Hashimoto, Osamu (1992a) Watashi (anata) datte rezubian ka mo shirenai (Maybe I [you] am/are lesbian), in *Kōkuko Hihyō* (Public Critique), July/August, pp. 46–62

Hashimoto, Osamu (1992b) *Renairon* (Love theory), Tokyo: Kōdansha Bunko (first print 1986)

Hashimoto, Osamu and Tsutamori, Tatsuru (1990) Toransu jendā ga furuku naru mae ni (Before transgender becomes old-fashioned), in *Toransu jendā genshō* (Transgender phenomena), Tsutamori Tatsuru ed., *Gendai no Esupuri* (L'Esprit d'Aujourd'hui; Today's spirit), Shibundō, August, pp. 5–47

Hashizume, Daisaburō (1992) Baishun no doko ga warui (What is bad about prostitution), in *Feminizumu no shuchō* (Assertions of feminism), Ehara Yumiko ed., Tokyo: Keisō Shobō, pp. 1–43

Hasogabe, Kiku (1913) Atarashiki onna no kaisetsu (An interpretation of new women), in *Seitō* (Blue Stockings) No. 1, furoku (supplement), pp. 36–45

Hasshii (1994) Mazu wa jibun o aishimashō (Let's begin by loving ourselves), in *Poko a Poko* (Little by Little) No. 3, November, pp. 23–6

Hattori Kōichi (1996) Ōsakafu o utsu! Dōseiai sabetsu jōrei e no torikumi: Ōsakafu jōrei o kaesaseta Hattori Kōichi shi ni kiku (Striking Osaka prefecture! Questioning regulations that discriminate against homosexuality: Listening to Mr Hattori Kōichi who made the regulations of Osaka prefecture change), in *Adon*, February, pp. 19–26

Hayashi, Iku (1990) *Kateinai rikon* (Divorce within the household), Tokyo: Chikuma Bunko

Hayashi, Yasuko (1993a) Rikon, sono kokoro no fūkei: Kare no bangohan ga tsukurenai (Divorce, scenery of its heart: I cannot make his evening meals), in *Kyōto Shinbun*, 27 December

Hayashi, Yasuko (1993b) Rikon, sono kokoro no fūkei: Seibetsu yakuwari bungyō e no kotei kannen (Divorce, scenery of its heart: Fixed ideas about sex role division), in *Kyōto Shinbun*, 28 December

Hayashi, Yasuko (1993c) Rikon, sono kokoro no fūkei: Itonami ga atte kekkon ga aru no (Divorce, scenery of its heart: I have my business, I have my marriage), in *Kyōto Shinbun*, 29 December

Hendry, Joy (1984) Shoes: The early learning of an important distinction in Japanese society, in *Europe interprets Japan*, Gordon Daniels ed., Tenterden: Paul Norbury Publications, pp. 215–22

Hendry, Joy (1986a) *Becoming Japanese: The world of the preschool child*, Manchester: Manchester University Press

Hendry, Joy (1986b) *Marriage in changing Japan: Community and society*, Rutland and Tokyo: Tuttle (original version 1981)

Hendry, Joy (1987a) Marriage and the family in modernising Japan, *Saeculum* Vol. 38, Heft 1, pp. 4–18

Hendry, Joy (1987b) *Understanding Japanese society*, London: Croom Helm

Hendry, Joy (1991) *Politeness and formality in Japanese social relations*, Stirling occasional papers on Japan, Stirling: Scottish Centre for Japanese Studies, University of Stirling

Hendry, Joy (1992a) The paradox of friendship in the field: Analysis of a long-term Anglo-Japanese relationship, in *Anthropology and autobiography*, Judith Okely and Helen Callaway eds, London: Routledge, pp. 163–74

Hendry, Joy (1992b) Generational diversity in a family life history: Two academic women, in *Japanese biographies: Life histories, life cycles, life stages*, Susanne Formanek and Sepp Linhart eds, Vienna: Verlag der ōsterreichische Akademie für Wissenschaften, pp. 113-25

Hendry, Joy (1992c) Individualism and individuality: Entry into a social world, in *Ideology and practice in modern Japan*, Roger Goodman and Kirsten Refsing eds, London and New York: Routledge, pp. 55–71

Hendry, Joy (1993a) *Wrapping culture: Politeness, presentation and power in Japan and other societies*, Oxford: Clarendon Press

Hendry, Joy (1993b) The role of the professional housewife, in *Japanese women working*, Janet Hunter ed., London and New York: Routledge, pp. 224–41

Herdt, Gilbert (1987) *The Sambia: Ritual and gender in New Guinea*, Fort Worth and Chicago: Holt, Rinehart & Winston

Herdt, Gilbert (1992) 'Coming out' as a rite of passage: A Chicago study, in *Gay culture in America: Essays from the field*, Gilbert Herdt ed., Boston: Beacon Press

Herold, Renate (1980) Liebe ohne Pille: Sexualität auf japanisch (Love without the pill: Sexuality the Japanese way), in *Die Frau* (Woman), Berlin: Erich Schmidt Verlag, pp. 119–27

Hibino, Makoto (1996) Tasha to no deai to iu tanoshimi o saihakken (Rediscovering the pleasure of meeting others), in *Kuia sutadiizu '96* (Queer studies '96), Kuia Sutadiizu Henshū Iinkai ed., Tokyo: Nanatsu Mori Shokan, pp. 203–6

Higuchi, Ayako (1993a) Jinbutsu retsuden 1: Hiratsuka Raichō (Personal biographies 1: Hiratsuka Raichō), in *Tanbi shōsetsu, gei bungaku bukkugaido* (Aesthetic novels: A gay culture book guide), Kakinuma Eiko and Kurihara Chiyo eds, Tokyo: Byakuya Shobō, pp. 276–9

Higuchi, Ayako (1993b) Jinbutsu retsuden 2: Yoshiya Nobuko to Monma Chiyo (Personal biographies 2: Yoshia Nobuko en Monma Chiyo), in *Tanbi shōsetsu: Gei bungaku bukkugaido* (Aesthetic novels: A gay culture book guide), Kakinuma Eiko and Kurihara Chiyo eds, Tokyo: Byakuya Shobō, pp. 280–2

Higuchi, Keiko (1984) *Tatta ichido no onna no jinsei* (A unique woman's life), Tokyo: Kōbunsha Bunko

Higuchi, Keiko (1986) *Onna no ko no sodatekata* (Bringing up girls), Tokyo: Kōbunsha Bunko (first publication 1978)

Higuchi, Keiko, Saitō, Shigeo and Itamoto, Yōko eds (1990) *Hanamuko gakkō* (The bridegroom school), Tokyo: Sanseidō

Hikage, Tadao (1987) Eizu kensa de shitta dōseiaisha no higeki (The hell of homosexuals that became known through AIDS tests), in *Fujin Kōron* (Public Discussion of Women), July, pp. 282–7

Hino, Reiko (1991) Kazoku no hōteki moderu to fūfu bessei undō: Sei sabetsu to hichakushutsushi sabetsu no shikaku kara (The legal model of the family and the movement for spouses having different names: From the viewpoint of sex discrimination and discrimination against illegitimate children), in *Joseigaku Nenpō* (Chronicle of Women's Studies) No. 12, October, pp. 63–74

Hinsch, Bret (1990) *Passions of the cut sleeve: The male homosexual tradition in China*, Berkeley: University of California Press

Hirano, Hiroaki (1991) 'Rasen no sobyō' wa dare o koroshita ka? (Who was killed by 'A spiral sketch'), in *Eiga Shinbun* (Film Newspaper) 1 June, pp. 6–7

Hirano, Hiroaki (1992) Otonagenai yakunin ya nē: Ōsakafu, shi hoken eisei tōkyoku to no 'ohanashiai' (Aren't they careless officials: 'A dialogue' with the hygiene and health offices of Osaka prefecture and city), in *OGC Nyūsu* (OGC News), 22 November

Hirano, Hiroaki (1993) *Iseiaisha wa, itsu, me o samasu?: Donkan to sakushu no kōzō* (When will heterosexuals wake up?: The structure of insensitivity and exploitation), Hirano Hiroaki, Matsubara (self produced pamphlet sold at Onna no Fesutibaru [Women's Festival] in Kyoto, March 1993)

Hirano, Hiroaki (1994) *Anchi-heterosekushizumu* (Anti-heterosexism), Tokyo: Pandora Books

Hiratsuka, Raichō (1914), Onna gakkō. . . (Women's school. . .), Introduction to Havelock Ellis, Joseikan dōsei renai (same-sex love between women), in *Seitō* (Blue Stockings), furoku (supplement), pp. 1–2

Hiratsuka, Raichō (1991) Genshi josei wa taiyō de atta: 'Seitō' hakkan ni saishite (In the beginning woman was the sun: On the occasion of the first publication of 'Blue Stockings'), in *Hiratsuka Raichō zenshū*, Kobayashi Tomie and Yoneda Sayoko eds, Tokyo: Iwanami Bunko, pp. 9–24 (first published in *Seitō* 1911)

Hiromi, Keiko (1992) Shataku watari aru nikki (Diary from a company housing estate), in *Waifu* (Wife) No. 236, July

Hirosawa, Yumi (1991) Nihon hatsu no rezubian gurūpu: 'Wakakusano Kai,' sono jūgonen no rekishi to genzai (The first lesbian group in Japan: 'Group of Young Grass,' its 15-year history and the present) in *Onna o aisuru onnatachi no monogatari* (Stories of women who love women), Bessatsu Takarajima No. 64, Tokyo: JICC Shuppan, pp. 111–19

Hirosawa, Yumi and Rezubian Ripōto Han (1991), Rezubian ripōto (Lesbian report), in *Onna o aisuru onnatachi no monogatari* (Stories of women who love women), Bessatsu Takarajima No. 64, Tokyo: JICC Shuppan, pp. 149–285

Hirschfeld, Magnus (1914) *Die Homosexualitätdes Mannes und des Weibes* (The homosexuality of the man and the woman), Berlin: Louis Marcus Verlagsbuchhandlung

Hisada, Megumi (1991) Genkiin no rezubian: 'Regumi no Gomame' tōjō! (Healthy lesbians: The appearance of 'Regumi no Gomame'), in *Onna o aisuru onnatachi no monogatari* (Stories of women who love women), Bessatsu Takarajima No. 64, Tokyo: JICC Shuppan, pp. 120–9

Hocquenghem, Guy (1978) *Homosexual desire*, London: Allison & Busby

Hollinghurst, Alan (1989) *The swimming pool library*, Harmondsworth: Penguin

Hollis, Martin (1985) Of masks and men, in *The category of the person: Anthropology, philosophy, history*, Michael Carrithers, Steven Collins and Steven Lukes eds, Cambridge: Cambridge University Press, pp. 217–33

Honda, Masuko (1991) 'S': Taai naku, shika mo kongenteki na ai no katachi ('S': Not love of the other but still a basic form of love), in *Imago* Vol. 2 No. 8: Rezubian (Lesbian), August, pp. 68–73

Hori, Yasuko (1913) Watashi wa furui onna desu (I am an old-fashioned woman), in *Seitō* (Blue Stockings), January, furoku (supplement), pp. 61–5

Horiba, Kiyoko ed. (1991) *'Seitō' josei kaihōron shū* (Collection of women's liberation discussions of 'Blue Stockings'), Tokyo: Iwanami Bunko

Humphreys, Laud (1971) *Tearoom trade: Impersonal sex in public places*, Chicago: Aldine Publishing Company

Ian, Marcia (1995) How do you wear your body?: Bodybuilding and the sublimity of drag, in *Negotiating lesbian and gay subjects*, Monica Dorenkamp and Richard Henke eds, London and New York: Routledge, pp. 71–92

Ichibangase, Yasuko (1971) *Sengo fujin mondai shi* (A post-war history of women), Tokyo: Kyōdō Tōgi

Ichikawa, Hiroyuki (1991) Anaru no kaikan o tsuikyū suru jinsei (A life in pursuit of anal pleasure), in *Hentai san ga iku* (There goes Mr/Ms Queer), Bessatsu Takarajima No. 146, Tokyo: JICC Shuppan, pp. 10–23

Ida, Makiko (1991) Tōkyō dōseiai saiban (Tokyo gay trial), in *Josei Sebun* (Woman Seven), 31 October

Idota, Hirofumi (1993) *Kazoku no hō to rekishi: Shi, koseki, sosen saishi* (Law and history of the family: Names, registration, ancestry, religious rites), Tokyo: Sekai Shisōsha

Ienaga, Saburō (1982) *Nihon rekishi sōsho: Taiheyō sensō* (Library of Japanese history: The Pacific War), Tokyo: Iwanami Shoten (nineteenth print)

Ihara, Saikaku (1976) *Comrade loves of the samurai*, Tokyo: Tuttle

Ihara, Saikaku (1990) *The great mirror of male love*, Paul Gordon Schalow transl., ed., Stanford: Stanford University Press

Ikeda, M.(1993) Media watching: Homo mo rezu mo nyūtai (Both gay men and lesbian women in the army), in *Adon*, March, pp. 34–5, after article in *Shūkan Jitsuwa* (Weekly True Stories)

Illich, Ivan (1982) *Gender*, New York: Pantheon Books

Imai, Yasuko (1994) The emergence of the Japanese *shufu*: Why a *shufu* is more than a 'housewife', in *US/Japan Women's Journal* (English supplement) No. 6, pp. 44–65

Imamura, Anne E. (1987) *Urban Japanese housewives: At home and in the community*, Honolulu: University of Hawaii Press

Inagaki, Taruho (1986) *Shōnenai no bigaku* (The aesthetics of paedophilia), Tokyo: Kawade Shobō Shinsha

Ino, Hiromi (1992) Josōsha wa mokuzen no ryōshin to tatakau (A male transvestite fights with his silent parents), in *Cross Dressing* No. 2, April, pp. 24–31

Inoue, Tadashi (1971) *'Sekentei' no kōzō :Shakai shinri e nokokoromi* (The structure of 'social appearance': An attempt at social psychology), Tokyo: NHK Bukkusu

Inoue, Teruko (1995) Renaikan to kekkonkan no keifu (A genealogy of views of love and marriage), in *Nihon no feminizumu* (Feminism in Japan) No. 6, Tokyo: Iwanami Shoten, pp. 54–75

Irokawa, Naho (1992) Sore wa zurui yo, Ueno san: Iseiaisha ni towarete iru koto (That is sly, Ms Ueno: What is asked of heterosexuals), in *Choisir* (Choose) Vol. 22, August, pp. 16–20

Ishii, Tatsurō (1991) *Isō no sekushuariti: Hito wa sei o koerareru ka* (Cross dressing sexuality: Can people overcome their sex?), Tokyo: Shinjuku Shobō

Ishikawa, Hiroyoshi (1984) Sekkusu wa koko made kaihō sareta: Rekishiteki henka to kokusaiteki ichi (Sex is liberated to here: Historical change and the international position), in *Nihonjin no sei* (Sex of the Japanese), Kyōdō Tsūshin 'Gendai shakai to sei' Iinkai, Ishikawa Hiroyoshi, Saitō Shigeo and Wagatsuma Hiroshi eds, Tokyo: Bungei Shunju

Itamoto, Yōko (1992a) Kekkonkan no henka (Changing views of marriage), in *Fujin hakusho 1992: Kyō no kazoku mondai* (White book on women 1992: Current family problems), Nihon Fujin Dantai Rengōkai ed., Tokyo: Horupu Shuppan, pp. 35–8

Itamoto, Yōko (1992b) Hanamuko gakkō kara mita dansei no sutoresu jōkyō (Male stress circumstances seen from the bride-groom school), in *Gendai no Esupuri* (L'Esprit d'Aujourd'hui; Today's Spirit) No. 300: Kazoku to katei no sutoresu (Stress of the family and the household), July, pp. 28–38

Itō, Bungaku (1986) *'Barazoku' henshūchō funsenki: Kokoro aru hito ni wa wakatte hoshii* (Notes on the desperate struggle of the chief editor of 'Barazoku': I wish people with a heart will understand), Tokyo: Daini Shobō

Itō, Bungaku (1993) Itō Bungaku no hitorigoto 214: Kimi no mawari no hito no koto mo kangaete hoshii (A few words by Itō Bungaku 214: Please think of the people around you), in *Barazoku* (Rose Clan) No. 240, January, pp. 140–1

Itō, Noe (1913) Atarashiki onna no michi (The way of the new woman), in *Seitō* (Blue Stockings) No. 1, furoku (supplement), pp. 20–2

Itō, Noe (1978a) Trennung (Separation), in *Frauen in der Revolution: Wilde Blumen auf unfreiem Feld* (Women in the revolution: Wild flowers in an unfree field), Terasaki Akiko and Ilse Lenz eds, transl., Berlin: Karin Kramer Verlag, pp. 33–40

Itō, Noe (1978b) Von einer Frau an ihren Ehemann (From a woman to her husband), in *Frauen in der Revolution: Wilde Blumen auf unfreiem Feld* (Women in the revolution: Wild flowers in an unfree field), Terasaki Akiko and Ilse Lenz eds, transl., Berlin: Karin Kramer Verlag, pp. 41–51

Itō, Satoru (1993) *Otoko futarigurashi: Boku no gei puraido sengen* (Two men living together: My gay pride declaration), Tokyo: Tarō Jirōsha

Iwai, Yasunari (1993) Kowai no wa byōki ka 'jinken' ka (Should we be afraid of disease or of 'human rights', in *Shokun!* (Gentlemen!), February, pp. 168–75

Iwao, Sumiko (1994) *The Japanese woman: Traditional image and changing reality*, New York: The Free Press

Izumi, Asato (1990) *B-kyū nyūsu zukan* (Illustrated B-class news), Tokyo: Shinchō Bunko

Izumo, Marō (1993) *Manaita no ue no koi* (Love as a carp on the cutting board), Tokyo: Takarajimasha

*Japan Times* (1997) Gays win suit against Tokyo, in *Japan Times*, 17 September

Josei no Jōhō o Hirogeru Kai ed. (1991) *Onnatachi no benrichō 1992–1993* (A service book for women 1992-1993), Tokyo: Jojo Kikaku

Kakefuda, Hiroko (1992a) *'Rezubian' de aru, to iu koto* (Being 'lesbian'), Tokyo: Kawade Shobō Shinsha

Kakefuda, Hiroko (1992b) Genjitsu to poruno to rezubain raifu (Reality, pornography and lesbian life), in *Nyū FeminizumuRebyū* (New Femimism Review) No. 3: Porunogurafii: Yureru shisen no seijigaku (Pornography: The politicology of the swaying gaze), Shirofuji Kayako ed., pp. 63–9

Kakefuda, Hiroko (1993) Motto 'onna no karada' o!: Rezubian noberu, porunogurafi, so shite . . . (More 'women's bodies'!: Lesbian novels, pornography, and . . . ), in *Tanbi shōsetsu: Gei bukku gaido* (Aesthetic novels: A gay book guide), Kakinuma Eiko and Kurihara Chiyo eds, Tokyo: Byakuya Shobō, pp. 320–1

Kakinuma, Chisato (1991) Pinku saron: Hassei sangyō no 'saiteihen' (Pink salon:'The lowest' of the ejaculation industry), in *Sekkusu to iu oshigoto* (The work called sex), Bessatsu Takarajima No. 124, Tokyo: JICC Shuppan, January (second print), pp. 66–71

Kamigata DJ Club (1992) *Midnight Minx* (Midnight Mix) No. 7, Ikeda, January (cassette-tape)

Kamigata DJ Club (1993) *Midnight Minx* (Midnight Mix) No. 10, Ikeda, March (cassette-tape)

Kamihara, Fumiko (1992) Kyō no fūfu kankei (Today's husband/wife relations), in *Fujin hakusho 1992: Kyō no kazoku mondai* (White book on women 1992: Current family problems), Nihon Fujin Dantai Rengōkai eds, Tokyo:Horupu Shuppan, pp. 39–45

Kamisaka, Fuyuko (1991) *Hitori de kurasu, hitori de ikiru* (Supporting oneself, living alone) Tokyo: Kōdansha

Kamisaka, Fuyuko (1992) *Dansō no reijin: Kawashima Shigeko* (A young woman in men's clothes: Kawashima Shigeko), Tokyo: Bunshun Bunko (first print 1988)

Kanda, Hisao (1992) Kateinai rikon to kodomo no sutoresu hannō (Divorce within the household and children's reaction to stress), in *Gendai no Esupuri* (L'Esprit d'Aujourd'hui / Today'sSpirit) No. 300: Kazoku to katei no sutoresu (Stress in the family and the household), July, pp. 81–91

Kandiyoti, Deniz (1994) The paradoxes of masculinity: Some thoughts on segregated societies, in *Dislocating masculinity: Comparative ethnographies*, Andrea Cornwall and Nancy Lindisfarne eds, London and New York: Routledge, pp. 197–213

Kanei, Sodeko ed. (1988), *Kazoku* (Family), Tokyo: Shinyōsha

Kanematsu, Sachiko (1987) *Tojirareta rirekisho: Shinjuku, sei o uru onnatachi no 30 nen* (A bound curriculum vitae: 30 years women selling sex in Shinjuku), Tokyo: Asahi Shinbunsha

Kanezuka, Sadafumi (1993) Kōmon wa ika ni shōhin ni natta no ka (To what extent has the anus become a commodity?), in *Ifū dōdō!: Waisetsu daishinkō* (Majestic!: Great progress of immorality), Bessatsu Takarajima No. 174, Tokyo: JICC Shuppan, pp. 154–64

Kanjō, Kiyoko (1992) *Kazoku to iu kankei* (Relations called family), Tokyo: Iwanami Shinsho

Kaoru (1992) Ā! Josō wa auto-doa ga saikō (Oh! Outdoor transvestism is the best), in *Himawari* (Sunflower) No. 9, April, pp. 44–5

Karasawa, Junichi (1992) Shiikuretto ripōto 1 (Secret report 1), in *June* No. 67, November, pp. 162–3

Kasuga, Kisuyo (1989) *Fushi katei o ikiru: Otoko to oya no aida* (Living in a single father's household: Between man and parent), Tokyo: Keisō Shobō

Katō, Harueko (1990) Shakaigakutekijosei kaihōronno atotori: Ueno Chizuko, Ehara Yumiko ryōshi no 1985–1989nen (The successors of sociological women's liberationtheory: The years from 1985 to 1989 of Ueno Chizuko and Ehara Yumiko), in *Jendā to sei sabetsu: Joseigaku kenkyū* (Gender and sex discrimination: Research of women's studies) No. 1, Tokyo: Keisō Shobō, pp. 150–63

Kawachi, Kazuko (1992) *Watashitachi no feminizumu: Ochiai Keiko to Nihon no onnatachi* (Our feminism: Ochiai Keiko and Japanese women), Tokyo: Kōdansha

Kawada, Kiyo (1915) Onna tomodachi (Female friends), in *Seitō* (Blue Stockings), March, pp. 73–88

Kawakoshi, Sodeko (1994) Danjobetsu gakunenbetsu bunseki (Analysis of differences between men and women and student years), in *Sei kōi ni taisuru daigakusei no ishiki* (The consciousness of university students of sexual activity), Yajima Zemi, Seiai Chōsa Kenkyūkai ed., Tokyo: Chūō Daigaku Bungakubu Shakaigakka, March, pp. 35–44

Kawamura, Nozomu (1994) *Sociology and society of Japan*, London and New York: Kegan Paul International

Kawano, Kiyomi (1990) *Sei gensō: Beddo no naka no senba e* (Sexual illusions: To the battlefield of the bed), Tokyo: Gakuyō Shobō

Kawara, Karito (1981) Onna de aru watashi ga suki da kara rezubian (Because I like being a woman I am lesbian), in *Onna Erosu* (Woman

Eros) No. 16, May 20, pp. 66–78

Kawarasaki, Kokutarō (1991) *Onnagata hanseiki* (Half a century of performing female characters in the Kabuki theatre), Tokyo: Shin Nihon Shuppansha

Kawashima, Takeyoshi (1974) *Kekkon* (Marriage), Tokyo: Iwanami Shinsho (first publication 1954)

Kawauchi, Hidetoshi (1992) Hanamuko gakkō no seitotachi (Pupils of the bridegroom school), in *Otoko ga abunai!?* (Are men in danger!?), Takarajima Bessatsu No. 112, Tokyo: JICC Shuppan, pp. 88–101 (first print 1990)

Keizai Kikakuchō ed. (1992) *Heisei yonnenban kokumin seikatsu hakusho: Shōshi shakai no tōrai, sono eikyō to taiō* (1992 white book on the nation's life: The advent of a society with small numbers of children, its effects and responses), Tokyo: Ōkurashō Insatsukyoku

Keizai Kikakuchō ed. (1993) *Heisei gonenban kokumin seikatsu hakusho: Yutaka na kōryū/Hito to hito no fureai no saihakken* (1993 white book on the nation's life: Abundant exchanges/The rediscovery of contacts between people), Tokyo: Ōkurashō Insatsukyoku

Keizai Kikakuchō Kokumin Seikatsukyoku ed. (1992) *Kokumin seikatsu o kaeru arata na omoyakutachi* (New chief actors changing the nation's life), Tokyo: Ōkurashō Insatsukyoku

Kelsky, Karen (1994) Postcards from the edge: The 'Office Ladies' of Tokyo, in *US/Japan Women's Journal* (English Supplement) No. 6, pp. 3–26

Kempny, Marian and Burszta, Wojciech J. (1994) On the relevance of common sense for anthropological knowledge, in *Social experience and anthropological knowledge*, Kirsten Hastrup and Peter Hervik eds, London and New York: Routledge, pp. 121–38

Khan, Badruddin (1992) Not-so-gay life in Karachi: A view of a Pakistani living in Toronto, in *Sexuality and eroticism among males in Moslem societies*, Arno Schmitt and Jehoeda Sofer eds, New York, London and Norwood, Harrington Park Press, pp. 93–105

Killick, Andrew P. (1995) The penetrating intellect: On being white, straight, and male in Korea, in *Taboo: Sex, identity and erotic subjectivity in anthropological fieldwork*, Don Kulick and Margaret Willson eds, London and New York: Routledge, pp. 76–106

King, Dave (1996) Cross-dressing, sex-changing and the press, in *Blending genders: Social aspects of cross-dressing and sex-changing*, Richard Enkins and Dave King eds, London and New York: Routledge, pp. 133–50

Kinsey, A.C., Pomeroy W.B. and Martin, C.E. (1948) *Sexual behavior in the human male*, Philadelphia, Saunders

Kitagawa, Joseph M. (1990) *Religion in Japanese history*, New York: Columbia University Press (first print 1966)

Kitahara, Dōmu (1991) Meichi Denki to sengo Nihon no SMshi (Meichi Denki and the history of sadomasochism in post-war Japan), in *Hentai san ga iku* (There goes Mr/Ms Queer), Bessatsu Takarajima No. 146, Tokyo: JICC Shuppan, pp. 48–64

Kitzinger, Celia and Coyle, Adrian (1995) Lesbian and gay couples: Speaking of a difference, in *The Psychologist*, February, pp. 64–9

Kokuhaku Rezu Kurabu (1992a) Rezubian shitagi chōsa '92 natsu (Lesbian underwear investigation, summer 1992), in *Kokuhaku Rezu Kurabu* No. 4, August, pp. 62–6

Kokuhaku Rezu Kurabu (1992b) Rezu giku no hajimaru wa ōoku de wa nai no shinsetsu (A new theory that the beginning of lesbian techniques was not in the shogun's harem), in *Kokuhaku Rezu Kurabu* No. 4, August, p. 103

Komashaku, Kimi (1982) *Murasaki Shikibu no messēji* (Messages of Murasaki Shikibu), Tokyo: Asahi Shuppansha

Komter, Aafke (1985) *De macht van de vanzelfsprekendheid* (The power of self-evidency), The Hague: VUGA

Komter, Aafke (1989) Hidden power in marriage, in *Gender and Society* No. 2, pp. 187–216

Kondo, Dorinne K. (1990) *Crafting selves: Power, gender, and discourses of identity in a Japanese workplace*, Chicago and London: University of Chicago Press

Kondo, Dorinne (1992) Multiple selves: The aesthetics and politics of artisanal identities, in *Japanese sense of self*, Nancy R. Rosenberger ed., Cambridge: Cambridge University Press, pp. 40–66

Kondo, Dorinne (1994) *Uchi no kaisha*: Company as family?, in *Situated meaning: Inside and outside in Japanese self, society, and language*, Jane Bachnik and Charles Quinn Jr eds, Princeton: Princeton University Press, pp. 169–91

Kuia Sutadiizu Henshū Iinkai ed. (1996a) Kuia hisutorii (Queer history), in *Kuia sutadiizu '96* (Queer studies '96), Kuia Sutadiizu Henshū Iinkai ed., Tokyo: Nanatsu Mori Shokan, pp. 18–35

Kuia Sutadiizu Henshū Iinkai ed. (1996b) *Kuia sutadiizu '96* (Queer Studies '96), Tokyo: Nanatsu Mori Shokan

Kuroyanagi, Toshiyasu (1992) *Samayoeru jendā: Seibetsu fukai shōkōgun no esunogurafii* (Wandering gender: An ethnography of the sex ambiguity syndrome), Tokyo: Gendai Shokan (first print 1987)

Kyōdō Tsōshin 'Gendai shakai to sei' Iinkai, Ishikawa, Hiroyoshi, Saitō, Shigeo and Wagatsuma, Hiroshi eds (1984) *Nihonjin no sei* (The sexuality of Japanese), Tokyo: Bungei Shunju

LaFleur; William R. (1992) *Liquid life: Abortion and Buddhism in Japan*, Princeton: Princeton University Press

Lam, Alice (1992) *Women and the Japanese management: Discrimination and reform*, London and New York: Routledge

Lam, Alice (1993) Equal employment opportunities for Japanese women: Changing company practice, in *Japanese women working*, Janet Hunter

ed., London and New York: Routledge, pp. 197–223
Leach, Edmund (1991) The social anthropology of marriage and mating, in *Mating and marriage*, Vernon Reynolds and John Kellets eds, Oxford, New York and Tokyo: Oxford University Press, Oxford, pp. 91–110
Lebra, Takie Sugiyama (1976) *Japanese patterns of behavior*, Honolulu: University of Hawaii Press
Lebra, Takie Sugiyama (1984) *Japanese women: Constraint and fulfillment*, Honolulu: University of Hawaii Press
Lebra, Takie Sugiyama (1992) Self in Japanese culture, in *Japanese sense of self*, Nancy R. Rosenberger ed., Cambridge: Cambridge University Press, pp. 105–20
Lebra, Takie Sugiyama (1993) *Above the clouds: Status culture of the modern Japanese nobility*, Berkeley: University of California Press
Lenz, Ilse (1990) Hausarbeit als Beruf und Berufung (Housekeeping as profession and calling), in *Nippons neue Frauen* (Japan's new women), Ruth Linhart and Fleur Wōss eds, Reinbeck: Rohwolt, pp. 73–92
Lepowsky, Maria (1990) Gender in an egalitarian society: A case study from the Coral Sea, in *Beyond the second sex: New directions in the anthropology of gender*, Peggy Reeves Sanday and Ruth Gallagher Goodenough eds, Philadelphia: University of Pennsylvania Press, pp. 171–223
Leupp, Gary P. (1995) *Male colors: The construction of homosexuality in Tokugawa Japan*, Berkeley, Los Angeles and London: University of California Press
LIB (1994) *Librariis lesborum amicorum: Rezubian no tame no dokusho annai* (A reading guide for lesbians), Kadoma: Kansai YLP
Linhart, Sepp (1984) Familie (Family), in *Japan-Handbuch* (Japan handbook), Horst Hammitzsch ed., Stuttgart: Franz Steiner Verlag, pp. 546-59
Lock, Margaret (1987) Protest of a good wife and wise mother: The medicalization of distress in Japan, in *Health, illness, and medical care in Japan: Cultural and social dimensions*, Edward Norbeck and Margaret Lock eds, Honolulu: University of Hawaii Press, pp. 130–57
Lock, Margaret (1988) New Japanese mythologies: Faltering discipline and the ailing housewife, in *American Ethnologist* Vol. 15 No. 1, February, pp. 43–61
Lock, Margaret (1992a) Symptoms of indolence: The rhetorics of middle age and menopause in Japan, in *Japanese biographies: Life histories, life cycles, life stages*, Susanne Formanek and Sepp Linhart eds, Vienna: Verlag der ōsterreichische Akademie fūr Wissenschaften, pp. 211–40
Lock, Margaret (1992b) The fragile Japanese family: Narratives about individualism and the postmodern state, in *Paths to Asian medical knowledge*, Charles Leslie and Allan Young eds, Berkeley: University of California Press, pp. 98–125
Lock, Margaret (1993a) The politics of mid-life and menopause: Ideologies for the second sex in North America and Japan, in *Knowledge, power, and*

*practice: The anthropology of medicine and everyday life*, Shirley Lindenbaum and Margaret Lock eds, Berkeley: University of California Press, pp. 330–63

Lock, Margaret (1993b) *Encounters with aging: Mythologies of menopause in Japan and North America*, Berkeley: University of California Press

Louis, Lisa (1992) *Butterflies of the night: Mama-sans, geisha, strippers and the Japanese men they serve*, New York and Tokyo: Tengu Books

Lumsden, Ian (1991) *Homosexuality: Society and the state in Mexico*, Toronto and Mexico, Canadian gay archives / Solediciones

Lunsing, Wim (Runshingu, W.) (1989) 'Fujin Kōron' Hagaki Tsūshin ni miru Nihon josei (Japanese women seen through postcard mail in *Fujin Kōron*), in *Fujin Kōron* (Public Discussions of Women), January, pp. 338–45

Lunsing, Wim (1994a) *Kono Sekai: Functions of places for gay men in Japan*, paper presented at the British Sociological Association (BSA) conference: 'Sexualities in Social Context' in Preston in March

Lunsing, Wim (1994b) *Japanese lesbian and gay movements: 1984–1994*, paper presented at the conference: 'Organizing Sexualities' in Amsterdam in June

Lunsing, Wim (Runjingu, W.) (1994c) 'Homo senshinkoku' Oranda ga boku o sodateta ('Gay frontline state' the Netherlands brought me up), in *Fujin Kōron* (Public discussions of women), February, pp. 342–8

Lunsing, Wim (1995) Japanese gay magazines and marriage advertisements, in *Journal of Gay and Lesbian Social Services* Vol. 3 No. 3, pp. 71–87, simultaneously published in *Gays and lesbians in Asia and the Pacific: Social and human services*, Gerard Sullivan and Laurence Wai-Teng Leong eds, Haworth: The Haworth Press, pp. 71–87, and New York, London and Norwood: Harrington Park Press, imprint of The Haworth Press

Lunsing (1997) 'Gay boom' in Japan: Changing views of homosexuality?, in *Thamyris: Mythmaking from Past to Present* Vol. 4, No. 2, pp. 267–93

Lunsing, Wim (forthcoming) Prostitution, dating, mating and marriage: Love, sex and materialism, in *Consumption and material culture in contemporary Japan*, John Clammer and Michael Ashkenazi eds, London: Kegan Paul International

Lunsing, Wim (1999a) Life on Mars: Love and sex in fieldwork on sexuality and gender in urban Japan, in *Sex, sexuality and the anthropologist*, Fran Markowitz and Michael Ashkenazi eds, Urbana and Chicago: University of Illinois Press

Lunsing, Wim (1999b) Japan: Finding its way?, in *The global emergence of gay and lesbian politics: National imprints of a worldwise movement*, Barry Adams, Jan Willem Duyvendak and André Krouwel eds, Philadelphia: Temple University Press

Lyman, Stanford M. and Scott, Marvin B. (1975) *The drama of social reality*, Oxford and New York: Oxford University Press

Lynch, Frederik R. (1992) Non-ghetto gays: An ethnography of suburban homosexuals, in *Gay culture in America: Essays from the field*, Gilbert Herdt ed., Boston: Beacon Press, pp. 165–201

McDonald, Gary B. (1992) Among Syrian men, in *Sexuality and eroticism among males in Moslem societies*, Arno Schmitt and Jehoeda Sofer eds, New York, London and Norwood: Harrington Park Press, pp. 43–54

McGough, James P. (1981) Deviant marriage patterns in Chinese society, in *Normal and abnormal behavior in Chinese culture*, Arthur Kleinman and Lin Tsun-Yi eds, Dordrecht: Reidel Publishing Company

McKinstry, John A. and McKinstry, Asako Nakajima (1991) *Jinsei Annai, Life's Guide: Glimpses of Japan through a popular advice column*, Armonk, New York and London: M.E. Sharpe Inc.

Malinowski, Bronislaw (1989) *A diary in the strict sense of the term*, London: The Athlone Press (first edition 1967)

Marra, Michele (1993) The Buddhist mythmaking of defilement: Sacred courtesans of medieval Japan, in *The Journal of Asian Studies* Vol. 52 No. 1, February, pp. 49–65

Martinez, D.P. (1992) NHK comes to Kusaki: Ideology, mythology, and documentary film-making, in *Ideology and practice in modern Japan*, Roger Goodman and Kirsten Refsing eds, London and New York: Routledge, pp. 153–70

Martinez, D.P. (1993) Women as bosses: Perceptions of the *ama* and their work, in *Japanese women working*, Janet Hunter ed., London and New York: Routledge, pp. 181–96

Marumo, Jun (1993) Kodomo ni chichioya ga hitsuyō ka (Do children need a father?), in *Fujin Kōron* (Public Discussions of Women), February, pp. 172–7

Maruyama Masao (1987) *Nihon no shisō* (Japanese thought), Tokyo: Iwanami Shinsho (first print 1961)

Maruyama, Masaya (1988), *Furin e no chiteki appurōchi* (An intellectual approach to illicit affairs), Tokyo: Janpanposuto

Masakami, Junichi (1992) Kekkon to gisō kekkon: Futsū no minasama e (Marriage and camouflage marriage: To all normal people), in *Kick Out* No. 1, August, pp. 15–17

Masuda, Koh ed. (1988) *Kenkyūsha's new Japanese/English dictionary*, fourth edition of 1974, Tokyo: Kenkyūsha

Matsubara, Junko (1988) *Kurowassan shōkōgun* (The Croissant syndrome), Tokyo: Bungei Shunju

Matsui, Midori (1993) Little girls were little boys: Displaced femininity in the representation of homosexuality in Japanese girls' comics, in *Feminism and the politics of difference*, Sneja Gunew and Anna Yeatman eds, St Leonards: Allen and Unwin, pp. 177–96

Matsuo, Hisako (1997) *Toransujendarizumu: Seibetsu no higan* (Transgenderism: On the other side of sex difference) Yokohama: Seori Shobō

Matsuoka, Hiroshi (1993) Sei kyōiku was kore de ii desu ka (Is sex education right as it is?), in *Seiron* (Sound Argument), March, pp. 192–202

Matsuura, Rieko (1987) *Nachuraru ūman* (Natural woman), Tokyo: Kawade Bunko

Mauss, Marcel (1985) A category of the human mind: The notion of person; the notion of self, in *The category of the person: Anthropology, philosophy, history*, Michael Carrithers, Steven Collins and Steven Lukes eds, Cambridge: Cambridge University Press, pp. 1–25

Mayoeru Sarariiman (nickname: Bewildered White-collar Worker) (1990), Kekkon shite kara tsui ni jikkō (After marriage the practice), in *Barazoku*, January, pp. 55–6

Mead, Margaret (1963) *Sex and temperament in primitive societies*, New York: Morrow Quill (first edition 1935)

Meguro, Yoriko (1987) *Kojinka suru kazoku* (Individualizing family), Tokyo: Keisō Shobō

Meigs, Anna (1990) Multiple gender ideologies and statuses, in *Beyond the second sex: New directions in the anthropology of gender*, Peggy Reeves Sanday and Ruth Gallagher Goodenough eds, Philadelphia: University of Pennsylvania Press, Philadelphia, pp. 101–12

Melhuus, Marit (1993) 'I want to buy me a baby!': Some reflections on gender and change in modern society, in *Carved flesh/cast selves: Gendered symbols and social practices*, Vigdis Broch-Due, Ingrid Rudie and Tone Bleie eds, Oxford and Providence: Berg, pp. 237–55

Metraux, Daniel A. (1988) *The history and theology of Soka Gakkai: A Japanese new religion*, Lewiston and Queenston: The Edwin Mellen Press

Michael, Robert T., Gagnon, John H., Laumann, Edward O. and Kolata, Gina (1995) *Sex in America: The most comprehensive, revealing report on our sexual behavior today and its surprising implications*, Boston, New York, Toronto and London: Little, Brown & Company

Mies, Maria (1983) Towards a methodology of feminist research, in *Theories of women's studies*, Gloria Bowles and Renate Duelli Klein eds, London and New York: Routledge, pp. 117–39

Mika and Torai (1993a) Mika to Torai no Kariforunia TS nikki (The transsexual diary of Mika and Torai in California), in *Queen* No. 76, February, pp. 42–51

Mika and Torai (1993b) Mika to Torai no Kariforunia TS nikki: K_hen (The transsexual diary of Mika and Torai in California: Second part), in *Queen* No. 77, April, pp. 54–63

Miller, Neil (1992) *Out in the world: Gay and lesbian life from Buenos Aires to Bangkok*, Harmondsworth: Penguin Books

Millet, Kate (1977) *Sexual politics*, London: Virago Press (first publication 1969)

Minami, Teishirō (1991) Sengo Nihon no gei mūbumento (The post-war gay movement in Japan), in *Impaction* No. 71: Tokushū: Gei riberēshon

(Special: Gay liberation), pp. 124–32
Minamoto, Junko (1991) Nihon no hinkon naru sei fūdo (The poor sexual climate in Japan), in *Nihonteki sekushuariti: Feminizumu kara no sei fūdo hihan* (Japanese sexuality: A feminist critique of the sexual climate), Yamashita Akiko ed., Kyoto: Hōkōkan, pp. 77–128
Mino (1992) Monogamii wa eizu o manen saseru ka?: Koibito nara sēfā sekkusu shinakute mo daijōbu? (Does monogamy spread AIDS?: Is it alright not to have safe sex when it is with your lover?), in *Sapporo Miitingu Nyūsuretā* (Sapporo Meeting Newsletter) No. 6, April, pp. 18–20
Mishima, Yukio (1949) *Kamen no kokuhaku* (Confessions of a mask), Tokyo: Shinchō Bunko
Mishima, Yukio (1953) *Kinjiki* (Forbidden colours), Tokyo: Shinchō Bunko
Miwa, Akihiro (1992) Otoko wa yowai mono, da kara itōshii (I love men because they are weak), in *Kōkoku Hihyō* (Public Critique), July / August, pp. 19–27
Miyauchi, Bundai (1994) Sei dōtokubetsu bunseki (Analysis according to sexual morals), in *Sei kōi ni taisuru daigakusha no ishiki* (Consciousness of university students on sexual activitiy), Yajima Zemi, Seiai Chōsa Kenkyūkai ed., Tokyo: Chūō Daigaku Bungakubu Shakaigakka, March, pp. 62–79
Mizuno, Mari (1992) *Sekando bājin shōkōgun* (Second virgin syndrome),Tokyo: Kōdansha
Moa Ripōto Han ed. (1983), *Moa ripōto: Nihon no joseitachi ga hajimete jibuntachi no kotoba de sei o katatta* (More report: Japanese women spoke for the first time of sex in their own words), Tokyo: Shūeisha
Moeran, Brian (1985) *Okubo diary: Portrait of a Japanese village*, Stanford: Stanford University Press
Moeran, Brian (1989) *Language and popular culture in Japan*, Manchester and New York: Manchester University Press
Mōhwald, Ulrich (1990) Keine Zeit fūr Familie: Zeitliche Aspekte der japanischen Familie (No time for family: Temporal aspects of the Japanese family), in *Japanstudien: Jahrbuch des deutschen Instituts fūr Japanstudien der Philipp-Franz-von-Sieboldt-Stiftung* (Japanese Studies: Chronicle of the German Institute for Japanese Studies the Philipp-Franz-von-Sieboldt Foundation) Vol. 2, pp. 147–75
Moon, Okpyo (1992) Confucianism and gender segregation in Japan and Korea, in *Ideology and practice in modern Japan*, Roger Goodman and Kirsten Refsing eds, London and New York: Routledge, pp. 196–209
Moore, Henrietta (1994a) *A passion for difference: Essays in anthropology and gender*, Oxford: Polity Press
Moore, Henrietta (1994b) The cultural construction of gender, in *The Polity reader of gender studies*, Oxford: Polity Press, pp. 14–21
Mori, Masumi (1992) Josei rōdōsha: Kintō hogo no josei rōdō jittai (Female

labourers: The reality of the protection of equality of female labour), in *Fujin Hakusho 1992: Ima no kazoku mondai* (White book on women 1992: Current family problems), Nihon Fujin Dantai Rengōkai ed., Tokyo: Horupu Shuppan, pp. 128–39

Morioka, Shinji (1979) Barairo no hikari ga itsu ka (One day the pink light), in *Barazoku* (The Rose Clan), July, pp. 23–9

Morishita, Misako (1991) S izen no koto (Before S), in *Imago* Vol. 2 No. 8, Tokushū: Rezubian (Special: Lesbian), August, pp. 84–91

Morita, Shinichi (1992a) Kamingu auto ni tsuite (On coming out), in *Dōseiai o kangaeyō: Ittai gei tte, nan ya nen* (Let us think about homosexuality: What on earth does gay mean?), hand-out at Osaka Daigaku Gakuensai, Sekushuariti and Jendā Kaihōdan Puapua ed., Osaka, 1–3 November

Morita, Shinichi (1992b) Ōsakafu seishōnen kenzen ikusei jōrei shikō kisoku ni tsuite (On the operation by Osaka prefecture of the regulations on healthy education of youngsters), in *Dōseiai o kangaeyō: Ittai gei tte, nan ya nen* (Let us think about homosexuality: What on earth does gay mean?), hand out at Ōsaka Daigaku Gakuensai, Sekushuariti and Jendā Kaihōdan Puapua eds, Osaka, 1–3 November

Morita, Shinichi (1993) Nikushimi o koete: Tokushū: Gei sabetsu (Overcoming of hate: Special: Gay discrimination), in *Poko a Poko* (Little by Little) No. 1, June, pp. 34–44

Morita, Shinichi (1994) Toransu sekushuaru: Otoko no nikutai ni tojikomerareta onna (Transsexual: Women trapped in a male body), in *Poko a Poko* (Little by Little) No. 3, November, pp. 62–73

Morley, John David (1985) *Pictures from the watertrade*, London: Flamingo

Morris, Brian (1994) *Anthropology of the self: The individual in cultural perspective*, London and Boulder: Pluto Press

Morsbach, Helmut (1973) Aspects of nonverbal communication in Japan, in *The Journal of Nervous and Mental Disease* Vol. 157 No. 4, pp. 262–77

Moses, Alice E. (1978) *Identity management in lesbian women*, New York: Praeger Publishers

Mouer, Ross and Sugimoto, Yoshio (1990) *Images of Japanese society: A study in the social construction of reality*, London and New York: Kegan Paul International

Munakata, Tsunetsugu and Tajima, Kazuo eds (1992) *Eizu to sekkusu ripōto, Japan: Kansen bakuhatsu no kizashi* (AIDS and sex report Japan: Signs of an explosion of infection cases), Tokyo: Nihon Hyōronsha

Murata, Tsutomu (1992) Dansei no futokutei sekkusu (Men's promiscuity), in Munakata Tsunetsugu and Tajima Kazuo eds, *Eizu to sekkusu ripōto Japan: Kansen bakuhatsu no kizashi* (AIDS and sex report Japan: Signs of an explosion of infection cases), Tokyo: Nihon Hyōronsha, pp. 75–91

Murayama, Chizuko (1992) Kyokugen no bōryoku 'gōkan' o karukuchi de menzai suru na (Do not pardon the extreme violence called 'rape' as a pleasantry), in *Asahi Jānaru* (Asahi Journal) Vol. 34 No. 13, 27 March, p.

89
Murray, Stephen O. (1992a) Components of gay community in San Francisco, in *Gay culture in America: Essays from the field*, Gilber Herdt ed., Boston: Beacon Press, pp. 107–46

Murray, Stephen O. (1992b) The 'underdevelopment' of modern/gay homosexuality in Mesoamerica, in *Modern homosexualities: Fragments of lesbian and gay experience*, Ken Plummer ed., London and New York: Routledge, pp. 29–38

Mutsuki, Kagerō (1991) Naze watashi wa shōjo no kutsu o nusunda no ka: Sērāfuku banzai (Why did I steal girls' shoes?: Long live sailor clothes), in *Hentai san ga iku* (There goes Mr/Ms Queer), Bessatsu Takarajima No. 146, Tokyo: JICC Shuppan, pp. 238–44

Nakada, Jun (1991) Subete no kihon wa mazo kara hajimaru (All basics start with being a masochist), in *Hentai san ga iku* (There goes Mr/Ms Queer), Bessatsu Takarajima No. 146, Tokyo: JICC Shuppan, pp. 65–77

Nakajima, Azusa (1990) *Bishōnengaku nyūmon* (An introduction into studies of the beautiful male youth), Tokyo: Shinshokan (first print 1986)

Nakajima, Keita (1991) Data toko shōbu: Kekkon (Data game: Marriage), in *Sabu*, November, pp. 42–5

Nakajima, Keita (1992) Data toko shōbu: Dōsei (Data game: Cohabitation), in *Sabu*, June, pp. 38–41

Nakajima, Takehiro (1992) *Okoge* (Fag hag), Tokyo: Magajin Hausu

Nakamura, Akira (1991) *Atarashii danjosō o motomete: 'Omoikomi' kara no itsudatsu* (In search of a new man/women image: Deviance from 'set ideas', Osaka: Gensōsha.

Nakane, Chie (1973) *Japanese society*, Harmondsworth: Penguin

Nakazawa, Shinichi and Yōrō, Takeshi (1992) Hito wa naze homo ni naru no ka (Why do people become gay?), in *Kōkoku Hihyō* (Public Critique) No. 152, July/August, pp. 4–18

Nanda, Serena (1990) *Neither man nor woman: The hijras of India*, Belmont: Wadsworth Publishing Company

Naoi, Michiko (1994) Women's changing status and status identification, in *Social stratification in contemporary Japan*, Kosaka Kenji ed., London and New York: Kegan Paul International, pp. 149–64

Naruse, Mineko (1977) Shizuka naru tatakai (A silent struggle), in *Wadatsumi no koe o towa ni: Dokushin Fujin Renmei jūnen no ayumi* (Voices of the ocean for eternity: Ten years of the Single Women's League), Dokushin Fujin Renmei Kinenshi Henshū Iinkai ed., Tokyo: Dokushin Fujin Renmei, pp. 34–5

Needham, Rodney (1979) *Symbolic classification*, Santa Monica: Goodyear Publishing Company Inc.

Neuss-Kaneko, Margret (1990), *Familie und Gesellschaft in Japan: Von der Feudalzeit bis in die Gegenwart* (Family and society in Japan: From the feudal times to the present), Munich: Verlag C.H. Beck, 1990

Neustupny, J.V. (1978) *Post-structural approaches to language: Language theory in a Japanese context*, Tokyo: University of Tokyo Press

Ninomiya, Shūhei (1991) *Jijitsukono kangaeru: Mō hitotsu no sentaku* (Thinking of common law marriage: An alternative choice), Tokyo: Nihon Hyōronsha

Ninomiya, Shūhei (1992a) Kazoku to hō (Family and law), in *Fujin Hakusho 1992: Kyō no kazoku mondai* (White book on women 1992: Today's family problems), Nihon Fujin Dantai Rengōkai ed., Tokyo: Horupu Shuppan, pp. 65–71

Ninomiya, Shūhei (1992b) Kekkon seido to raifusutairuno jiyū (The marriage system and the freedom of lifestyles), in *Hikon o ikitai: Kongaishi no sabetsu o tou* (I want to live single: Questioning discrimination against extra-marital children), Yoshizumi Kyōko ed., Tokyo: Aoki Shoten, pp. 219–51

Nishi, Pasukaru (1992) Pari no hekotachi (Slaves of Paris), in *Za Gei* (The Gay), January

Nonomura, Kōji (1986) Gunpuku no seishun 6: Senba no dorei (Youth in a military uniform 6: A slave of the battlefield), in *Barazoku* (The Rose Clan) No. 165, October, pp. 126–44

Ochiai, Keiko (1990) *Gūzen no kazoku* (Family by coincidence), Tokyo: Chūō Kōronsha

Ōe, Kenzaburō (1989) *Seiteki ningen* (Sexual humans), Tokyo: Shinchō Bunko (original publication 1968)

Ōgoshi, Aiko (1991) Feminizumu wa ai to sei o katareru ka (Can feminism talk of love and sex?), in *Nihonteki sekushuariti: Feminizumu kara no sei fūdo hihan* (Japanese sexuality: A feminist critique of the sexual climate), Yamashita Akiko ed., Kyoto: Hōkōkan, pp. 129–202

Ogura, Chikako (1988) *Sekkusu shinwa kaitai shinsho: Sei genshō no shinsō o tsuku* (New book dismantling sex myths: Piercing the depths of sexual phenomena), Tokyo: Gakuyō Shobō

Ogura, Chikako (1989) *Matsuda Seiko ron* (Matsuda Seiko theory), Tokyo: Tottori Shinsha

Ogura, Chikako (1991) *Onna no jinsei sugoroku* (A game of goose of women's lives), Tokyo: Chikuma Shobō (first print 1990)

Ogura, Tō (1993) Gei no rakuen 'inran sauna' no reigi sahō (Rules of politeness in the gay garden of Eden, 'the lecherous sauna'), in *Eizu o ikiru hon* (Book for living with AIDS), Bessatsu Takarajima No. 172, Tokyo: JICC Shuppan, pp. 233–40

Ōhama, Hōei (1988) *Nihon no eizu: Sekaiteki shibyō to no tatakai* (AIDS in Japan: The struggle against a global lethal disease), Tokyo: Saimaru Shuppankai

Ōhayashi, Masako (1991) *Warui onna ka shira: Watashi no shiawasesagashi no tabi* (Am I a bad women?: My voyage in search of happiness), Tokyo: Iisuto Puresu

Ohnuki-Tierney, Emiko (1987) *The monkey in the mirror: Symbolic transformations in Japanese history and ritual*, Princeton: Princeton University Press

Ohnuki-Tierney, Emiko (1993) *Rice as self: Japanese identities through time*, Princeton: Princeton University Press

Oikawa, Taku (1993) Nichōmebyō: Gei sekkusu no otoshiana (Nichōme disease: A pitfall of gay sex), in *Imago* Vol. 4 No. 12, pp. 165–77

Okano, Haruko (1991) Weiblichkeitssymbolik und Sexismus in alten und neuen Religionen Japans (The symbolics of femininity and sexism in Japan's old and new religions), in *Japan: Ein Land der Frauen?* (Japan: A woman's country?), Elisabeth Gōssman ed., Munich: Iudicium Verlag, pp. 117–29

Ōkubo Sawako (1977) Danketsu shiyō, zenkoku no hai missu: Dokushin fujin no jittai chōsa (Let's unite, high misses of the whole country: Research into the actual situation of single women), in *Wadatsumi no koe o towa ni: Dokushin Fujin Renmei j_nen no ayumi*, (Voices of the ocean for eternity: Ten years of the Single Women's League), Dokushin Fujin Renmei Kinenshi Henshū Iinkai ed., Tokyo: Dokushin Fujin Renmei, pp. 16–22

Ōkubo Sawako (1987) Dokufuren wa jikka? (Is the Single Women's League a parental home?) in *Hanayaka ni shinguru raifu: 20nen o kinen ni shite* (A bright single life: Remembering twenty years), Dokushin Fujin Renmei 20nen Kinenshi Henshū Iinkai ed., Tokyo: Dokushin Fujin Renmei, p. 73

OLP (1994) Onna o aisuru onnatachi no tame no akutibitii: OLP e no sasoi (Activities for women who love women: An invitation to OLP), *OLP Newsletter* No. 1, September, pp. 2–3

OLP (1997) OLP for active lesbians, in *Tsunagaru tame no kamu auto* (Coming out in order to relate), Ochiya Kumiko, (Two articles from *OLP Newsletter* of January and February, published in a separate pamphlet)

Ōmura, Atsushi (1995a) Sei tenkan, dōseiai to minpō (jō) (Transsexuality, homosexuality and the civil law [part 1]), in *Jurisuto* (The Jurist) No. 1080, 1 December, pp. 68–74

Ōmura, Atsushi (1995b) Sei tenkan, dōseiai to minpō (ge) (Transsexuality, homosexuality and the civil law [part 2]), in *Jurisuto* (The Jurist) No. 1081, 15 December, pp. 61–9

Onitsuka, Tetsurō (1993) Komyuniti wa tsukuritai, de mo gettō wa iranai . . . (I want to build a community, but I don't need a ghetto . . . ), in *Musubikko* (Connecting child), November, pp. 14–15

Onitsuka, Tetsurō (1996) Gei ribu to eizu akutibizumu (Gay lib and AIDS activism), in *Kuia sutadiizu '96* (Queer studies '96), Kuia Sutadiizu Henshū Iinkai ed., Tokyo: Nanatsu Mori Shokan, pp. 124–37

Onna no Sei to Sei o Kangaeru Bunkakai (1991) *Dansei no sei ishiki ni kansuru ankēto chōsa: Otoko no sei to sei* (Questionnaire on the sexual consciousness of men: The life and sex of men), Osaka: Nihon Joseigaku Kenkyūkai

Onodera, Akiko (1982) Nani ga fukushi nan darō (What is welfare?), in *Shinguru Mazā: Kekkon o erabanakatta onnatachi no sei to sei* (Single mothers: The life and sex of women who did not choose marriage), Ikegami Chizuko ed., Tokyo: Gakuyō Shobō, pp. 20–32

Ortmanns, Annelie (1993) Rollenbilder im Wandel: Mann und Frau in japanischen Sozialkundebūcher von 1945 bis 1993 (Role images on the move: The man and the woman in Japanese sociology books from 1945 until 1993), in *Japanstudien:Jahrbuch des deutschen Instituts fūr Japanstudien der Philipp-Franz-von-Siebold-Stiftung* Band 5, pp. 182–309

Ortner, Sherry (1974) Is female to male as nature is to culture?, in *Woman, culture and society*, Michelle Rosaldo and Louise Lamphere eds, Stanford: Stanford University Press, pp. 67–88

Orwell, George (1949) *Nineteen eighty-four*, London: Secker & Warburg

Ōshima, Fukayuki (1994) Danjobetsu bunseki (Analysis of male/female differences), in *Sei kōi ni taisuru daigakusha no ishiki* (Students' consciousness of sexual activity), Yajima Zemi, Seiai Chōsa Kenkyū-kai ed., Tokyo: Chūō Daigaku Bungakubu Shakaigakka, March, pp. 17–34

Ōshima, Yumiko (1992) *Tsurubara tsurubara* (Rambler, rambler), Tokyo: Kadokawa Shoten, Asuka Comics

Ōsugi, Sakae (1978a) Die freie Liebe, nach der ich mich sehne (The free love I am longing for), in *Frauen in der Revolution: Wilde Blumen auf unfreiem Feld* (Women in the revolution: Wild flowers in an unfree field), Terasaki Akiko and Ilse Lenz eds, transl., Berlin: Karin Kramer Verlag, pp. 61–4

Ōsugi, Sakae (1978b) Geschichte, wie ich einen Geist gesehen habe (The story of how I saw a ghost), in *Frauen in der Revolution: Wilde Blumen auf unfreiem Feld* (Women in the revolution: Wild flowers in an unfree field), Terasaki Akiko and Ilse Lenz eds, transl., Berlin: Karin Kramer Verlag, pp. 65–89

Ōta, Tenrei (1987) *Daisan no sei: Sei wa hōkai suru no ka* (The third sex: Is sex collapsing?), Tokyo: Ningen no Kagakusha (reprint of *Daisan no sei: Sei no hōkai?* [The third sex: The collapse of sex?], Tokyo: Myōgi Shuppan 1957)

Ōta, Toshiko (1992) Masukomi ni miru hikon no oya, kongaishi sabetsu (The discrimination against unmarried parents and illegitimate children in the mass media), in *Hikon o ikitai: Kongaishi sabetsu o tou* (I want to live an unmarried life: Questioning discrimination against illegitimate children), Yoshimizu Kyōko ed., Tokyo: Aoki Shoten, pp. 103–99

Oya Fukō (nickname: Unfilial) (1993) Jibun mo higai mōsō ni (Me too in delusion of persecution), in *Barazoku* (The Rose Clan) No. 243, April, p. 111

Ōzaki, Eiki (1993) Seiyoku!: Wakiagaru yokubō inran sauna wa tōgenkyō!? (Sexual desire!: Is the lecherous sauna where desire boils up a Shangri-La!?) in *Gei no omochabako* (A gay toy box), Bessatsu Takarajima Ex, Tokyo: JICC Shuppan, p. 56

Pai Hsien-yung (1990) *Crystal boys*, San Francisco: Gay Sunshine Press

Pe san to Tomo ni Nyūkyo Sabetsu o Kanagaeru Kai and Kokusai Kyojūnen Kinen Ōsaka Renraku Kai (1991) *Sumitai nen, kono machi ni: Pe Kon Iru ikka e no nyūkyo sabetsu jiken o tou* (I want to live in this town: Questioning the housing discrimination against the family of Pe Kon Il), Osaka

Pharr, Susan J. (1981) *Political women in Japan: The search for a place in political life*, Berkeley: University of California Press

Pharr, Susan J. (1990) *Losing face: Status politics in Japan*, Berkeley: University of California Press

*Popeye* (1993) Imechen to iu yori betsujin: Tsutamori Tatsuru san (Another person rather than a change of image: Mr Tsutamori Tatsuru), in *Popeye* No. 400, 17 February, pp. 94–5

Probyn, Elspeth (1993) *Sexing the self: Gendered positions in cultural studies*, London and New York: Routledge

Psathas, George (1980) Early Goffman and the analysis of face-to-face interaction in 'Strategic Interaction', in *The view from Goffman*, Jason Ditton ed., London: Macmillan, pp. 52–79

Rabinow, Paul (1977) *Reflections on fieldwork in Morocco*, Berkeley: University of California Press

Raymond, Janice (1994) *The transsexual empire: The making of the she-male*, New York: Teachers College Press

Raymond, Janice (1996) The politics of transgenderism, in *Blending genders: Social aspects of cross-dressing and sex-changing*, Richard Ekins and Dave King eds, London and New York: Routledge, pp. 215–23

Reed, David (1992) The Persian boy today, in *Sexuality and eroticism among males in Moslem societies*, Arno Schmitt and Jehoeda Sofer eds, New York: Harrington Park Press, pp. 61–6

Reinharz, Shulamit (1983) Experiential analysis: A contribution to feminist research, in *Theories of women's studies*, Gloria Bowles and Renate Duelli Klein eds, London and New York: Routledge, pp. 162–91

Rezubian Feminisuto Sentā (1981) Porunogurafi wa onna e no bōryoku de aru (Pornography is violence against women), in *Onna Erosu* No. 16, 20 May, pp. 5–19

Rich, Adrienne (1993) Compulsory heterosexuality and lesbian existence, in *The lesbian and gay studies reader*, Henry Abelove, Michèle Aina Barale and David M. Halperin eds, New York and London: Routledge, pp. 227–54

Riviere, P.G. (1971) Marriage: A reassessment, in *Rethinking kinship and marriage*, Rodney Needham ed., London and New York: Tavistock Publications, pp. 57–74

Robertson, Jennifer (1991) *Native and newcomer: Making and remaking of a Japanese city*, Berkeley: University of California Press

Robertson, Jennifer (1992) Doing and undoing 'female' and 'male' in Japan:

The Takarazuka Revue, in *Japanese social organization*, Takie Sugiyama Lebra ed., Honolulu: University of Hawaii Press, pp. 165–93

Robertson, Jennifer (Robātoson, Jenifā)(1993) 'Dōseiai' no butaijō, butaigai ni okeru hyōgen (Expressions of 'homosexuality' on and off stage), in *Mugendai* (Infinity) No. 94, August, pp. 133–8

Robins-Mowry, Dorothy (1983) *The hidden sun: Women of modern Japan*, Boulder: Westview Press

Rosaldo, Renato (1986) From the door of his tent: The fieldworker and the inquisitor, in *Writing culture: The poetics and politics of ethnography*, James Clifford and George A. Marcus eds, Brekeley, Los Angeles and London: University of California Press, pp. 77–97

Rosenberger, Nancy R. (1992) Tree in summer, tree in winter: Movement of self in Japan, in *Japanese sense of self*, Nancy Rosenberger ed., Cambridge: Cambridge University Press, pp. 67–92

Ross, Michael W. (1983), *The married homosexual man: A psychological study*, London and New York: Routledge and Kegan Paul

Saeki, Junko (1992) *Bishōnen tsukushi* (Beautiful boys to the full), Tokyo: Heibonsha

Sagawa, Issei (1991) Fetchiteki hanzai: Watashi wa fetisshu ni kanojo o tabeta (Fetishist crime: I ate her as a fetish), in *Hentai san ga iku* (There goes Mr / Ms Queer), Bessatsu Takarajima No. 146, Tokyo: JICC Shuppan, pp. 258–71

Saitō, Ayako (1991) Baisekushuaru ga kataru: Onna to no ai, otoko to no kairaku (A bisexual talks: Love with women, lust with men), in *Onna o aisuru onnatachi no monogatari* (Stories of women who love women), Bessatsu Takarajima No. 64, Tokyo: JICC Shuppan, pp. 80–5

Saitō, Ayako (1993) *Rubii furūtsu* (Ruby fruits), Tokyo: Sōyosha

Saitō, Ayako and Fushimi, Noriaki (1993) *Taiwa: Kairaku no gijutsu* (Dialogue: Techniques of pleasure), Tokyo: Gakuyō Shobō

Saitō, Shigeo (1983) *Tsumatachi no shishūki* (Housewives' autumn), Tokyo: Kyōdō Tsūshinsha (first print 1982)

Sanday, Peggy Reeves (1990) Introduction, in *Beyond the second sex: New directions in the anthropology of gender*, Peggy Reeves Sanday and Ruth Gallagher Goodenough eds, Philadelphia: University of Pennsylvania Press, pp. 1–19

Sankar, Andrea (1986) Sisters and brothers, lovers and enemies: Marriage resistance in Southern Kwangtung, in *The many faces of homosexuality: Anthropological approaches to homosexual behavior*, Evelyn Blackwood ed., New York: Harrington Park Press, pp. 69–82

Sansom, G.B. (1961) *A history of Japan: 1334–1615*, Stanford: Stanford University Press

Sansom, G.B. (1978) *Japan: A short cultural history*, Stanford: Stanford University Press (first print 1931)

Sasabe, Taketoshi and Katsura, Ryōtarō (1990) *Kazoku to fukushi: Gendai kazoku fukushi kenkyū josetsu* (Family welfare: An introduction into research on contemporary family welfare), Tokyo: Kaiseisha

Sasano, Michiru (1995) *Coming out!*, Tokyo: Gentōsha

Saso, Mary (1990) *Women in the Japanese workplace*, London: Hilary Shipman

Satō, Bunmei and Kaibara, Hiroshi (1990) *Koseki* (Legal registration), For beginners shiriizu, irasutohan orijinaru (For beginners series, original illustrated edition), Tokyo: Gendai Shokan

Satō, Fumiko (1982) Annetto ga ima o ikiru koto no imi (The significance of Annette being alive today), in *Shinguru mazā: Kekkon o erabanakatta onnatachi no sei to sei* (Single mothers: The life and sex of women who did not choose marriage), Ikegami Chizuko, Tokyo: Gakuyō Shobō, pp. 63–79

Satō, Ikuya (1992) *Fiirudowāku: Sho o motte machi e deyō* (Fieldwork: Let's take our books and go into town), Tokyo: Shinyōsha

Satō, Masaki (1996) Shōjo manga to homofobia (Girl's comics and homophobia), in *Kuia sutadiizu '96* (Queer studies '96), Kuia Sutadiizu Henshū Iinkai ed., Tokyo: Nanatsu Mori Shokan, pp. 161–9

Saunders, A. Dale (1964) *Buddhism in Japan: With an outline of its origins in India*, Philadelphia: University of Pennsylvania Press

Sawabe, Hitomi (1990) *Yuriko, Dasubidāniya: Yuasa Yoshiko no seishun* (Farewell, Yuriko: The youth of Yuasa Yoshiko), Tokyo: Bungei Shunju

Sawada, Akio (1992) Feminizumu no mashō (Feminism's devilishness), in *Shokun!* (Gentlemen!) January, pp. 221–9

Sawaragi, Noi (1991) Hebi metarisuto to bondōji mania (Heavy metallists and bondage mania), in *Hentai san ga iku* (There goes Mr/Ms Queer), Bessatsu Takarajima No. 146, Tokyo: JICC Shuppan, pp. 224–37

Schalow, Paul Gordon (1989) Male love in early modern Japan: A literary depiction of the 'youth', in *Hidden from history: Reclaiming the gay and lesbian past*, Martin Bauml Duberman, Martha Vicinus and George Chauncy eds, New York: New American Library Books, pp. 118–28

Schmitt, Arno (1992) A critique of John Boswell's writings on Muslim gays, in *Sexuality and eroticism among males in Moslem societies*, Arno Schmitt and Jehoeda Sofer eds, New York, London and Norwood: Harrington Park Press, pp. 169–78

Schooler, Carmi and Smith, Karen C. (1978) Women as mothers in Japan: The effect of social structure and culture on values and behavior, in *Journal of Marriage and the Family*, August, pp. 613–20

Schrijvers, Joke (1985) *Mothers for life: Motherhood and marginalization in the North Central province of Sri Lanka*, Delft: Eburon

Schrijvers, Joke (1993) Motherhood experienced and conceptualized: Changing images in Sri Lanka and the Netherlands, in *Gendered fields: Women, men and ethnography*, Diane Bell, Pat Caplan and Wazir Jahan Khan eds, London and New York: Routledge, pp. 143–67

Schuyf, Judith (1994) *Een stilzwijgende samenzwering: Lesbische vrouwen in*

*Nederland, 1920-1970* (A silent conspiracy: Lesbian women in the Netherlands, 1920-1970), Amsterdam: Stichting Beheer IISG

Sechiyama, Kaku (1992) Yori yoi sei no shōhinka e mukete (Towards a better commercialization of sex), in *Feminizumu no shuchō* (Assertions of feminism), Ehara Yumiko ed., Tokyo: Keisō Shobō, pp. 45–91

Sei, Shōnagon (1962) *Makura no sōshi* (The pillow book), Ikeda Kikan ed., comm., Tokyo: Iwanami Shoten

Sennyo, Mako (1996) Genzai Nihon de TG ga chokumen suru mondaiten (Problems a transgender is confronted with in contemporary Japan), in *Kuia sutadiizu '96* (Queer studies '96), Kuia Sutadiizu Henshū Iinkai ed., Tokyo: Nanatsu Mori Shokan, pp. 99–107

Senya, Tsugio (1986a) Joshin dantai (A women's heart, a man's body), in *Barazoku* (The Rose Clan) No. 165, October, pp. 106–17

Senya, Tsugio (1986b) Shiroi jōyoku (White passion), in *Barazoku* (The Rose Clan) No. 165, October, pp. 118–25

Shiba, Fumiko (1993a) Shōwa rokujō nendai rezubian būmu: Ano koro, rezu wa osshare datta (The lesbian boom of the 1980s: At the time, lesbians were trendy), in *Tanbi shōsetsu: Gei bungaku bukku gaido* (Aesthetic novels: A gay culture book guide), Kakinuma Eiko and Kurihara Chiyo eds, Tokyo: Byakuya Shobō, pp. 290–1

Shiba, Fumiko (1993b) Maboroshi no rezu 'kaze' zasshi (The illusive lesbian 'wind' magazine), in *Tanbi shōsetsu: Gei bungaku bukku gaido (Aesthetic novels: A gay culture book guide)*, Kakinuma Eiko and Kurihara Chiyo eds, Tokyo: Byakuya Shobō, pp. 304–5

Shibatani, Atsuhiro (1990) *Hansabetsuron: Mukonkyōsei no paradokkusu (gyakusetsu)* (Anti-discrimination theory: The paradox of unfoundedness), Tokyo: Akashi Shoten

Shibuya, Michiyo (1990) Kibun wa baishun (The feeling is that of prostitution), in *Nyū Feminizumu Rebyū* (New Feminism Review) No. 1: Renai tekunorojii: Ima renai tte nani? (Love technology: What is love today?), Ueno Chizuko ed., pp. 255–60

Shida, Sabeji (1992) Nausika Konpurekkusu: Renai dekinai otokotachi (The Nausicaa Complex: Men who cannot find love), in *Marco Polo*, September, pp. 112–15

Shigekawa, Haruki (1990) *Shinguru pearento: Otoko no kaji, otoko no henkaku* (Single parent: Men doing the household, men who change), Tokyo: Kōunsha

Shiina, Masae (1994), Coping alone: When work separates families, in *Japan Quarterly*, January / March, pp. 26–34

Shimazu, Yoshiko (1992) Hikon no haha to sono kodomo: Sono rekishi to genzai (The unmarried mother and her children: Their history and their present situation), in *Hikon o ikitai: Kongaishi sabetsu o tou* (I wish to live single: Questioning discrimination against extra-marital children), Yoshizumi Kyōko ed., Tokyo: Aoki Shoten, pp. 178–218

Shimazu, Yoshiko (1994) Unmarried mothers and their children in Japan, in *US-Japan Women's Journal* (English supplement) No. 6, pp. 83–100

Shiono, Hiroshi, Maeda, Yasu, Hirai, Yoshio and Aoyama, Yoshimitsu eds (1993) *Shōroppō, Heisei rokunenban* (Concise six codes of law: 1994 edition), Tokyo: Yōhikaku

Sieber, Joan E. (1993) The ethics and politics of sensitive research, in *Researching sensitive topics*, Claire M. Renzetti and Raymond Lee eds, Newbury Park: Sage, pp. 14–26

Sievers, Sharon L. (1983) *Flowers in salt: The beginnings of feminist consciousness in modern Japan*, Stanford: Stanford University Press

Signorile, Michelangelo (1994) *Queer in America: Sex, the media and the closets of power*, London: Abacus

Singer, Bennett L. and Deschamps, David eds (1994) *Gay and lesbian stats: A pocket guide of facts and figures*, New York: The New Press

Smith, Dorothy E. (1990) *Texts, facts, and femininity: Exploring relations of ruling*, London and New York: Routledge

Smith, Robert J. (1983) *Japanese society: Tradition, self and the social order*, Cambridge: Cambridge University Press

Smith, Robert J. and Wiswell, Ella Lury (1982) *The women of Suye mura*, Chicago and London: University of Chicago Press

Sofer, Jehoeda (1992) Testimonies of the holy land: Israeli and Palestinian men talk about their sexual encounters, in *Sexuality and eroticism among males in Moslem societies*, Arno Schmitt and Jehoeda Sofer eds, New York, London and Norwood: Harrington Park Press, pp. 105–21

Sōmuchō Tōkeikyoku ed. (1992) *Nihon no tōkei* (Statistics of Japan), Tokyo: Ōkurashō Insatsukyoku

Sōmuchō Tōkeikyoku ed. (1996) *Heisei 7nendo kokusei chōsa chūshutsu sokuhō* (1995 population census of Japan results prompt sample tabulation), Tokyo: Ōkurashō Insatsukyoku

Strathern, Marilyn (1992a) *Reproducing the future: Anthropology, kinship and the new productive technologies*, Manchester: Manchester University Press

Strathern, Marilyn (1992b) *After nature: English kinship in the late twentieth century*, Cambridge: Cambridge University Press

Sugii, Shizuko (1990) *Sekushuaru harasumento shohōsen: Shokuba no atarashii danjo kankei, bengoshi kara no adobaisu* (Prescriptions for sexual harassment: New male / female relations in the workplace, a lawyer's advice), Tokyo: Adoa Shuppan

Sugiura, Yoshiaki and Sugiura, Takaaki (1992) Watashitachi, sukusuku to gei ni natchatta ne (We became gay in no time, didn't we), in *Kōkoku Hihyō* (Public Critique), July / August, pp. 28–35

Sunaya, Chizuko (1992) Josōsha no otto o motsu shufu no tachiba kara horumon ni tsuite kataru: Dekireba ataerareta sei o mattō shite kudasai . . . (Talking about hormones from the standpoint of the housewife who has a transvestite husband: If possible, please perform in agreement with the sex you have been born with . . . ), in *Himawari* (Sunflower) No. 9, Spring, pp. 68–70

Taira, Kazuaki (1993) Raifu hisutorii: 'Shindosa' no kaimei (Life history: The solution to 'tiresomeness'), in *Poko a Poko* (Little by Little) Vol. 0: pure sōkangō (pre-first number), January, pp. 30–9

Tajima, Yōko (1992) *Ai to iu na no shihai* (Domination in the name of love), Tokyo: Tarō Jirōsha

Takaguchi, Satosumi (1991) *Rakkii kun (Kōun danshi) 1* (Lucky boys 1), Tokyo: Kōdansha

Takaguchi, Satosumi (1993) *Rakkii kun (Kōun danshi) 2* (Lucky boys 2), Tokyo: Kōdansha (first print 1992)

Takakura, Daisuke (1992) Sabu yarō kōkengaku: Sei ni kansuru gojō no shitsumon (Opinions of macho men: Fifty questions on sex), in *Sabu*, February, pp. 139–54

Takamizawa, Shigeru (1979) Amerikan ripōto 5: Ōjiirōmu no rankōshiin, San Furanshisuko no yoru o saguru (American report 5: Promiscuous scenes in the OG room: Investigating nightlife in San Francisco), in *Barazoku* (The Rose Clan) No. 78, July, pp. 105–9

Takamure, Itsue (1991) *Nihon koninshi* (The history of marriage in Japan), Nihon Rekishi Shinsho, Tokyo: Tōbundō

*Takarajima* (1993) Kamingu auto shita gei kappuru! (A gay couple that came out!), in *Takarajima*, 9 March, No. 267, pp. 30–1

Takehara, Yoshinobu (1993) Ore no 'kamu auto' (My 'coming out'), in *Choisir* (Choose) Vol. 27, March, p. 29

Takemiya, Keiko (1977–84) *Kaze to ki no uta* (Le poème du vent et des arbres; The poem of the wind and the trees), part 1–17, Tokyo: Shōgakukan, Flower Comics

Tamura, Tarō (1988) Homo no kekkon, rikon, hikon o kangaeru: Kekkon suru wa yasuku, rikon suru wa gatashi (Thinking about the marriage, divorce and singleness of gay men: Marrying is easy, divorce is difficult), in *Barazoku* (The Rose Clan), April, pp. 114–21

Tamura, Zenjū (1989) Shin burujoakei kekkon no jidai: 30sai ni shite hirogaru otoko no sentaku (The times of the new bourgeois marriage: The choice of men broadens at thirty), in *Akurosu* (Across) No. 184, July, pp. 44–58

Tanaka, Kazutaka ed. (1991) *In and out of By-sexual: Kaizokuban* (Ins and outs of By-sexual: A pirated version), Tokyo: JICC Shuppan

Tanaka, Mitsu (1975) *Inochi no onnatachi e: Torimidashi ūman ribu ron* (That women may live: Disorderly theories of women's liberation), Tokyo: Tabata Shoten (first print 1972)

Tanaka, Yōko (1992) Tanshin funin no sutoresu (The stress of living apart for reasons of employment), in *Gendai no Esupuri* (L'Esprit d'Aujourd'hui/Today's spirit) No. 300: Kazoku to katei no sutoresu (Stress in the family and the household), July, pp. 70–80

Tani, Kayoko (1982) *Onna hitori ikiru: Dokushin sabetsu no naka o ikinuku chie*

(Women living alone: The wisdom to survive in the middle of discrimination of singles), Kyoto: Mineruba Shobō

Tani, Kayoko (1993) Ohaka no arikata o kangaeru (Thinking about the situation of graves), in *Seiron* (Sound Argument), March, pp. 208–11

Tanigawa, Tamae (1993) Josei no shōnenai shōkō ni tsuite II: Shikisha no kenkai to feminizumu ni okeru kanōsei (On the yearning of women for boys: The viewpoint of leaders and the possibility of feminism), in *Joseigaku Nenpō* (Chronicle of Women's Studies) No. 14, October, pp. 66–79

Tanigawa, Tamae (1995) Josei no shōnenai shōkō ni tsuite III: Yaoi ronsō kara (On the yearning of women for boys III: from the Yaoi discussion), in *Joseigaku Nenpō* (Chronicle of Women's Studies) No. 16, pp. 36–51

Taniguchi, Shōko (1992) Tasha e no kamu auto to sabetsu, henken (Coming out towards others and discrimination), in *Dōseiai kenkyū josetsu: Dōseiaisha to iseiaisha no hikaku chōsa yori* (An introduction into the study of homosexuality: From a comparative investigation of homosexuals and heterosexuals), Yajima Zemi ed., Uhauha Hakusho 1991, Tokyo: Chūō Daigaku Bungakubu Shakaigakka, October, pp. 76–86

Tanimura, Shiho (1990) *Kekkon shinai ka mo shirenai shōkōgun* (The maybe-I-will-not-marry syndrome), Tokyo: Shufu no Tomosha

Tapinc, Huseyin (1992) Masculinity, femininity, and Turkish male homosexuality, in *Modern homosexualities: Fragments of lesbian and gay experience*, Ken Plummer ed., London and New York: Routledge, pp. 39–49

Taudin-Chabot, Jeanette A. (1981) Die japanische Frauenrechtsbewegung von 1868 bis heute – ein Ūberblick (The Japanese women's movement from 1868 until today – an overview), in *Beitrāge zur Japanologie* (Contributions to Japanese Studies) Band 17: Die Japanerin in Vergangenheit und Gegenwart (The Japanese woman in past and present), Vienna: Universitāt Wien, pp. 255–72

Taylor, Charles (1985) The person, in *The category of the person: Anthropology, philosophy, history*, Michael Carrithers, Steven Collins and Steven Lukes eds, Cambridge: Cambridge University Press, pp. 257–81

Taylor, Clark L. (1986) Mexican male homosexual interaction in public contexts, in *The many faces of homosexuality: Anthropological approaches to homosexual behavior*, Evelyn Blackwood ed., New York: Harrington Park Press, pp. 117–36

Tazaki, Hideaki (1993a) *Sekkusu nan te kowakunai: Kairaku no tame no 7tsu no ressun* (Who is afraid of sex?: Seven lessons in pleasure), Tokyo: Kawade Shobō Shinsha

Tazaki, Hideaki (1993b) *Eizu nan te kowakunai* (Who is afraid of AIDS?), Tokyo: Kawade Shobō Shinsha

Teruoka, Yasutaka (1992) *Nihonjin no ai to sei* (The love and sex of Japanese), Tokyo: Iwanami Shinsho (first print 1989)

Tobin, Joseph (1992) Japanese preschools and the pedagogy of selfhood, in *Japanese sense of self*, Nancy R. Rosenberger ed., Cambridge: Cambridge University Press, pp. 21–39

Tomonari, Junichi (1991) Nihon no hentai no rūtsu o sagase: Rondon wa hentai no machi da (Looking for the roots of Japanese queerness: London is the town of queerness), in *Hentai san ga iku* (There goes Mr / Ms Queer), Bessatsu TakarajimaNo. 146, Tokyo: JICC Shuppan, pp. 210–23

Tōgō, Ken (1981) *Yokujō no kisu o doko ni suru ka* (Where shall we put our kisses of passion?), Tokyo: Sanichi Shobō

Tōgō, Ken (1984) *Tenkei aishoka 1* (The heavenly bibliophile 1), Tokyo: Kōyō Shuppan

Torai, Masae (1992) Beikoku seitenkan jijō: Saishūkai shūjutsu hen (The situation of sex change in America: About the last surgery), in *Queen* No. 70, February, pp. 48–58

Torai, Masae (1996) *Onna kara otoko ni natta watashi* (I who changed from a woman into a man), Tokyo: Seikyūsha

Toshitani, Nobuyoshi (1994) The reform of Japanese family law and changes in the family system, in *US/Japan Women's Journal* (English supplement) No. 6, pp. 66–82

Tsuji, Akio (1992) *Kekkon sabetsu: 'Buraku yue ni'* (Marriage discrimination: 'Because you are of *buraku* origin'), Osaka: Kaih_ Shuppansha

Tsuji, Tetsuya (1989) Seiai ni okeru ryōsei sabetsu (Discrimination of both sexes in sexual love), in *Gendai no Esupuri* (L'Esprit d'Aujourd'hui / Today's Spirit) No. 262: *Kappuruzu* (Couples), May, pp. 77–88

Tsumura, Akiko and Kita, Akemi (1994) Koyō ni okeru danjo byōdō to rōdō kumiai (The equality of men and women in hiring and labour unions), in *Rōdōryoku no joseika: 21seiki e no paradaimu* (The feminization of the labour force: A paradigm for the 21st century), Takenaka Emiko and Kuba Yoshiko eds, Tokyo: Yōhikaku Sensho, pp. 179–216

Tsunoda, Yukiko (1992) *Sei no hōritsugaku* (The juris prudence on sex), Tokyo: Yōhikaku Sensho (first print 1991)

Tsuru and Kame (1993) Gakusai josō kontesuto rupo (A report of a transvestite contest at a university festival), in *Queen* No. 76, February, pp. 84–7

Tsutamori, Tatsuru ed. (1990a) *Gendai no Esupuri* (L'Esprit d'Aujourd'hui / Today's Spirit) No. 277: Toransu Jendā Genshō (Transgender phenomena), August

Tsutamori, Tatsuru (1990b) *Otoko datte kirei ni naritai* (Men want to be pretty), Popeye Books, Tokyo: Magajin Hausu, Tokyo

Tsutamori, Tatsuru (1991) Oiwai gitai to tokudai no hanataba ga matte iru (Simulated celebrations and outsize bouquets are waiting), in *Cross Dressing* No. 1, 15 December, pp. 42–5

Tsutamori, Tatsuru (1992) *Soshite, boku wa, otoko ni natta* (And I became a man), Tokyo: Magajin Hausu

Tsutamori, Tatsuru (1993) *Otoko de mo naku, onna de mo nai: Shinjidai no andorojinasutachi e* (Neither man nor woman: To the androgynous people of the new times), Tokyo: Keisō Shobō

Tuan, Yi-Fan (1982) *Segmented worlds and self: Group life and individual consciousness*, Minneapolis: University of Minnesota Press

Tyler, Stephen E. (1986) Post-modern ethnography: From document of the occult to occult document, in *Writing culture: The poetics and politics of ethnography*, James Clifford and George A. Marcus eds, Berkeley, Los Angeles and London: University of California Press, pp. 77–97

Uchikoshi, Yukio (1995) Uchikoshi Yukio-san no raifu historii (The life history of Uchikoshi Yukio), in *Gei no 11gatsusai tengoku: Hōkokushū* (The celestial gay November festival: Report collection), Kyōdai 11Gatsusai Gei Purojekuto Jikko Iinkai eds, pp. 5–23

Uemura, Kuniko (1988) *Sei no hōkai* (The destruction of sex), Tokyo: Nihon Jitsugyō Shuppansha

Ueno, Chizuko (1988a) *Onna asobi* (Women's play), Tokyo: Gakuyō Shobō

Ueno, Chizuko (1988b) The Japanese women's movement: The counter-values to industrialism, in *The Japanese trajectory: Modernization and beyond*, Gavan McCormack and Yoshio Sugimoto eds, Cambridge: Cambridge University Press, pp. 167–85

Ueno, Chizuko (1989) *Sukāto no shita no gekijō: Hito wa dō shite pantii ni kodawaru no ka* (Theatre in the skirt: Why do people adhere to panty hoses?), Tokyo: Kawade Shobō Shinsha

Ueno, Chizuko (1990a) *Kafuchōsei to shihonsei: Marukusushugi feminizumu no chihei* (Patriarchy and capitalism: The horizon of Marxist feminism), Tokyo: Iwanami Shoten

Ueno, Chizuko (1990b) Kekkon sensō sabaibaru sakusen (Tactics for surviving the marriage war), in *Hanamuko Gakkō* (Bridegroom school), Higuchi Keiko, Saitō Shigeo and Itamoto Yōko eds, Tokyo: Sanseidō

Ueno, Chizuko ed. (1990c) Ankēto: Anata wa naniha? (Questionnaire: What sort are you?), in *Nyū Feminizumu Rebyū* (New Feminism Review) Vol. 1: Renai tekunorojii: Ima renai tte nani? (Love technology: What is love today?), pp. 266–73

Ueno, Chizuko (1991a) *Onna to iu kairaku* (The pleasure of womanhood), Tokyo: Keisō Shobō (first print 1986)

Ueno, Chizuko (1991b) Famiri aidentiti no yukue: Atarashii kazoku gensō (Where family identity goes: New family illusions), in *Kazoku no shakaishi: Henbō suru kazoku* (Social history of the family: Transfiguring family), Tokyo: Iwanami Shoten, pp. 2–38

Ueno, Chizuko (1991c) *Sekushi Gyaru no daikenkyū: Onna no yomikata, yomarekata, yomasekata* (Great studies of the sexy girl: How women read, are read and let themselves be read), Kappa Science, Tokyo:

Kōbunsha
Ueno, Chizuko (1992) Sekushuariti wa shizen ka (Is sexuality nature?), in *Bungei* (Art and Literature), Autumn, pp. 323–30
Ueno, Chizuko (1993) *Middonaito kōru* (Midnight call), Tokyo: Asahi Shinbunsha (first edition 1990)
Ueno, Chizuko (1995) Sei no seijigaku (The politics of sex), in *Jendā no shakaigaku* (The sociology of gender), Inoue Toshi, Ueno Chizuko, *et al.* eds, Tokyo: Iwanami Shoten, pp. 1–26
Ueno, Chizuko and Dentsū Nettowāku Kenkyūkai (1989) *'Joen' ga yo no naka o kaeru: Datsu sengyū shufu (enjoisuto) no nettow_kingu* (Women's networking is changing the world: The networking of housewives breaking out [enjoyers]), Tokyo: Nihon Keizai Shinbunsha (first print 1988)
Ueno, Chizuko, Ogura, Chikako and Oda, Motoko (1992), Nihon no feminizumu wa ima, dō natte iru no ka? (Now what is happening with Japanese feminism?), in *Wakaritai anata no tame no feminizumu nyūmon* (An introduction to feminism for those who want to understand), Series: Bessatsu Takarajima No. 85, Tokyo: JICC Shuppan, pp. 42–57 (first print 1988)
Ugoku Gei to Rezubian no Kai (Akō) ed. (1992) *Gei ripōto: Dōseiaisha wa kōgen suru* (Gay report: Homosexuals speak out), Tokyo: Tottori Shinsha
Umechika Fōramu 'Anta mo watashi mo higaisha no kai' (1990) *Soko no ke soko no ke Ōsaka shiyakusho ga tōru* (In whatever manner Osaka city hall continues), Osaka: Nihon Kikanshi Shuppan Sentā
Umeyama, Asuka (1994) Danjokanbetsu bunseki (Analysis of differences between men and women), in *Sei kōi ni taisuru daigakusei no ishiki* (The consciousness of university students of sexual activity), Yajima Zemi, Seiai Chōsa Kenkyūkai ed., Tokyo: Chūō Daigaku Bungakubu Shakaigakka, March, pp. 45–61
Valentine, James (1990) On the borderlines: The significance of marginality in Japanese society, in *Unwrapping Japan*, Eyal Ben-Ari, Brian Moeran and James Valentine eds, Manchester: Manchester University Press, pp. 36–57
Valentine, James (1997) Skirting and suiting stereotypes: Representations of marginalised sexualities in Japan, in *Theory, Culture and Society*
Vogel, Suzanne Z. (1978) Professional housewife: The career of urban middle-class Japanese women, in *The Japan Interpreter* No. 12, pp. 16–43
Wada, Naoko (1991) Nihon no senpai rezubiantachi (Japanese lesbian predecessors), in Onna o aisuru onnatachi no monogatari (Stories of women who love women), Bessatsu Takarajima No. 64, Tokyo: JICC Shuppan, pp. 74–9
Wade, Peter (1993) Sexuality and masculinity in fieldwork among Columbian blacks, in Gendered fields: Women, men and ethnography, Diane Bell, Pat Caplan and Wazir Jahan Khan eds, London and New York:

Routledge, pp. 199–214
Waifu Henshūbu ed. (1989) Anchi Kurowassan shōkōgun: Kekkon shinai onnatachi no sugao (Against the Croissant syndrome: The unpainted faces of women who do not marry), Tokyo: Shakai Shisōsha
Warren, Carol A.B. (1988) Gender issues in field research, Qualitative research methods series 9, Newbury Park: Sage
Warren, Hans (1986a) Geheim dagboek, derde deel: 1949–1951 (Secret diary, third part: 1949–51), Amsterdam: Bert Bakker (first print 1983)
Warren, Hans (1986b) Geheim dagboek, vierde deel: 1952–1953 (Secret diary, fourth part: 1952–53), Amsterdam: Bert Bakker (first print 1984)
Warren, Hans (1987) Geheim dagboek, vijfde deel: 1954–1955 (Secret diary, fifth part: 1954–55), Amsterdam: Bert Bakker (first print 1985)
Warren, Hans (1991) Geheim dagboek, negende deel: 1971–1972 (Secret diary, ninth part: 1971–72), Amsterdam: Bert Bakker
Watanabe, Mieko (1990) Nihon ni okeru josei dōseiai no nagare: Atogaki ni kaete (The flow of female homosexuality in Japan: Epilogue), in Ūman rabingu: Rezubian ron sōsei ni mukete (Loving women: Towards the creation of lesbian theory), Watanabe Mieko et al. transl., eds, Tokyo, Gendai Shokan, pp. 184–9
Watanabe, Mieko et al. transl. eds, (1990) Ūman rabingu: Rezubian ron sōsei ni mukete (Loving women: Towards the creation of lesbian theory), Tokyo: Gendai Shokan
Watanabe, Tsuneo (1989) Datsu dansei no jidai: Andorojinesu o mezasu bunmeigaku (The times of deserting manhood: Cultural studies aiming at androgyny), Tokyo: Keisō Shobō (first print 1986)
Watanabe, Tsuneo (1991) Meikyū no erosu to bunmei: Ryōdō suru jendā, jiga, sekaikan no shinrigaku (Erotics and culture in a labyrinth: A psychology of floating gender, selves and worldviews), Tokyo: Shinyōsha
Watanabe, Tsuneo and Iwata, Junichi (1987) La voie des éphèbes: Histoire et histoires des homosexualités au Japon (The way of the youth: History and stories of homosexuality in Japan), Paris: Editions Trismégiste
Watanabe, Yōko (1991) Shizen to tatakau (Fighting nature), in Onna ga kodomo o umitagaranai wake (Why women do not want to have children), Yoshihiro Kiyoko ed., Tokyo: Bansei Shobō, pp. 125–35
Weber, Claudia (1990) Chancengleichheit per Gesetz (Equality of opportunity by law), in Nippons neue Frauen (Japan's new women), Ruth Linhart and Fleur Wōss eds, Reinbeck: Rohwolt, pp. 104–25
Weeks, Jeffrey (1983) Coming out: Homosexual politics in Britain from the nineteenth century to the present, London, Melbourne and New York: Quartet Books (first print 1977)
Weeks, Jeffrey (1991a) Sexuality, London and New York: Routledge (first print 1986)
Weeks, Jeffrey (1991b) Sexuality and its discontents: Meanings, myths and modern sexualities, London and New York: Routledge (first print 1985)

White, James W. (1970) The Sōkagakkai and mass society, Stanford: Stanford University Press

White, Merry (1987) The Japanese educational challenge: A commitment to children, New York: The Free Press

Whitehead, Harriet (1981) The bow and the burden strap: A new look at institutionalized homosexuality in native North America, in Sexual meanings: The cultural construction of gender and sexuality, Sherry B. Ortner and Harriet Whitehead eds, Cambridge: Cambridge University Press, pp. 80–115. Also in: The lesbian and gay studies reader, Henry Abelove, Michèle Aina Barale and David M. Halperin, London and New York: Routledge, 1993, pp. 498–527

Whitehead, Tony Larry (1986) Breakdown, resolution and coherence: The fieldwork experiences of a big, brown, pretty talking man in a West Indian community, in Self, sex and gender in cross-cultural fieldwork, Tony Larry Whitehead and Mary Ellen Conaway eds, Urbana and Chicago: University of Illinois Press, pp. 213–39

Whitehead, Tony Larry and Brown, Judith (1986) Gender-related issues in carrying out rapid team fieldwork in the Cameroon: in Self, sex and gender in cross-cultural fieldwork, Tony Larry Whitehead and Mary Ellen Conaway eds, Urbana and Chicago: University of Illinois Press, pp. 196–210

Whitehead, Tony Larry and Price, Laurie (1986) Summary: Sex and the fieldwork experience, in Self, sex and gender in cross-cultural fieldwork, Tony Larry Whitehead and Mary Ellen Conaway eds, Urbana and Chicago: University of Illinois Press, pp. 289–304

Whittle, Stephen (1996) Gender fucking or fucking gender?: Current cultural contributions to theories of gender blending, in *Blending genders: social aspects of cross-dressing and sex-changing*, Richard Enkins and Dave King eds, London and New York: Routledge, pp. 196–214

Wieringa, Saskia (1987) *Uw toegenegen Dora D.: Reisbrieven* (Your devoted Dora D.: Travel letters), Amsterdam: Uitgeverij Furie

Wittig, Monique (1992) *The straight mind and other essays*, Boston: Beacon Press

Wōss, Fleur (1981) Die Frau im Amida-Buddhismus: Von 'Boten der Hōlle' zum bevorzugten Erlōsungsobjekt: The woman in Amida Buddhism: From 'missionaries from hell' to favorite salvation objects), in *Beitrāge zur Japanologie* (Contributions to Japanese studies) Vol. 17: Die Japanerin in Vergangenheit und Gegenwart (The Japanese woman in past and present), Vienna: Universitāt Wien, pp. 27–45

Wōss, Fleur (1990) Konfliktlōsung extrem: Selbstmord im weiblichen Lebenslauf (The extreme solution of conflict: Suicide in female lifecourses), in *Nippons neue Frauen* (Japan's new women), Ruth Linhart and Fleur Wōss eds, Reinbeck: Rohwolt, pp. 170–91

Xiao, Ming Xiong (1984) *Zhongguo Tongxingai Shilu* (A veritable history of

homosexuality in China), Hong Kong: Samshasha
Y.A. (1993) Watakushi wa kekkon shite imasu (I am married), in *Labrys* No. 3, p. 24
Yamada, Keiko (1993) Onna sankai no ie (Three times a household for women), in *Waifu* (Wife) No. 240, March, pp. 10–16
Yamada, Yuichi (1992) Bijinesuman no sutoresu to kitaku kyōfu shōkōgun (Stress of businessmen and the syndrome of returning-homephobia), in *Gendai no Esupuri* (L'Esprit d'Aujourd'hui/Today's Spirit) No. 300: Kazoku to katei no sutoresu (Stress of the family and the household), July, pp. 115–24
Yamagishi, Ryōko (1991–2) *Hiizure dokoro no tenshi* (The angel from the sun), in Yamagishi Ryōko zenshō Nos. 1–8, Tokyo: Kadokawa Shoten (sixteenth to eighteenth print)
Yamaguchi, Yōko (1985) *Hyakunin no otokotachi* (Hundred men), Tokyo: Bungei Shunju
Yamashita, Akiko (1991) Sei shinryaku, sei bōryoku no rekishi to kōzō (The history and structure of sexual aggression and sexual violence), in *Nihonteki sekushuariti: Feminizumu no sei fūdo hihan* (Japanese sexuality: A feminist critique of the sexual climate), Yamashita Akiko ed., Kyoto: Hōkōkan, pp. 3–76
Yamashita, Etsuko (1991) *'Josei no jidai' to iu shinwa* (The myth of 'women's times'), Tokyo: Seikyūsha
Yamashita, Noriko (1992) *Kamen fūfu: Watashi ga otto to wakareru riyū* (A masked couple: Why I separated from my husband), Tokyo: Shōdensha
Yamauchi, Noboru (1991) Dōseseiaisha ni okeru renai kōkan no heni (Changes in spaces for love of homosexuals), in *Gendai fūzoku '92: Renai kūkan* (Modern customs '92: Love spaces), Gendai Fūzoku Kenkyūsho ed., pp. 61–7
Yamazaki, Misao (1993) Call No. 5, in *Sabu*, April, pp. 39–56
Yoshida, Akimi and Fushimi, Noriaki (1992) Isai mendan: Tsuintōkusu (A personal talk of great talents: Twintalks), in *June* No. 62, January, pp. 151–6
Yoshihiro, Kiyoko (1987) *Hikon jidai* (The times of not marrying), Tokyo: Sanseidō
Yoshihiro, Kiyoko (1988) *Otokotachi no hikon jidai* (The times of men who do not marry), Tokyo: Sanseidō
Yoshiya, Nobuko (1924) *Hana monogatari* (A flower tale), Tokyo: Kokushokan Kōkai
Yoshizawa, Natsuko (1992) Utsukushii mono ni okeru byōdō: Feminizumu no gendaiteki hihan (Equality in beautiful things: A contemporary critique of feminism), in *Feminizumu no shuchō* (Assertions of feminsim), Ehara Yumiko ed., Tokyo: Keisō Shobō, pp. 93–132
Yoshizumi, Kyōko (1992) Kongai shussei to mibun tōroku seido: Nihon, Suēden, Amerika no sankoku hikaku (Birth outside marriage and the

identity registration system: A comparison of the three countries Japan, Sweden and America, in *Hikon o ikitai: Kongaishi sabetsu o tou* (I want to live single: Questioning discrimination against children born outside marriage), Yoshizumi Kyōko ed., Tokyo: Aoki Shoten, pp. 122–77

Yukidaruma (nickname: Snowman) (1993) Boku ga, asshu no hitotachi no kekkon ni tsuite kangaeru . . . (What I think of marriages of gay men . . . ), in *Magazine DON!*, Tokushō: Kekkon (Special: Marriage), August, pp. 5–6

Yukio (1992) Watakushi no hisoka na tanoshimi (My secret pleasure), in *Sabu*, July, pp. 182

Za Gei Henshūbu (1992) Daigokai *Za Gei* ankēto (The fifth *The Gay* questionnaire), in *Za Gei*, July, pp. 42–52

# Magazines, *Minikomishi*, *Dōjinshi* and Newspapers

*Adon*, *Akurosu* (*Across*), *Anan*, *Asahi Jānaru* (*Asahi Journal*), *Asahi Shinbun* (Asahi Newspaper)

*Badi* (Buddy), *Barazoku* (The Rose Clan), *Behold* (*Bihōrudo*), *Brutus* (*Burūtasu*), *Bungei* (Art and Culture)

*Choisir* (*Showajiiru*, Choose), *Chotto Rezubian* (A Little Bit Lesbian), *Crea* (*Kurea*), *Cross Dressing* (*Kurosu Doresshingu*)

*De Volkskrant* (The People's Newspaper)

*Ejanaika* (So what?)

*Faito Bakku* (*Fight Back*), *Frau* (*Furau*, Woman), *Fujin Kōron* (Public Discussions of Women)

*Gekkan Kadokawa* (Monthly Kadokawa), *Gekkō Bunka* (Moonlight Culture), *G-men*

*Himawari* (Sunflower)

*Josei Jishin* (Woman's Own), *Josei Sebun* (Woman Seven), *June*

*Kick Out*, *Kokuhaku Rezu Kurabu* (Confessing Lesbian Club), *Kōkoku Hihyō* (Public Critique), *Kuiin* (*Queen*), *Kurowassan* (*Croissant*)

*Labrys* (*Raburisu*)

*Magazine DON!*, *Marco Polo* (*Maruko Poro*), *Men's Nonno* (*Menzu Nonno*), *Musubikko* (Connecting Child)

*Nonno*, *NRC Handelsblad* (NRC Newspaper)

*OGC Nyūsu* (OGC News), *Okazu* (Side-dish), *OLP no Newsletter* (OLP Newsletter), *Onna Erosu* (Woman Eros)

*Poko a Poko* (Little by Little), *Popeye* (*Popai*), *Poporo* (*Popolo*, People)

*Regumi Tsūshin* (Regumi Newsletter)

*Sabu* (Macho), *Samuson* (*Samson*), *Sapporo Miitingu Nyūsuretā* (*Sapporo Meeting Newsletter*), *SAY*, *Seiron* (Sound Argument), *Seitō* (Blue Stockings), *Shokun!* (Gentlemen!), *S & M Sunaipā* (SM Sniper), *SM Hishōsetsu* (SM Secret Novels), *SM Tōkō Supesharu* (SM Contributions Special)

*Takarajima* (Treasure Island), *Takarazuka Revue*, *Tarzan* (*Tāzan*), *The Gay Times*, *The Guardian*, *Together*

*Wife* (*Waifu*)

*XX* (*Kusukusu*)

*Yagō* (Illicit Affairs), *Yomiuri Shinbun* (Yomiuri Newspaper)

*Za Gei* (*The Gay*)

**Japanese Studies**
**General Editor: Yoshio Sugimoto**

Beyond Common Sense: *Wim Lunsing*
Beyond Computopia: *Tessa Morris-Suzuki*
Changing Japanese Suburbia: *Eyal Ben-Ari*
Constructs for Understanding Japan: *Yoshio Sugimoto and Ross E. Mouer*
Consumption and Material Culture in Contemporary Japan: *Michael Ashkenazi and John Clammer*
A Cultural History of Post-war Japan: *Shunsuke Tsurumi*
Difference and Modernity: Social Theory in Contemporary Japanese Society: *John Clammer*
Diversity in Japanese Culture and Language: *John C. Maher and Gaynor Macdonald*
Enterprise Unionism in Japan: *Hirosuke Kawanishi*
Foreign Workers and Law Enforcement in Japan: *Wolfgang Herbert*
Group Psychology of the Japanese in Wartime: *Toshio Iritani*
Hibakusha Cinema: Hiroshima, Nagasaki and the Nuclear Image in Japanese Film: *Mick Broderick*
The Human Face of Industrial Conflict in Post-war Japan: *Hirosuke Kawanishi*
Images of Japanese Society: *Ross E. Mouer and Yoshio Sugimoto*
An Intellectual History of Wartime Japan: *Shunsuke Tsurumi*
Japanese Childcare: An Interpretive Study of Culture and Organization: *Eyal Ben-Ari*
Japanese Encounters with Postmodernity: *Johann P. Arnason and Yoshio Sugimoto*
Japanese Models of Conflict Resolution: *S.N. Eisenstadt and Eyal Ben-Ari*
Kanji Politics: *Nanette Gottlieb*
Lives of Young Koreans in Japan: *Yasunori Fukuoka*
Migrant Workers in Japan: *Hiroshi Komai*
Negotiating Identity in Contemporary Japan: *Ching Lin Pang*
The Origin of Ethnography in Japan: *Minoru Kawada*
The Rise of the Japanese Corporate System: *Koji Marsumoto*
Science, Technology and Society in Post-war Japan: *Shigeru Nakayama*
Social Psychology of Modern Japan: *Munesuke Mita*
Social Stratification in Contemporary Japan: *Kenji Kosaka*
Social Theory and Japanese Experience: *Johann P. Arnason*
Sociology and Society of Japan: *Nozomu Kawamura*